P9-DVK-241

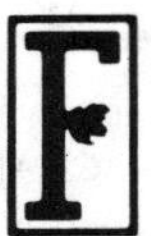

Also by Augustus A. White III, M.D.

THE CLINICAL BIOMECHANICS OF THE SPINE, second edition (with M.M. Panjabi)

SYMPOSIUM ON IDIOPATHIC LOW BACK PAIN (coedited with S.L. Gordon)

YOUR ACHING BACK

A Doctor's Guide to Relief

Augustus A. White III, M.D.

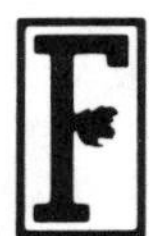

A FIRESIDE BOOK

Published by Simon & Schuster

New York London Toronto Sydney Tokyo Singapore

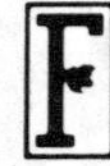

Simon and Schuster/Fireside
Rockefeller Center
1230 Avenue of the Americas
New York, New York 10020

Designed by Irving Perkins Associates
Manufactured in the United States of America

3 5 7 9 10 8 6 4 2
7 9 10 8 PBK

Library of Congress Cataloging in Publication Data
White, Augustus A.
Your aching back : a doctor's guide to relief / August A. White III.
p. cm.
"A Fireside book."
Includes bibliographical references (p.) and index. 1. Backache.
I. Title.
RD771.B217W49 1990
617.5'64—dc20 90-9879
CIP

ISBN 0-671-68933-9 (hardcover)
0-671-71000-1 (paperback)

Terms from the American Academy of Orthopaedic Surgeons' Glossary of
Spinal Terminology reprinted with permission.

Dedicated with enthusiasm
to all my family, friends, and patients
past, present, and future

Dear Reader:

The advice and suggestions presented here represent my best opinion based on updated contemporary scientific and clinical knowledge, as well as the experience gleaned from my practice of twenty-nine years. While I fully believe that the information is useful and the advice is the same as I would give to my family, my friends, and myself, nevertheless there can be no guarantees about your back condition. It could get better or worse with time. If you choose to follow the advice presented here, *you* must assume full responsibility.

There may be instances where my opinion differs from what you have been told by your own physician. He or she has examined you and knows your unique situation. When there is a discrepancy, follow the advice of your own doctor, in whom you have confidence, or, if you are unsure, consult another doctor. The information and advice provided here is accurate and reliable for *most* people, but any individual patient can be an exception.

Sincerely,
A.A. White III, M.D.

Contents

Acknowledgments

MOST EVERY endeavor has a prime mover. The prime mover in this project is A. Barry Merkin. Barry has guided me with great skill through the preliminaries and the process of this endeavor. He has been a constant source of friendship, encouragement, and wise advice.

Ms. Laura Yorke has worked with imagination, understanding, and sensitivity in the editing of this work. She has been careful to preserve the tone, the spirit, and the individuality of the presentation.

Pat Lynch and Sue Lee are two gifted medical illustrators who have a great ability to understand ideas and their intended nuances. To this understanding they add their abilities as artists and teachers to produce dynamic, instructive illustrations.

A number of family members and friends have taken time from busy schedules to review and critique various chapters. They have made helpful and important suggestions about clarification, content changes, and translations from medical jargon. These very helpful people are Montague Cobb, M.D., Jackie Derosier, Nancy Hindlian, Paul Johnson, Peter Jokl, M.D., Ellen Jones, Jennifer Kelsey, Ph.D., Robert Leach, M.D., George Lewinnek, M.D., Willie Naulls, Adrienne Rabkin, Anita White, and Vivian White.

For this edition there have been some very thorough, second, helpful, and insightful readers. My gratitude is extended to the following colleagues who conscientiously provided important editorial critique: Kay Bendix, Mark Bernhardt, M.D., Michele Finnell, R.N., Richard Hynes, M.D., Brian McCarthy, M.D., Louis Meeks, M.D., Dennis McGowan, M.D., and Michael Yaszemski, M.D.

Several other friends and colleagues have helped in a variety of important aspects of this project. They are Paul Curtis, M.D., Anthony Davis, Ph.D., Charles Epps, M.D., William Fielding, M.D., Toby Hayes, Ph.D., Carl Hirsch, M.D., Rev. Harry Hoehler, Daniel E. Hogan, Don King, M.D., J. Antony Lloyd,

Henry Mankin, M.D., Alf Nachemson, M.D., Al Poussaint, M.D., Manohar Panjabi, D. Tech, Mitchell T. Rabkin, M.D., Victor Richards, M.D., Suzanne Schwartz, Wayne Southwick, M.D., and Daniel Tosteson, M.D.

As colleagues and editors, Linda Clark and Brad Miner have helped considerably in a number of administrative and informational activities related to the completion of this work.

Marge McBride has been tremendously helpful in gathering information from the medical literature. Here also is grateful acknowledgment of the fact that this project simply could not have been done without the excellent help of Kashine Dolan and Suzanne Hunerwadel, who put together many drafts of the manuscript.

I would like, as well, to express my thanks to the many patients who have drawn my attention to the need for the information herein. They have allowed me to share in the gratification they have derived from having accurate information about their back problems.

I would also like to express my appreciation to the many residents and medical students whose astute questions have inspired me to try to think more probingly about what is known about back pain, and to consider the best means for clearly and practically expressing that knowledge.

I would also like to express my gratitude to institutions that have contributed significantly to the contents of this book: the Manassas School in Memphis, Tennessee, the Northfield Mount Herman School, Brown University, Stanford University, University of Michigan Medical Center, San Francisco's Presbyterian Medical Center, Yale Medical Center, the 85th Evacuation Hospital in Vietnam, Fort Ord Army Hospital in Monterey, California, University of Goteborg and Karolinska Institute in Sweden, the National Institutes of Health in Bethesda, Maryland, the American Academy of Orthopaedic Surgeons, the Orthopaedic Research Society, the International Society for the Study of the Lumbar Spine, the Cervical Spine Research Society, Harvey Cushing Library, the Countway Library in Boston, Massachusetts, the Weston and Wellesley Public Libraries, the Massachusetts Institute of Technology, Beth Israel Hospital, and the Harvard Medical School.

Introduction

Raison d'Être

During my twenty-nine years as a physician, I have found low back pain to be one of the most complex and troubling problems to handle. If that's so for me, it's doubly or triply true for my patients, the backache sufferers themselves. It is for you, my backache sufferers, that this book is written and dedicated.

I'm writing this book to tell those of you with back problems what scientific and clinical research has substantiated to be *true* about backache. Unfortunately, as many of you may have already discovered, there's a tangle of confusion and misunderstanding surrounding low back pain. And sometimes the diagnosis, or the treatment, is just plain wrong. I will try to be clear and simple, but I won't withhold important concepts and facts just because they are technical or complex. I think it's to your benefit to be exposed to all the relevant and current knowledge on this topic.

I'm working on the assumption that, all things being equal, it's better to know the truth. This book has several purposes. It will help you understand the cause and prevention of back pain. The contents are selected so as to inform you as to what you can expect once you get a backache. It will tell you about the diagnosis and treatment of back problems and provide information to help you to decide among treatment options. There are numerous specific tips to help you ease the difficulties associated with a bad back. Knowing the facts is your best ammunition. For many of you the knowledge and understanding provided here will spell relief from your problems.

This book contains the necessary information to keep you "out of trouble," should you get a backache. Forewarned is forearmed.* Finally, I want you to get this message and theme:

* I've provided some *checklists* designed to summarize specific key information that you may want or need at a particular time.

"Things take time. . . ." Please be assured that you won't have backache forever. You will gradually get better. Be patient. You will gradually get better.

How to Read This Book

People should read books however they please. Nevertheless, here are some thoughts that will help you get the most out of this book. I suggest that you skim through the entire book very quickly. You can even limit yourself to the pictures and captions the first time through. This will give you an overview, a perspective of what the book may do for you, and a preview of the various treatment strategies available for dealing with your particular back problem. I would then suggest that you read the book again, this time carefully picking out the parts of special interest to you. These parts should be read in depth and studied. Having done that, you should read the whole thing through once more. This will allow you another opportunity to pick up on points that may be especially meaningful for you. If there are times when you get a bit more information than is absolutely necessary, be patient. I decided that it would be better to overestimate your interest and inquisitiveness than to underestimate it.

The annotated bibliography at the end of the book is almost completely from the medical literature. The most important new references have been included. The articles vary in the amount of technical terminology they use. However, those readers interested in delving deeper into a particular topic presented in this book will be put well on their way by the references listed. Most public libraries can now provide medical literature through interlibrary loan programs. These references are also a way of reminding you that you're not just getting "one man's opinion"; there is a lot of evidence to back up the information that is being offered to help you.

I wish you the best. I *know* that the information here will help you *some*—and I *trust* that it will help you a *great deal!*

YOUR ACHING BACK

Chapter I

Who Suffers?

TRY LISTING the names of ten adult friends at random. If seven of them are backache victims, and only three are free of the sufferings addressed in this book, they're a set of typical persons. If you are one of the seven unfortunates (and the fact that you're opening this book means you probably are), the problem becomes acutely personal in terms of pain and inconvenience. However, the probabilities are that if this is a new backache, you will be just fine within the next four to five weeks.

In any case, you're not alone. In the Western world, epidemiological studies reveal that back pain afflicts a staggering sixty to eighty percent of the population. Out of every ten people under forty-five who have chronic medical conditions limiting their activities, four are back and spine pain victims. Backache takes a backseat only to headache as the most common medical complaint, and is second only to the common cold as a reason for missed work. In fact, absence from the workplace due to disabling back pain has soared.

There was a fourteen-fold increase in the prevalence of low back pain in the United States between 1970 and 1981, and even more of an increase in England and Sweden. Unfortunately, five percent of the population will complain of low back pain in a given year. Furthermore, sciatica, pain in the leg, may be associated with back pain. It is known that forty percent of all adults will have sciatica at some point in their lives.

A sore back becomes even more sobering when you realize how often it can become chronic, debilitating, and life-diminishing. If you're laboring under a difficult back, you don't have to be reminded of this—but consider: If you're a worker who is absent from work for more than six months with a bad back, statistics show you have only a fifty percent chance of ever regaining full productivity. After a year, your chances dip to twenty-five percent. Add the high cost of treatment and you have a more graphic portrait of the social and financial sufferings involved. The average bad-back episode will run you $4,300, and the diagnosis and treatment of backaches in the United States costs $5 billion every year. If we count up loss of productivity, cost of disability payments, Workmen's Compensation, and lawsuits, the figure soars to about $14 billion. **You should not leave this pessimistic paragraph without being reassured that over eighty-five percent of people with an acute backache will be over it in a month's time.**

Here's one more way you can grasp the magnitude of the financial problem. The U.S. Postal Service is one of the largest employers in the country. There was a time when we paid 20¢ for a first-class postage stamp. Guess how much of that 20¢ was applied to the medical care, compensation, and related expenses of postal employees with backache? About five percent—0.9¢—nearly *one cent!*

The purpose of dragging in statistics like these is not to depress you, but rather to convince you, if you need convincing, that back pain is a major social problem. What cannot be expressed in numbers, although it is of equal or greater importance, is the profound human suffering and compromise in quality of life that the back pain sufferer experiences.

The question that may occur to you at this point is, why? Why is the human back such a vulnerable, annoying, and frequently painful part of the anatomy? Has it always been thus? Certainly the spine has been a preoccupation for centuries—as attested to by sayings such as "He's a spineless person" and "She really has her back up about it," or "He's got a yellow streak down his back" and "She's carrying the team on her back." Shakespeare aficionados will recall the insinuating words of Iago, who whispers to Desdemona's father: "Your daughter and the Moor [Othello] are now making the beast with two backs"—Elizabethan jargon for "having sex." Perhaps echoing the Elizabethans, Jamaican men complaining of impotence will say they have lost the strength of their backs. Treachery, we know, is conveyed as a "stab in the back," and paranoia in the phrase "They're laughing behind my back." We could go on cataloguing spinal expressions in art and life, but if you're lying on a painful back or "with your back against the wall" you'll probably want to get to the treatment/prevention chapter pretty quickly.

Some researchers have reflected that we humans have only recently evolved into two-legged creatures, and that staying on all fours might have saved us from backaches. There are several problems with this theory. One is that the treatment implied, reversion to four-legged locomotion, would require some radical life-style changes, perhaps driving shoemakers out of business or placing undue market demands on glove and knee-pad manufacturers. Besides, animals have back pain too; they just don't complain about it. Most important, the hypothesis doesn't fit the anatomic and evolutionary facts: Our spines are perfectly suited to an upright stance and don't differ significantly from those of our hominid ancestors. Finally, even though there are sexual problems associated with backache (Chapter VIII), back problems could not play a part in the process of evolution because the genes can be readily passed on well before the onset of backache, which is usually in one's thirties.

If we are to look for reasons, we'd do better to examine the quality of our lives—especially what we do with our backs. Frankly, even an extensive analysis of all the data does not provide a simple, clear answer. Nevertheless, you will certainly get a better understanding, so read on!

WHO'S AT RISK?

Of course, if you're a backache sufferer, your interest in this book is more apt to be personal than sociological. How do the back statistics apply to you? What category of back sufferer do you fall into? What are your risks—and how can you reduce them? One of the goals of this book is to provide this information, along with *specific* recommendations for managing your back on the job and at home. The following facts, gathered from epidemiological studies, can help you calculate your risks—for we now know that sex, age, occupation, leisure activities, and life-style all influence the state of your back.

Age

Back pain patients tend to be between thirty and fifty-five years old. Why? Very simply, the discs between the vertebrae of your lower back change in the normal course of aging. The young disc is elastic and full of fluid, but starting at about age thirty, it gradually becomes dry or scarred and its mechanics change, making it more likely to fragment, move out of place, or cause pain. This is analogous to a jelly doughnut. When it's fresh, the pastry is pliable, resilient, and the center contains jelly. As it ages, the outer portion hardens, becomes more brittle, cracks, and flakes. The jelly in the middle dries out.

The puzzle, however, is that while all discs undergo this transformation, not all cause pain—and certainly all do not herniate.

Actually, back-pain risk decreases for men after age fifty, but this is not so for women. This is because the problem of osteoporosis begins to occur in women and causes backache. In the next section, gender-related issues in low back pain are discussed.

Sex

Epidemiological studies suggest that males are slightly more prone to herniated discs (this is a situation in which a part of the disc moves out from its normal position between the vertebral bodies, causing severe back and/or leg pain) and more likely to undergo surgery than females with problems of equal severity. Perhaps differences in occupation, athletics, and amount of driving, rather than genetics, account for the male's greater weakness. Or perhaps men simply tolerate pain badly and are thus more afflicted and therefore more likely to end up with the most rigorous treatment.

On the female side, elderly women are at highest risk for osteoporosis, a loss of bone density that weakens the vertebrae and sometimes causes them to collapse. The relative risks are even greater (3:1) for a woman who has had more than two full-term pregnancies. Hormonal changes after menopause are thought responsible, and there is evidence that estrogen-replacement therapy—together with adequate vitamin D and sunlight, dietary calcium, vigorous physical activity, and exposure to fluorides—can be of help in the treatment of osteoporosis.

Full-term pregnancy is notoriously hard on the lower back. For one thing, it brings with it mechanical problems, such as increased weight and a protruding abdomen, that combine to shift the mother-to-be's center of gravity forward and put stress on her back. But, perhaps more to the point, a hormone called *relaxin*, produced during the later stages of pregnancy, can cause the ligaments in the pelvis and lumbar spine to relax, undermining the back's mechanical strength. After her child is born and requires trips to an appropriate changing table and so on, the new mother should learn the proper biomechanics of lifting, described in Chapter II.

There is also a type of arthritis of the lumbar spine (low back) associated with an abnormal forward displacement of the vertebra (degenerative spondylolisthesis), which is four times more common in women than in men. Sorry folks, but the reason for this remains to be discovered.

Heredity

One kind of back problem, *intervertebral disc disease* (see Chapter III), seems to run in families. Ditto for slipped vertebrae, the almost unpronounceable name of which is *spondylolisthesis* (SPON-dil-low-la-THEE-sis).

A few racial differences show up here. American whites, for example, are more prone to spondylolisthesis than American blacks—and Eskimos have about a ten times greater tendency to develop the disease than whites. The basis of this seems to be an anatomic difference in the lower part of the lumbar spine.

There is evidence that herniated disc problems "run in families." There may be a hereditary predisposition in the chemical makeup of the disc that makes it more likely to fragment and move out of its normal anatomic position and cause nerve irritation.

Occupation

You can't do very much about your sex, age, or race, but you can change your job, or some of its tasks, when necessary—which is fortunate, since your job may affect your back more than anything else.

People who spend at least half their job time driving a motor vehicle are *three times* more likely than the average worker to suffer a herniated disc. This fact has some cogent and interesting associated observations. A key issue here is that of road vibrations. Most vehicles vibrate in a range of 4.5 to 5.0 Hz (cycles per second). The first resonant frequency (that frequency likely to cause perturbation or damage) of our spines is in the same range. Laboratory tests have shown that vibrating the spine at this frequency range can damage the spine and cause disc herniation. Vibration in this range has also been shown experimentally to increase the production of pain-causing substances. To put it simply, most cars, buses, and trucks vibrate at 4.5 to 5.0 cycles per second, and this is a range that can damage the spine and cause back pain and disc herniation. The reader should know that some Swedish and Japanese cars do not vibrate at 4.5 to 5.0 cycles per second.

Sedentary occupations in general are bad news for your back, as sitting puts great pressure on the disc between the vertebrae. When it comes to driving, then, we have prolonged sitting without changing position and—what is probably more important—a spine constantly jarred by vibrations. Cabbies, truck drivers, bus drivers, train conductors, beware: Your job could be hazardous to your back. Chapter VI will give you some advice that should help you, should you be one of these at-risk people.

It takes about five years for sedentary occupations or damaging leisure pursuits to do their evil work on your back. Weekend sitting, for example, has been linked to herniated disc disease in males, a fact that football widows may find useful ammunition. Obviously, most office jobs fall into the sedentary category—so secretaries, accountants, lawyers, academicians, computer programmers, and middle managers alike would do well to change position, stand, walk to appointments, and relax from time to time.

However, if you get off your backside to spare your back, don't turn around and lift your typewriter, either. Jobs involving heavy lifting, pulling, or carrying probably lead to lumbar disc disease. Sudden unexpected bouts of lifting, as when you're helping a friend move his piano and he lets go, appear to be followed by complaints of acute back pain in doctors' offices. Certainly in heavy-labor jobs, the weight lifted, frequency of lifting, improper lifting, and body mechanics all go hand in hand with low back pain. Is it any coincidence that heavy-industrial workers, farmers, and nurses and nurse's aides are more often afflicted with bad backs than most of us? On the basis of my experience, I'd also have to put firemen, policemen, and emergency medical technicians, who must perform extensive lifting quickly and without proper positioning, in the high-risk class.

Another note: Twisting injuries are often blamed for back pain and disc damage, and future occupational studies should consider this.

One noteworthy condition that appears to be an occupational hazard is degenerative disc disease of the lumbar spine. The term is unfortunate, as it sounds as though we were moldering away and falling apart inside. Actually, lumbar disc degeneration is probably little more than normal wear changes in the spine. On the X ray, the doctor sees a narrowed disc space and some *osteophyte* (bony outgrowth or spur) formation. As people age, these changes tend to show up on the X rays of half of all women and about seventy percent of the men—but mechanical stress does appear to hasten the process. Miners, dockworkers, and outdoor laborers such as farmers and road workers are at risk, while sedentary workers appear not to be.

A similar problem is arthritis of the facet joints. See figures 2–2, 3–5, and 3–9 to understand facets, facet joints, and facet joint capsules. Two facets go together, alone with a capsule, to form a facet joint. Arthritis of the facet joints is a condition that can come on with age, though it can occur independently of degenerative disc changes. Degenerative changes in the facet joints are frequently observed in miners and even more frequently in obese people.

In summary, here's how Dr. Gunnar Anderson of Sweden has mapped out the occupational danger signals for your back:

- Physically heavy work
- Static work postures
- Frequent bending and twisting
- Lifting and forceful movements
- Repetitive work (such as assembly-line occupations)
- Vibrations

In Chapter V, you'll learn how to minimize the wear and tear on your back at home and on the job.

Sociological Risks

Back in the sixties, we doctors cared for a number of patients who complained of back pain associated with a new dance craze called the twist. To a rock and roll beat of Chubby Checker and others, the twist dancer held his upper torso relatively fixed while rotating the pelvis as vigorously as possible about the long axis of the body. Nowadays, twist injuries are as rare as smallpox, though one wonders about the effects of *Saturday Night Fever* gyrations, break dancing, dirty dancing, and acrobatics on the lumbar spine.

In a more sober vein, some studies have linked the tendency to report sick from work to lower educational level, lower intelligence, and lower socioeconomic status. Workers with a low sense of self-importance or those who describe their jobs as boring, dissatisfying, and repetitious are also more apt to stay in bed with backaches. These fellow humans should not be patronized, but must be treated with compassion and careful attention to the quality of their work life. Of course, pain can be a signal of depression. The onset of back pain can also be related to life situational stresses, such as a promotion, a vacation, an honor, the loss of a friend, mate, or a job, or the necessity to move. Recently, psychiatrists have been reporting that a sadomasochistic patient may complain of spine pain in the hopes of obtaining a surgical procedure. Like the notorious "Munchausen's syndrome" patient, who seeks and achieves a collection of abdominal scars, these patients are usually found to be free of disease when their backs are needlessly opened up.

Cultural factors play a role in back pain, or lack of it. Backache appears to be far less common in cultures in which the squatting position is common. Squatting curves the spine into a slightly flexed position, in contrast to the Western mode of standing and sitting, where the spine curves in the opposite, slightly extended direction. One study comparing X rays of individuals from a squatting culture with those from a sitting culture noted less evidence of disc degeneration in those from the squatting culture. A second theory is that people in developing countries are less prone to back problems because they work harder, walk more, and are less sedentary generally. Still, evidence for both theories remains meager, but thought provoking.

Body Build and Posture

"For heaven's sake, stand up straight, or you'll get a bad back!" your parents may have innocently instructed you. Well, parental dogmas notwithstanding, most studies maintain that there is no real connection between voluntary posture and back pain. A flat back and a slumped back are equal in the eyes of the spine. Moderate scoliosis, or sideways curvature of the spine, is probably unrelated to back pain, though severe lumbar lateral (sideways) curvature probably is hard on your back.

An interesting study allowed by an outdated tradition helps to prove this point. In certain women's colleges in the Eastern United States, posture was carefully evaluated, to the point of obtaining standing nude photographs to permit an unencumbered evaluation of posture. A careful study of these pictures of the classes of 1957, 1958, and 1959, and a review of the department of physical education's written evaluation, dictated the following conclusion: Posture, neither good nor bad, was in any way associated with a higher or lower incidence of low back pain over a twenty-five-year period.

Also contrary to folklore, moderate differences—as much as three-fourths of one inch—in leg length are inconsequential to your back.

As for body build, most studies support the contention that there's no strong correlation between height, weight, body build, and backache. Yet, all researchers can't agree all of the time: A few studies have shown a tendency for tall and obese people to develop backache.

Miscellaneous

A Vermont study turned up the unexpected fact that people with chronic coughs and bronchitis frequently suffer from herniated disc disease, and now more recent research has implicated cigarette smoking in disc disease. Here is yet another health negative for smokers. There is pretty good evidence that nicotine interferes with the blood flow to the vertebral body and around the disc. This may cause abnormalities in the normal biological functions of the disc, as well as back pain.

The size and shape of your spinal canal may predispose you to develop sciatica (leg pain and weakness that may or may not be

Below is an outline that summarizes the major epidemiological factors and provides a sense of their relative import.

RELATIONSHIP OF CERTAIN RISK FACTORS TO LUMBAR DISC DISEASE OR LOW BACK PAIN

Well-established risks

- Driving motor vehicles more than two hours a day
- Exposure to vibrations
- Cigarette smoking
- Standing, carrying, pushing, pulling, twisting, bending
- Lifting (especially if associated with twisting or with knees straight or arms extended)

Suggested risks

- Use of jackhammers
- Cross-country skiing
- Emotionally stressful work
- More than two full-term pregnancies
- Working as a nurse or nurse's aide
- Sedentary occupations
- Leg-length discrepancy greater than 2.5 cm. (1 inch)

Factors not constituting risks

- Race (white/black)
- Baseball, golf, bowling, tennis
- Height
- Weight

associated with back pain). When the canal is small or trefoil-shaped, the nerves that can cause sciatica are more easily irritated.

Perhaps you've concluded, after perusing the last few pages, that the most likely candidate for back pain is a socially maladjusted male truck driver who is tall and does a lot of loading and unloading during a working day. So much the worse for him if he has a family history of low back pain, is divorced, drinks and smokes to excess, and belongs to a lower socioeconomic stratum. If he isn't particularly proud of his work, and spends his weekends vegetating in front of the TV, give him up as a hopeless back pain invalid! Well, this sort of composite portrait is an improper use of statistics, of course, since each individual defies easy categorization. Many a TV-addicted, sedentary, depressed truck driver has never had a backache in his life. Of course, this characterization is presented to emphasize some points. I certainly mean no disrespect to these frequently helpful and lifesaving fellow humans of the highways.

Yet all of the life-style factors we've mentioned *can* translate themselves into an aching back, and it's best to start with a good, hard look at yourself and your life. Don't despair: Soon we'll tell you what you can do *for* your back.

Chapter II

Basic Back Mechanics

"The spinal column is a long chain of bones. The head sits at the top and you sit on the bottom."

—Anonymous

You may think anatomy too complicated, boring, or scary to contemplate in any depth, particularly if your own is acting up. But take heart. Many philosophers since classical times have extolled the beauty of the human anatomy, and I happen to agree with them.

But what is more to the point, you can't operate your car properly if you don't know its instrument panel, and you may consider this chapter an abbreviated owner's manual for the spine, if you like. Some of the information in this chapter may strike you as unduly technical and unsuitable for bedtime reading. By all means, skim over it if you're in a hurry to get to the real basics of back care, and use this chapter as a reference guide or dictionary.

Does your doctor ever refer to specific anatomical structures that sound to your ears like distant galaxies or exotic topographical points? Well, this chapter can help you interpret your doctor's conversation (though you should feel free to ask him or her to explain things in plain English!) and understand something about your troubling back as well.

THE SPINAL COLUMN

The human spine is one of the most fascinating and elegant mechanical structures in the animal kingdom. It consists of twenty-four *vertebrae* plus the *sacrum* (the triangular bone between the lowest lumbar—lower back—vertebrae and the tailbone) and the coccyx, or tailbone. The rigid vertebrae, separated by elastic ligaments, form the *spinal canal,* wherein the *spinal cord* and nerve roots lie (Figure 2–1). The whole structure is balanced and controlled by a complex series of muscles.

What does the spinal column do—and what makes it so fancy, anyway? Well, first of all, it can move in many different directions with speed and agility. Secondly, it can stiffen yet remain supple enough to withstand and cushion powerful mechanical forces. Finally, it performs the crucial job of protecting the vital spinal cord and nerves. You might suppose that the ideal way to shield the spinal cord would be with a straight bony rod, much as the skull protects the brain. But such a spine would neither allow motion nor possess the necessary protective energy-absorbing properties.

So what we have instead is a curvaceous spine, if you will, which permits flexibility with strength and stability, plus superior shock-absorbing capacity. Your spine curves forward at the neck (the cervical spine) and lower back (lumbar spine), while at the midback (thoracic spine) and the bottom of the spine (sacral region) it curves slightly backwards. You may not have been aware of it, but you've probably already admired the graceful curve of the lumbar region in the opposite sex.

What we call the "functional spinal unit" consists of two adjacent vertebrae and their intervening soft tissues, ligaments, discs, and muscles. Nowadays some exciting research is going into defining the full mechanical behavior of these units—their stiffness, flexibility, reaction to various stresses, and so on. As these data are validated they can be translated into mathematical formulas and stored in a computer. Then the computer can construct the entire human spine and provide information about its expected mechanical behavior under different pressures, including those that could cause failure or injury.

This futuristic mathematical model won't be like a living

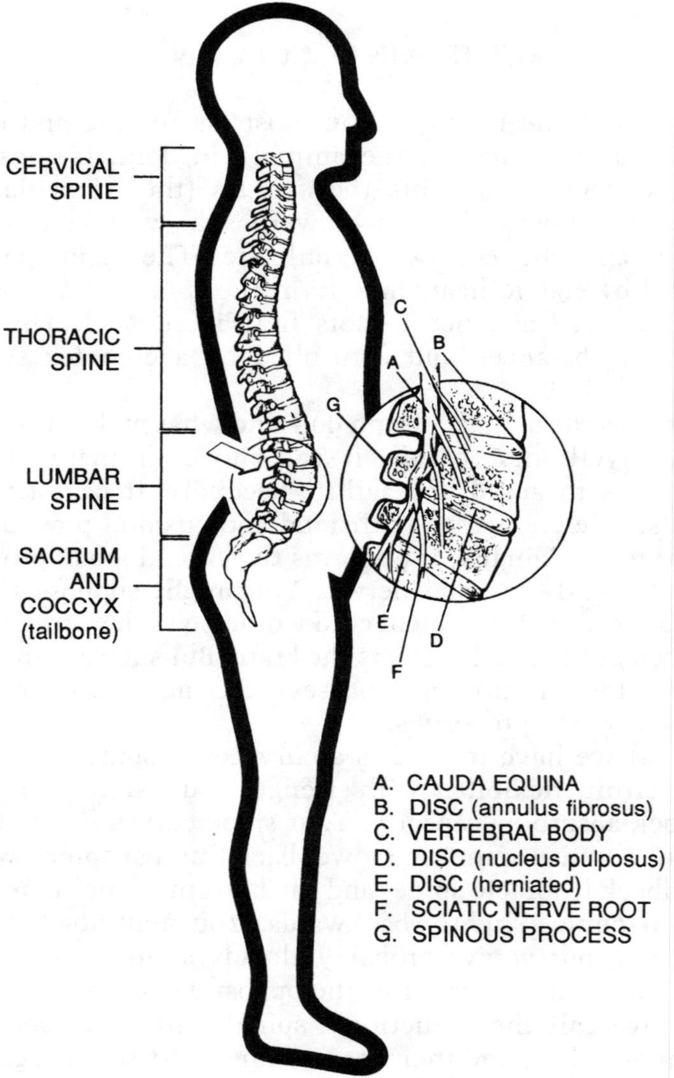

FIGURE 2–1 This anatomic picture is the key to an understanding of the anatomy of the spine, disc disease, and its associated leg pain. The upper portion of the spine is known as the neck or the cervical spine, the midportion is the midback or thoracic spine, to which the ribs are attached, and the lower region of the spine, featured in this book, is the lumbar spine or the low back. As you can see, the nerves run from the spinal canal down toward the leg. (Courtesy of *Wellbeing,* the medical magazine of Boston's Beth Israel Hospital.)

spine, nor will it be a replica of a particular patient's back; it will be a reliable portrayal of the spine's mechanics. As such it could give information more effectively than actual experiments can. This model may provide some breakthrough information to help your aching back in the future.

Meanwhile, let's examine exactly what *your* spine is made of and how nature has designed it.

The Lumbar Spine

Since this book focuses on the lumbar spine—considered the source of low back pain—let's start here.

The bone is made up of what is called the *vertebral body* (Figure 2–1), a cylindrical bone in which blood, fat, bone marrow, and certain fluids lie. At both ends of the vertebral body are the *vertebral end plates* (Figure 2–2), which are prone to fracture (often unrecognized) and are therefore one source of back pain. Connecting the back bony part of the vertebral body at either side of the spinal canal are tubelike portions of bone called *pedicles* (Figure 2–2). The spine takes its name from the *spinous processes* (Figure 2–1), those familiar knobs you feel beneath your skin at the midline. The base of the spinous processes and the *lamina* (Figure 2–6B), a thin plate of bone, complete the spinal canal's ring.

The spine, like the rest of you, possesses joints, which are unfortunately susceptible to the same diseases as the joints of your fingers, hips, or knees. The *facet joints* are a case in point (Figure 2–5). If all this seems a bit dry and academic, don't worry. It will add up to a new understanding between you and your back.

The Disc

Between the vertebrae is the famous—or infamous—disc, a tough bunch of fibers and cartilage with a jellylike center, like a jelly-filled doughnut (Figure 2–3). Believe it or not, the intervertebral discs constitute about one-third the length of your spine and are the largest organs in your body without their own blood supply. In fact, you grow taller at night, as the discs swell; in the daytime, you shrink back to your "normal" height as the discs' accumulated water is forced out. This swelling is even more marked in the weightless state, as our astronauts found out to their discomfiture. During space flights they actually "grew" as much as two inches taller.

But since you, the reader, probably don't need to worry about zero-gravity conditions, let's get back to what concerns you. There's evidence that biochemical changes in the disc can increase its moisture content, causing pain. Since emotional stress is reported to change body chemistry, some researchers have wondered whether this is the mechanism whereby stress produces backache. Could the effects of mental strain on disc swelling provide a partial solution to the old philosophical problem of how the mind affects the body? Maybe.

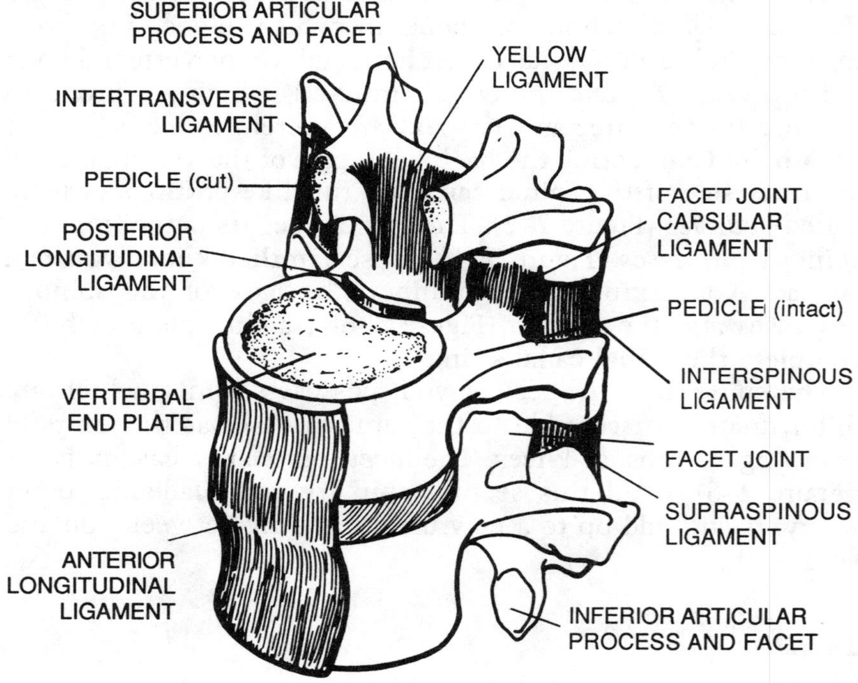

FIGURE 2–2 *Ligaments of the spine.* In addition to the disc, there are about seven other ligaments that connect one vertebra to the next. The ligaments help to control the motion of the spine and prevent excessive motion. Because of their elasticity, a certain amount of motion is allowed. (Reproduced with permission from White, A.A., and Panjabi, M.M.: *Clinical Biomechanics of the Spine,* J.B. Lippincott, 1990, second edition.)

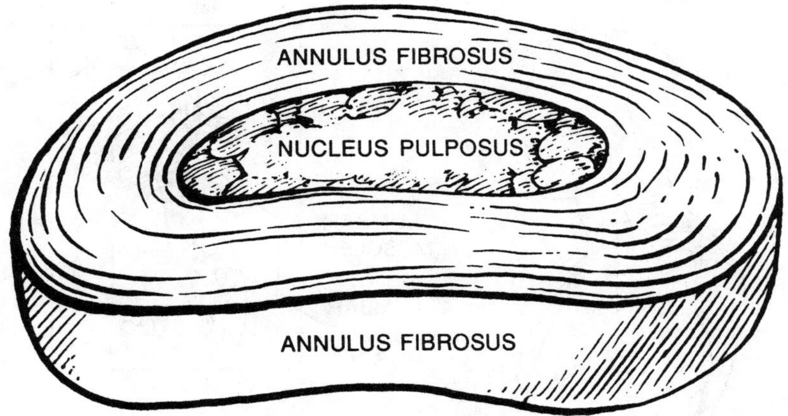

FIGURE 2–3 *The intervertebral disc.* Here we see an isolated drawing of the intervertebral disc. The central portion is the nucleus pulposus, which contains a large amount of water. The concentric layered rings are known as the annulus fibrosus. These structures change with age. The nucleus tends to dry out and the annulus tends to become disorganized and less elastic. Any combination of the nucleus and the annulus can become displaced into the spinal canal, causing pain in the back and/or leg.

In any case, much of the spine's strength comes from the disc, especially its main structure, the *annulus fibrosus* ("ring of fibers" in Latin). The annulus fibrosus, composed of tough collagen, fits directly into the bone around the vertebral end plate, providing mechanical strength. The disc's other beauty is its elegant design for energy absorption, as the spine's "shock absorber," which we'll discuss further in the biomechanics section of this chapter.

Facet Joints

The gliding joints between the vertebrae are called the *facet joints* or *facet articulations* (Figure 2–5). You couldn't move your spine without them, but, sadly, they can be every bit as troublesome as the joints in the rest of your body, lending themselves to the whole spectrum of arthritic diseases. (More about this in Chapter III.) The bony protuberances of these joints are covered on one side with smooth, slick cartilage, like the gristle in a chicken bone. Part of their lining is composed of

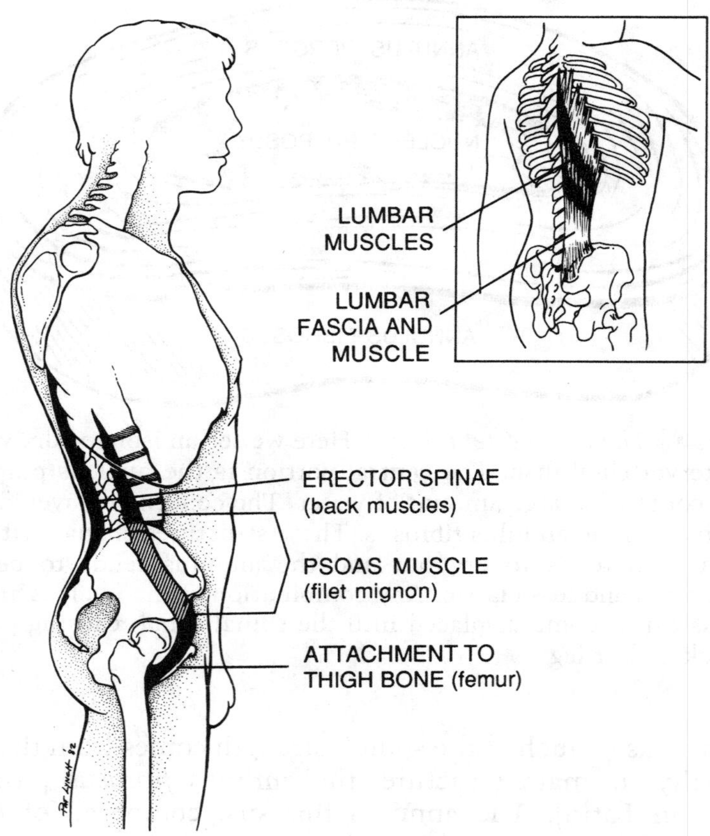

FIGURE 2–4 It is very important to understand this picture. First of all, it shows the important erector spinae muscles (see muscles and fascia in insert), which are the firm, prominent muscles that you can feel in the lower part of your back on either side of the midline. These are the muscles that can be so painful when they get tensed and cramped up in spasms. (Spasms are intensely contracted, painful muscles.) On the front of the spine there is the psoas muscle, which attaches to the front and sides of the lower back and goes down and across the hip joint to attach to the near part of the thighbone (femur). When strains are imposed on this muscle, tremendous forces are exerted on the lumbar spine. These forces can be very irritating to the low back. In a number of places in the book you will find these muscles to be a key factor in back pain. I hope that we've made the anatomy clear to you, as it will help you to understand and relieve your backache.

sensitive synovial tissue that nourishes and lubricates the joints and that can become irritated or inflamed and cause back pain.

Your spine's mechanics depend heavily on the little facet joints, as the angles of their sliding surfaces determine the way your spine moves. So their special mechanics probably play a role in back pain or lack of it.

Ligaments

Ligaments, as you may know, are strong bands of fibrous tissue that bind bones, or other body parts, together (Figure 2–2). We won't discuss all your back's ligaments in detail, but a few are very pertinent, or at least problematic, to backache sufferers. One is the *posterior longitudinal ligament,* which, as its name suggests, runs down the length of the column behind the vertebral bodies. Because it's narrower at the level of the disc, some doctors have proposed that it increases the danger that the disc may protrude back into the spinal canal and cause nerve irritation. More about this later.

Another potentially troubling ligament is the *ligamentum flavum* (yellow ligament), a generous bunch of highly specialized fibers running along the back of the spine at the base of the spinous processes, connecting the bony back parts of the vertebrae (*laminae*). The yellow ligament is the most elastic structure in the human body. Alas, this ligament loses its elasticity as you grow older, and it can bulge into the spinal canal. The result? A frequently painful narrowing or crowding that doctors call *spinal stenosis.*

Muscles

The back muscles are quite complex. The basic biomechanical principle is that your abdominal muscles are crucial to your spine's stability. The major players are the abdominal muscles, the iliopsoas, and the erector spinae muscles (Figure 2–4). The abdominal muscles, not shown in the illustration, are made up of two to three layers of flat muscles that cover the front and sides of the abdomen (lower trunk). The iliopsoas muscle runs along the front of the spine from the lumbar area to just below

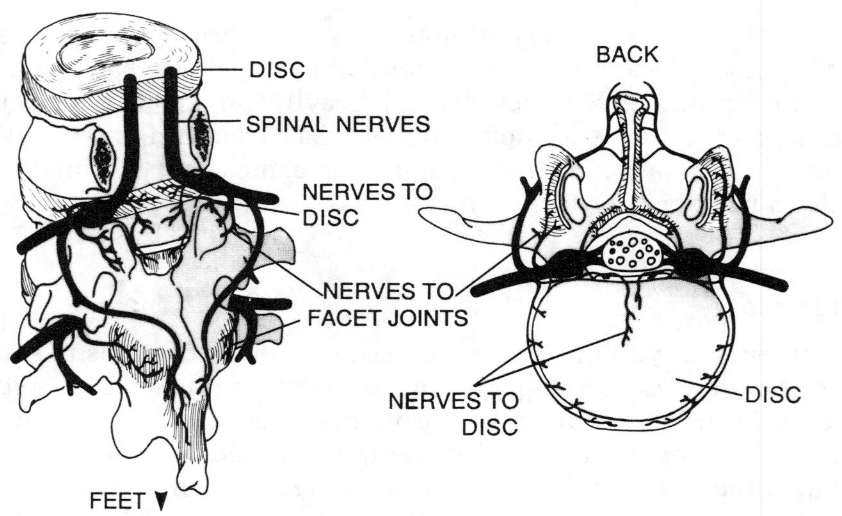

FIGURE 2–5 This picture demonstrates that there is a generous nerve supply to most of the anatomic structures in the lumbar spine. To the left, we have a look at the back of the spine, with one of the structures removed to show the nerves. On the right, there is a cross-section (horizontal or axial section) of the spine, which gives us a look right down the spinal canal. This is the kind of view we see on a CAT scan. The major important structures shown here are the nerves to the capsule of the facet joints and the nerves to the intervertebral disc. However, we must remember that almost any of the structures can be a source of spine pain, because there is an ample nerve supply to them. (Reproduced with permission from White, A.A., and Panjabi, M.M.: *Clinical Biomechanics of the Spine,* J.B. Lippincott, 1990, second edition.)

the hip joint (in the steer, it provides the delicate filet mignon steak); the erector spinae muscle runs down the back along both sides of the spine. Both play a major role in spinal support and biomechanics.

Covering all these muscle tissues is a specialized fibrous tissue called *fascia,* which has been thought by some to be a source of back pain syndromes. In Japan surgeons have actually removed part of this sheath of fascia in the hopes of relieving pain. The procedure has never been popular in the United States; however, there is considerable interest in fibrositis and fibromyalgia, which some physicians think may be causes of back pain. These conditions are reviewed in the next chapter.

Nerves

Ah, let's not forget nerves, the bane of back pain sufferers. Most of the structures we've just discussed—the fibers of the disc, the posterior longitudinal ligament, parts of the facet articulations,

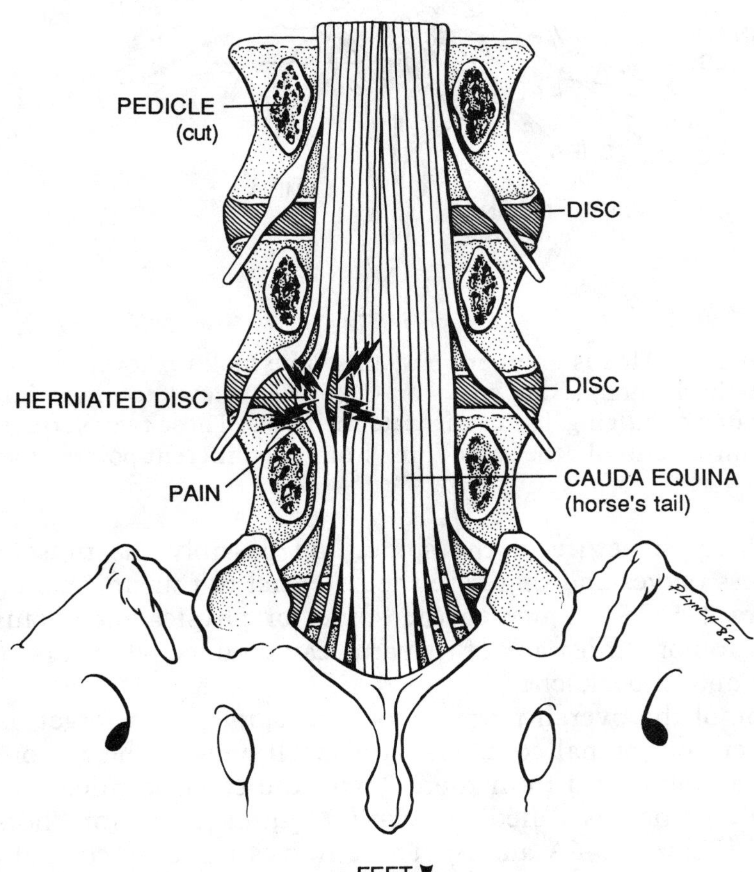

FIGURE 2–6A This is a posterior view of the lumbar spine with all of the bone removed and the dura opened up. The purpose is to demonstrate that lots of nerves are coming through here. The picture shows that a bulging or herniated disc in the area can irritate the nerve going out into the leg and/or the combined group of nerves known as the cauda equina.

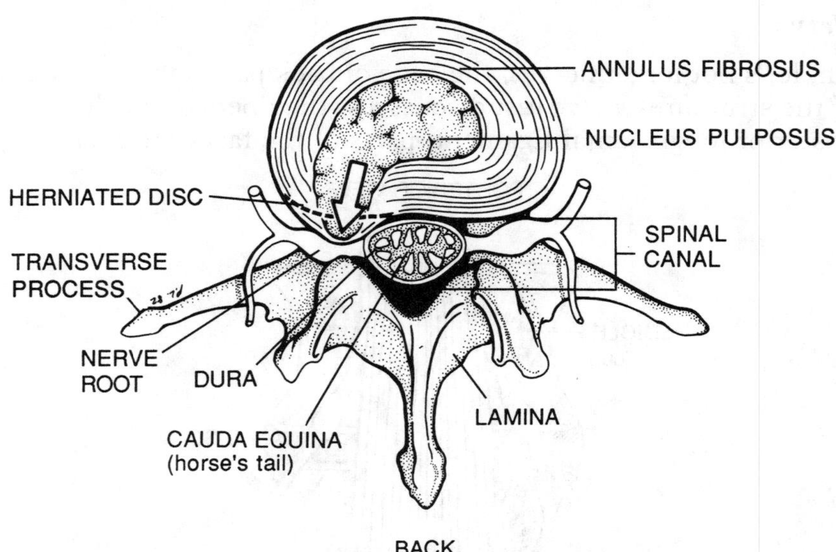

FIGURE 2–6B This is another view, this time looking down the spinal canal (horizontal, axial view, or CAT scan view) to show how a herniated or bulging disc can irritate the nerve. These two pictures are showing essentially the same thing from two different points of view.

the bony structure of the spine, and possibly the muscles—possess nerves and therefore the potential to transmit pain (see Figure 2–5). So injury to the spine, or physical or chemical irritation of almost any of its parts, can produce what this book is all about: backache.

One of the overall purposes of your spine, don't forget, is to protect your spinal cord. The cord itself ends at the top of the lumbar spine, and from there down, the canal is filled with a bundle of nerves called the *cauda equina* (Latin for "horse's tail") (Figures 2–6A and B). These nerves not only control the muscles of the legs, bladder, bowel, and sexual function, but also carry sensation from the hips and legs to the spinal cord and brain. So when the cauda equina's canal is encroached upon by any other structure—a problem known as spinal stenosis—back and leg pain may ensue. By the way, if you wanted to insult someone in Latin you could refer to him as a cauda equina. It means horse's tail, but that's pretty close to being a horse's ——.

The Sacroiliac Joint

Remember the words of the song, "Get a little movement in your sacroiliac"? In fact, there is some motion possible in this joint, which thirty or forty years ago was the number one scapegoat for back pain. Recently, though, there has been a backlash, and the sacroiliac—located between the sacrum and the ilium, or large pelvic bone—receives too scant attention. Certainly, many of our patients point to just that region when they localize their backache.

Because it's a synovial joint, with a membrane prone to irritation and inflammation, it can be affected by any kind of arthritis. One type of arthritis known as *ankylosing spondylitis* can provoke deformity, a rigid spine, severe pain, and inflammation, sometimes followed by actual bony growth across the sacroiliac. More about ankylosing spondylitis, and other kinds of arthritis, in Chapter III.

SPINE MECHANICS

Well, now that you know the rudiments of your back's anatomy, it's time for a primer in back mechanics: how all its parts actually work. Like the preceding anatomy lesson, you can refer to this biomechanics guide as you go along, if you don't feel like reading it through like *Gone With the Wind.* However, you may find it quite intriguing, especially if you have a mechanical bent.

Mechanical laws are reliable and consistent when we're dealing with automobiles or road-building. Though they can help us a good deal, when we apply them to biological systems they don't work out quite so precisely. Unfortunately, the physical behavior of bones and ligaments is quite different from that of inorganic materials like steel. For example, an engineer can design a bridge if he knows the span, the weather conditions, the bridge materials, the number and weight of the vehicles that will cross it, and so on. Now, if you imagine the bridge to be constructed out of biological materials, the task becomes much less predictable. The materials won't all have the same strength; if the loads of the vehicles are increased or decreased the bridge becomes weaker or stronger; if one structure becomes damaged (diseased) it may suddenly fail without warning.

The point to take home with you is this: Dead metals follow clear engineering laws, but you probably would not want to have an inert, fixed steel spine. Biological systems, in contrast, are in a state of constant change. That means they can *adapt* or *respond* to changes in the environment, including disease and injury. It's ultimately helpful that your living bone ligaments are more mercurial and adaptive than the parts of a bridge. They have the ability to heal. If you absorb this section well, you should learn to manage your back better and even improvise a few back-care tricks in addition to the ones listed in Chapter V.

You may be surprised to learn that much of the pioneering work in biomechanics was, in fact, done on the spine; most of it concerned the collection of data on vertebral strength. Why? Well, because of two of the "four horsemen," war and disease. When fighter pilots had to escape from a doomed aircraft, they were ejected basically by an explosion under their seats, which, needless to say, applied considerable impact to both derriere and spine. So tolerance limits of the vertebrae to the forces applied to them was the obvious knowledge to seek.

The other early work, by Swedish researchers led by the late Professor Carl Hirsch and subsequently his protégé, Professor Alf Nachemson, was motivated by more humanitarian and clinical aspects of survival. The pervasiveness of low back pain, its depressing impact on job absenteeism, and its high cost to society lent impetus to the emerging science of orthopaedic biomechanics of the spine. And here is what we've learned:

Posture

It would make a fascinating master's thesis to analyze cocktail parties and other social events by observing the posture of the participants, pondering, perhaps, the relative influences of biology and culture. Whom might you notice? Perhaps someone with a spinal deformity like scoliosis (sideways curvature of the spine)—of which the Hunchback of Notre Dame is the literary example. Or, an erect military person; an athlete; a dancer; a short man who is stretching; a tall woman slouching. An assertive person who is leaning over his interlocutor; a timid person cowering; a seductive woman in a tight sweater who is standing so as to show off her charms; a come-hither male lounging in tight pants. All of the partygoers have their characteristic posturing, and I recommend posture analysis as a pastime to take your mind off your backache at a party.

But posture has its medical side, too. As we've said, the spine has its natural physiological curves. As long as these curves are neither exaggerated by excessive or inappropriate muscle activity, nor deformed by laziness and slack muscles, we have normal posture. Good posture is a matter of holding the shoulders level and slightly back and carrying the chin slightly tucked in, while moderately flattening the lumbar lordosis ("swayback") by rotating the pelvis forward (Figure 2–7).

In the relaxed standing posture, the muscles shouldn't have to work too vigorously—for it's the job of the spine's ligaments to hold it in the proper position, allowing the muscles relative "R & R" (rest and relaxation) while we stand. But the erector spinae muscles down the back of the spine and, to some extent, the abdominal muscles, contract in the standing position, while the psoas major ("filet mignon") muscle contributes a little, too. When it comes to sitting, our muscles do the same job, though the erector spinae muscles must work a little harder.

Movement

When a prospective spinal-fusion patient asks, "How much will I be able to bend after surgery?" he's usually concerned with something we doctors call *flexion,* or bending forward (Figure 2–8). Whenever you bend forward, the bending or rearrangement of your lumbar vertebrae accomplishes the first sixty degrees of the movement, then your hip joint takes care of an additional twenty-five degrees. If you have a spinal fusion, usually two adjacent lumbar segments are fused, eliminating about ten to fifteen degrees of flexion motion. However, because of hip motion and the motion of the remaining unfused vertebral segments, restricted motion is hardly noticed in most patients.

A second important motion of the spine is *extension:* This is the medical term for arching your back, bending it backwards as a diver does (Figure 2–8). It's crucial not only to lovers everywhere but also to dancers and athletes—especially gymnasts, divers, football players, wrestlers, boxers, and tennis players. Here our erector spinae muscles really count.

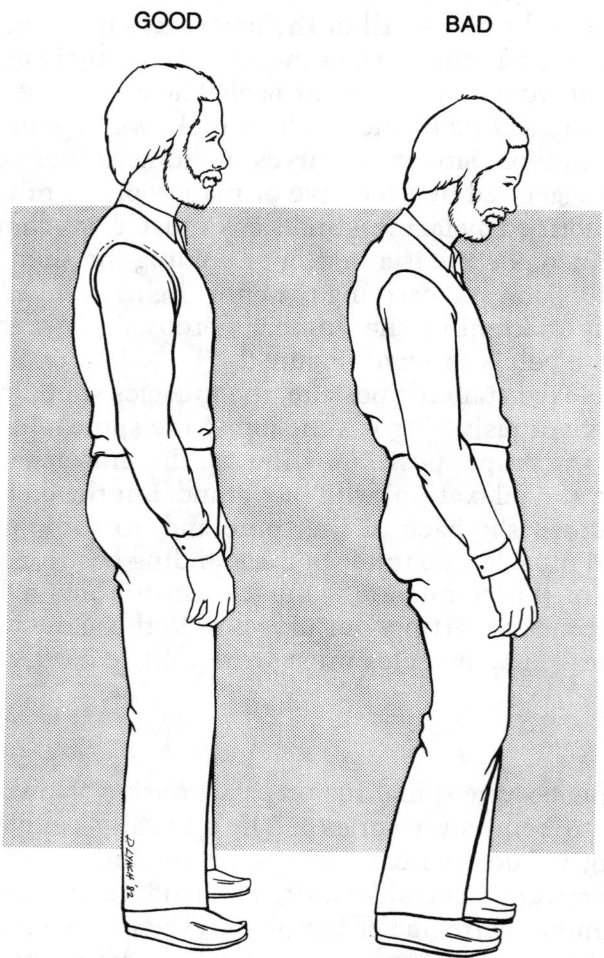

FIGURE 2–7 Here we see "good" and "bad" posture. The point is that the spine on the left is in the less "swayback" or extended position; that is, it's more straight. The spine in this position tends to be better balanced and distributes the forces in a more even manner. Theoretically, this is a less painful, more therapeutic position for the ailing back. There is room for legitimate disagreement on this issue. The posture issue may be no more than aesthetics. When the spine is extended in the "swayback" position shown on the right, there may be excessive forces and irritation of the posterior joints. There may also be disc bulging, which can be irritating to the nearby nerves.

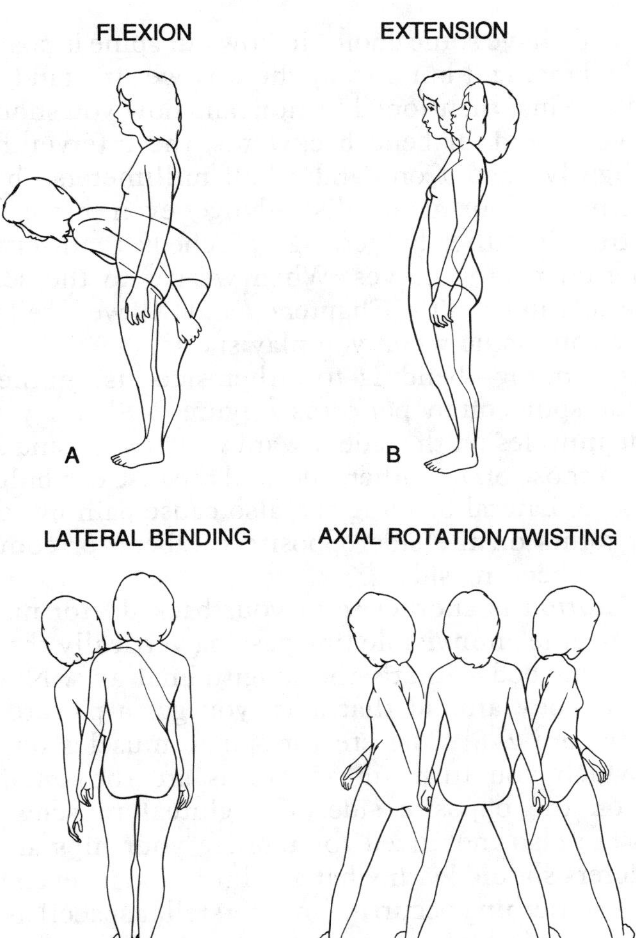

FIGURE 2–8 The purpose of this diagram is to clearly define several terms used throughout the book so that there is no confusion or misunderstanding. A) *Flexion.* The loads on the spine in this position are very large, and diseased spines are certainly likely to be irritated by this position. B) *Extension.* This is the extension or the "swayback" position; this too can be painful to the diseased spine because of irritation of the posterior (facet) joints and disc bulging. C) *Lateral Bending.* This can sometimes be painful on one or both sides due to irritation of the facet joints. D) *Axial Rotation or Twisting.* In a number of instances in the book we will talk about twisting motions, axial rotations, or torsional loading on the spine. These are key movements in a number of sports.

Now, we do have some choice in how our spine is positioned—not just by bracing it but also by the way we sit, stand, and play sports. We've just mentioned flexion, and now you should know that as we extend, or bend backwards, the intervertebral disc bulges slightly—about one and a half millimeters—backward. And degenerated or worn discs bulge even more, possibly making trouble either by getting "pinched" themselves or by impinging on nearby nerves. When we get to the section on backache do's and don't's (Chapters V and IX), we'll tell you how to protect your spine when you play sports.

Lateral bending—bending to either side—is another movement your spine often performs (Figure 2–8). As you might guess, the muscles on the side toward which you bend are more active than those on the other side, and the disc can bulge on the bending side. Lateral bending can also cause pain by stretching the facet joints on the side opposite the bend or compressing those on the bending side.

Axial rotation is another term your back doctor may throw around. Imagine an invisible line passing vertically through the center of your body—that's the longitudinal axis. Now if you rotate your body around that axis, you get a picture of axial rotation (Figure 2–8). The erector spinae muscles on the side toward which you turn are active, as are the small rotator muscles on the opposite side. The gluteal muscles in your buttocks are also mobilized to stabilize your hips and pelvis. Back sufferers should learn what axial rotation is (even if it does sound like something occurring in interstellar space!), because it applies a particularly dangerous stress to the disc (see page 234).

SOURCES OF MECHANICAL PROBLEMS

Muscle Spasm

When the spinal parts are irritated or diseased, the related back muscles—especially the erector spinae—sometimes go into spasm. Perhaps this is intended as a splinting mechanism to prevent further injury, and to reduce motion and diminish irritation. Anyone who's ever had a "muscle cramp," or any skier, runner, or swimmer who's suffered a "charley horse," knows the agony of muscle spasm. Our introduction to the way the muscles constantly monitor the spine's movements should prepare us for the fact that pitching a ball, or even climbing out of the bathtub, could irritate a sick spine and throw a sensitive muscle into spasm. Any contraction or stretching can produce spasm in a vulnerable muscle, and that's why rest, heat, braces, massage, and medications that relax you and your muscles have been a reliable nostrum for low back pain for years.

Disc Mechanics

Here's where we get to what, for many of you, is the crux of backache. If you read the first part of this chapter, you already know that the disc is a tough, fibrous, layered organ with a gelatinous center that absorbs a great deal of water in its young, healthy state. And, just as inexorably as we get smile lines and our hair turns gray, our discs become less resilient, less mobile, less fluid, and narrower as we get older. Of course, this natural disc aging need be no more pathological than gray hair. But as your discs can sometimes give you a hard time, a basic course in disc mechanics, shock absorbing and weight bearing, is essential. So here goes.

Most of the disc-pressure studies done on living human beings were initially performed on rather heroic Swedish medical students who agreed to have needles inserted through their backs and spinal canals into the center of the intervertebral disc. From their humane and entrepreneurial volunteerism we've learned a lot about different mechanical pressures on the disc. (These subjects and others did, in fact, receive a tax-free payment for their time and efforts. To my mind, however, this does not detract from the courage they demonstrated.)

For the moment, one all-important fact pops out: When you sit, the forces on your lumbar spine are almost fifty percent greater than when you stand. Lying on your side? The lumbar spine is subjected to forces twenty-five percent *less* than standing pressures. And lying supine (on your back) with your hips and knees bent is best of all, since the forces on the disc are a bare third of what they are standing.

Now, we've already mentioned that as fluid pressure builds up inside the disc, the disc becomes stiffer and less energy-absorbent—even possibly painful and subject to injury. When we lie in bed at night, less force is exerted on the intervertebral disc, as we might expect. But as a result, it absorbs more fluid. This may be the answer to the perplexing problem of morning back pain for those who notice that their spines hurt most when they get out of bed in the morning. All of which has a bearing on back care, as we'll see in Chapter V. The nocturnal disc-fluid accumulation re-equilibrates itself in two hours or less.

As your automobile gets older, its shock absorbers tend to wear out; and the same is true, more or less, of your discs. As their shock-absorbing powers wane, various mechanical problems may occur. Modern clinical scientists have not yet figured out why some aging discs become painful and others do not. Several new theories suggest that chemical irritants associated with the degenerative changes may be the culprits. Here we'll mention how some of your daily activities—which have names you probably never expected—can affect the disc.

Vertical compression loading: Picture stacking weights on top of your disc, which is essentially what happens when you pick up your child, your groceries, your briefcase, or your paycheck. Compression loading won't actually make the disc herniate, but it can make it bulge into the spinal canal, and degenerated discs bulge more than normal ones. The most frequent compression-loading injury is fracture of the vertebra's end plate, which, by the way, often doesn't show up on an X ray.

Torsional loading: Think of this one as a twist to the disc. If you were to twist a wire by holding one end firm and turning the other along the up-and-down axis, you'd have torsion. When it comes to your back, perhaps the most serious mechanical threat comes from lifting something heavy while twisting the back. Doctors' offices are full of patients who relate the onset of back pain to this ominous lift-with-a-twist movement, often describing a loud snap or pop that most likely means a rupturing disc. It comes as no surprise that twisting sorts of sports like bowling, golf, and baseball produce a fair share of back pain and sciatica patients.

The Psoas Muscle

One of the basic mechanical principles of back function is the fact that a tense, highly stressed psoas muscle tends to irritate the back, and a relaxed one does not. This is because the muscle originates from the front of the lumbar spine and attaches to the thighbone (the femur) just past the hip joint. This is shown in Figure 2–4. You should understand that a relaxed psoas muscle is good for the bad back, and I will be demonstrating this repeatedly in Chapters VIII and IX.

The Yellow Ligament

This ligament, lying just in back of the spinal canal, deserves some comment here (Figure 2–2). In the very early phases of a motion, only a slight force permits extensive stretching of this ligament, but as the motion continues, more force is needed. In the later phase, the ligament becomes very taut, and continued loading—for instance, working for an extended period in a flexed, forward posture, as in gardening—can permanently stretch or rupture it. The same is true of all the back's other ligaments. And when the very elastic yellow ligament loses its elasticity it sometimes bulges into the canal, contributing to back and leg pain—usually in conjunction with the bulging of other structures. When this occurs, we call it spinal stenosis.

Abdominal Muscle Mechanics

You probably don't realize how important your abdomen is to your back. Why? Well, when we hold the spine erect or bend slightly forward, the back muscles must contract and exert tremendous forces to maintain balance and equilibrium. And these muscles must work at considerable mechanical disadvantage, because they apply their forces close to the center of motion (remember your high-school physics lessons on levers and pulleys?). The result is that strong forces are applied to the discs, vertebrae, and other elements, and the spine is very sensitive to anything that shifts the center of gravity forward and adds to its mechanical disadvantage. Obesity, pregnancy, and carrying a heavy object in front of you are three noteworthy examples (Figure 2–9, 3–10, and 5–3 respectively).

However, your spine has an excellent ally in the abdomen. Strong abdominal muscles that create good turgor in the trunk (stomach and chest) can share some of the spine muscles' work. Then there's less pressure on the spine, and less danger of damage or irritation. It's important to note that in both health and disease, but particularly disease, the spine is highly sensitive

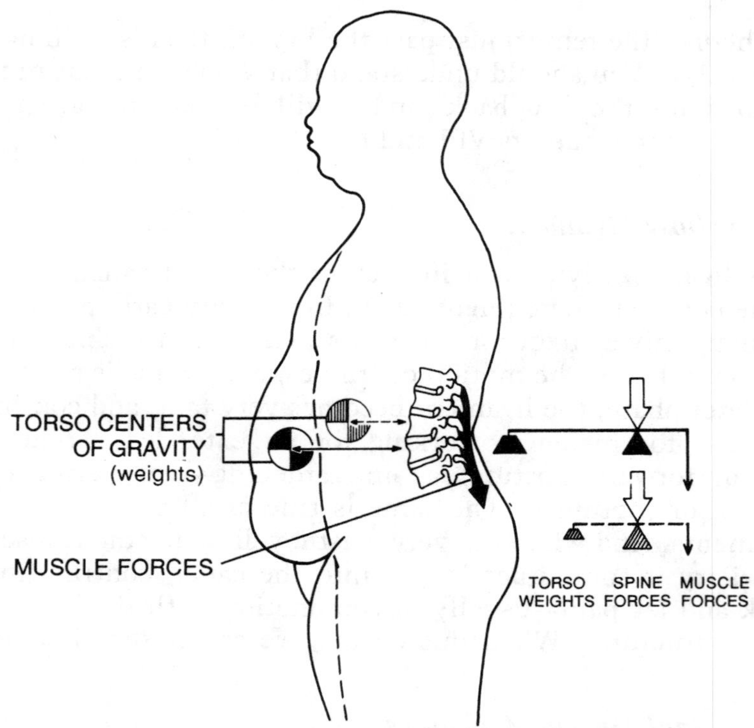

FIGURE 2–9 This figure shows how obesity shifts the center of gravity forward. This figure allows us to compare the different forces operating on the spine in a fat man and a thin man. The erector spinae muscles represented by the dark area in back of the spine must contract and exert forces to hold the person erect. In a fat person, the center of gravity is moved forward; in the diagram, this is indicated by the circle with dark sections, which is shifted more anteriorly. In this case, the erector spinae muscles must work harder and exert a greater force to keep the spine erect. When this occurs, there is a great deal more force and pressure within the structures of the spine at both the facet joints and at the disc. This is irritating even to a normal spine, and certainly it can cause difficulty to an abnormal spine.

If we look at the center of gravity that is closer to the spine, as shown by the circle with the gray quadrants, we see that the erector spinae muscles don't have to work quite as hard to counterbalance the center of gravity; the forces within the spine are not as great and therefore not as irritating or painful. This is one of the important reasons that staying as lean as possible is thought to be helpful for those with back problems. (Reproduced with permission from White, A.A., and Panjabi, M.M.: *Clinical Biomechanics of the Spine,* J.B. Lippincott, 1990, second edition.)

to even the most subtle mechanical factors. This fact will help you to look after your bad back, as we'll see when we get to Chapter V.

Now that you know everything (well, just about everything) about your spine's anatomy and mechanics, you're almost ready to tackle your bad back. Here you've learned how it's all put together, and how it functions. In the next chapter, you'll find out about some of the ways in which this exquisitely complex part of you can go awry.

Chapter III

Why Does My Back Hurt?

HERE'S WHAT you've been waiting for. This chapter lists just about all the known medical causes of low back pain. Use the following information as a convenient reference, but don't lose any sleep worrying about serious or mysterious diseases. Some of the disorders you'll read about here are indeed ominous-sounding. Rest assured that most of the really bad diseases occur very rarely, and that more prosaic diseases are likely to be causing your malaise. While I can't urge you strongly enough to get proper diagnosis and treatment of any pain that stays with you for more than three or four weeks, take comfort in the knowledge that even persistent backaches seldom spell dire disease.

This long inventory notwithstanding, we must face the disquieting fact that the exact cause of backache all too frequently remains incognito. As a matter of fact, in the strict scientific sense, modern medical science can definitively diagnose the cause in only about fifteen percent of the acute cases. (Beware the "practitioner" who quickly examines you and says, "I know exactly what is wrong and I will cure you.") On the positive side, modern clinical skills are quite effective in diagnosing herniated discs, certain types of arthritis, infections, tumors, and spinal stenosis when they cause low back pain. We doctors are actually better at managing your back problem than we are at finding its exact cause. Now, onward.

DISC DISEASES

Disc Degeneration

An unfortunate term, but don't let it dismay you. As you've already learned, your intervertebral discs inexorably age—gracefully or ungracefully—just as the rest of you does. In the case of your disc, aging means that it gradually loses water, becoming less springy, smaller, and less effective as a shock absorber from about age thirty on (Figure 3–1). After age forty, it can also become calcified, and on rare occasions a bony fusion forms across the disc.

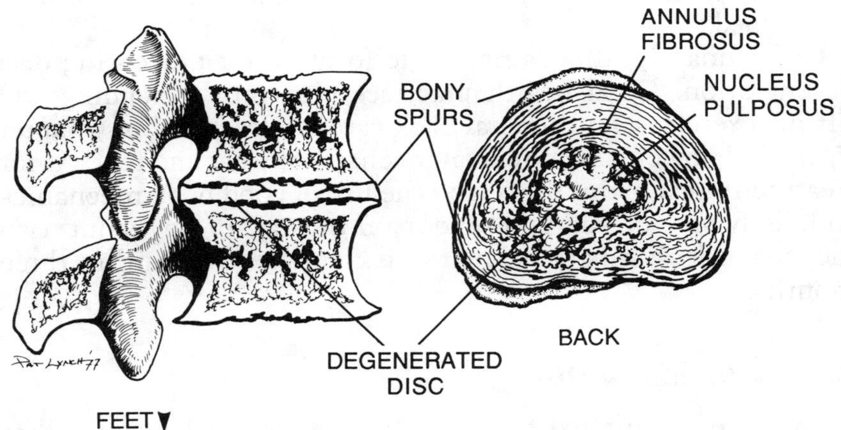

FIGURE 3–1 Cross-section of the vertebra that shows, diagrammatically, the severe degeneration of a disc. The picture on the left is the cut that goes right down through the middle of the two vertebrae. Looking at this side view, the part closest to the viewer has been removed so that you are looking down to the middle of the cross-section. We see these changes as a virtually normal process of aging. However, in some people it seems to be associated with a great deal of back pain. Patients may have symptoms of simple back pain, or back and leg pain. If you compare the disc shown here with the more normal disc in Figure 2–3, you can appreciate the changes of degeneration. (Reproduced with permission from White, A.A., and Panjabi, M.M.: *Clinical Biomechanics of the Spine,* J.B. Lippincott, 1990, second edition.)

We don't understand why some degenerating discs cause a lot of trouble for their owners, while others that look virtually identical on an X ray or physical exam are completely painless. As we'll see, episodes of low back pain *without* sciatica, or irritation of the sciatic nerve (from your buttocks to your foot), can sometimes foreshadow actual sciatic symptoms caused by disc herniation. More about this in the next subsection.

It's not easy to be sure that an X-ray finding of disc degeneration can be considered the cause of your low back pain. Usually, it's blamed when there's no other apparent cause and when there's a localized area of wear that seems to have progressed beyond the disc itself. The diagnosis is made with an X ray and sometimes a *discography,* a moderately painful test in which a special dye is injected into the disc before the "picture" is snapped.

Unfortunately, there's no magic formula for preventing disc degeneration. Good health practices plus proper bending and lifting, exercises, and general back care, as described in Chapter V, can help by cutting down on mechanical wear and tear. As for treatment, rest, painkillers, and the use of good body mechanics should have you upright and pain-free again in about two months or less; ninety percent of patients recover within three months.

Sciatica/Herniated Disc

If you've ever suffered from *sciatica,* you're probably familiar with its annoying symptoms in your lower back and legs: numbness or abnormal sensitivity (when even a light touch is painful), tingling, or "pins and needles" in the leg.

The sciatic nerve runs from your buttocks down your leg to your foot, and when something presses against it you end up with sciatica and the aforementioned kinds of pain. The sciatic nerve lies close to the intervertebral disc. When part of the disc bulges or gets dislodged from between the vertebrae—a condition called *disc herniation*—it impinges on the nerve (see Figures 2–6A and B and the glossary). The first documented case was reported in England in 1911, and, sadly, the patient died. Nowadays, of course, no one dies of lumbar disc disease, though it can make you quite uncomfortable. In 1934, two Harvard professors, Mixter, a neurosurgeon, and Barr, an orthopaedic surgeon, completed their classic report on disc herniation, documenting the disease clinically and by microscopic description. Thanks to them, we can now tell you a good deal about how your disc is behaving when it acts up.

Before moving on, here's the answer to the question patients often ask: What causes the disc to herniate? Here's a scientific answer. Engineers studied human disc specimens and produced herniation by flexing, laterally bending, and applying a sudden compression load (Figure 3–2). Obviously, the situation shown in the diagram is not the way it happens in real life. However, bending forward and then to one side associated with sudden lift (compression) could "do the job." We also know that a disc can herniate gradually and as a result of other types of forces and movements.

How can you tell if you have disc disease? This and the following seven paragraphs will tell you how we diagnose a disc herniation. You'll usually feel significant low back pain *before*

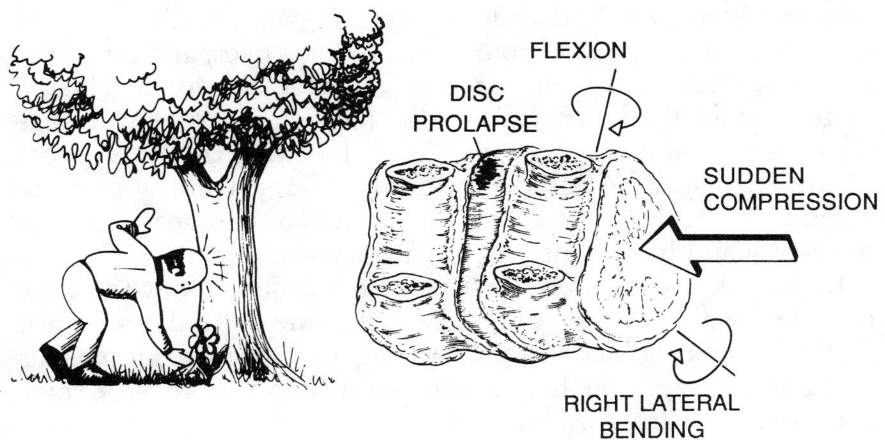

FIGURE 3–2 A mechanism of disc herniation is shown here, somewhat facetiously, but the point can be made. Using fresh human spine specimens with the posterior bone removed, the specimen was manipulated as shown in the figure. It was flexed, bent forward, bent to the right side, and then a sudden compression was applied to it. The man in the picture who is bumping his head against the tree, theoretically, is at risk for rupturing his disc on the left side and developing sciatica, or left leg pain. (Reproduced with permission from White, A.A., and Panjabi, M.M.: *Clinical Biomechanics of the Spine,* J.B. Lippincott, 1990, second edition.)

the onset of leg symptoms. It may start as severe pain or a superficial ache, and often coughing, sneezing, or straining at the stool will make the pain shoot down your leg all the way into your toes. Or sometimes the leg pain, especially if you're an athlete, may start by mimicking a charley horse or pulled muscle. The misery of sciatica may run the gamut from sharp, precise pain to hazy aches, and patients describe it in myriad ways. You may find that bending or twisting around aggravates your symptoms.

An important part of your clinical evaluation is the physical examination conducted by your doctor. The entire physical exam will not be reviewed, but a few salient points will provide a useful background to you as you encounter this aspect of your evaluation. The physician will look for changes in your reflexes—that is, the knee jerk and ankle jerk. This will be tested with the use of a neurologic camera which taps your leg just below the knee joint and taps the large tendon immediately behind your ankle. The strength of certain muscles in your leg will also be tested. This is done by testing your ability to resist certain manipulations of your toes, ankles, knees, and hips. It is also important that the straight leg test be done. This is performed as you lie supine and the physician carries your legs through several manipulations. Please be aware that this aspect of the exam can sometimes temporarily aggravate your pain. Though painful, this causes no particular damage and is a necessary and important part of the examination.

Regular X rays, which don't give us a good peek at the disc, can't really diagnose the disease. And beware of needless X rays: A routine set of spine X rays in a young woman, for example, has a radiation effect on her ovaries equivalent to chest X rays administered daily for sixty days.

Magnetic Resonance Imaging (MRI), because of its safety and image quality, when available, has almost completely replaced myelography and computer tomography (CT scans) as the technology of choice to diagnose a herniated disc. This is a rapidly developing technology that is likely to develop numerous additional capabilities. It has been discovered that the intravenous administration of a contrast medium gadolinium-diethelene triaminepentacetic acid (DPTA) combined with MRI, brings out anatomic detail and may help in recognizing the distinction between scar tissue and recurrent disc herniation.

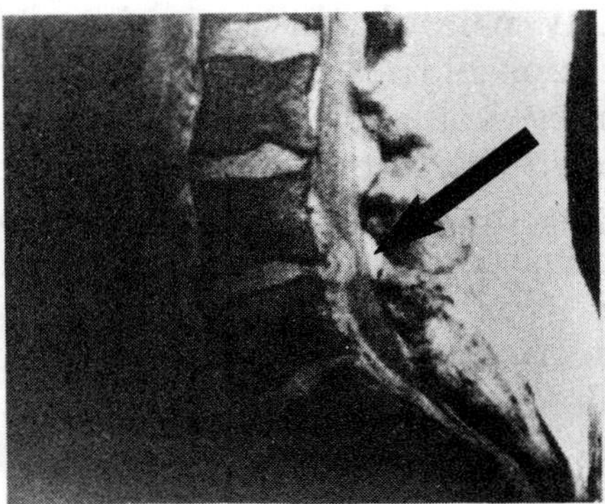
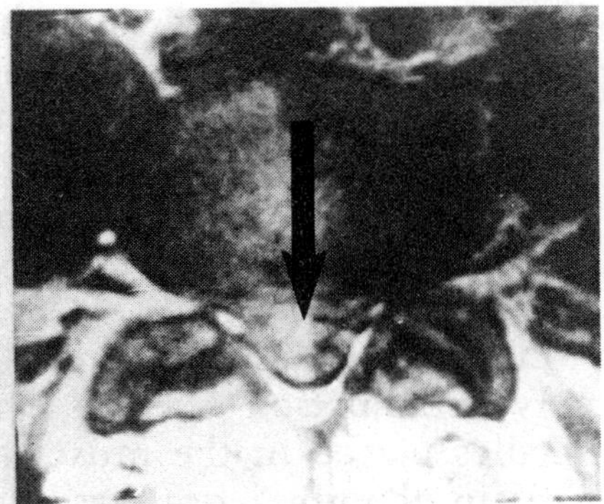

FIGURE 3–3 A) This is a lateral view of MRI scan. Note large protrusion posterior to the disc space between L4 and L5 (arrow). B) This is a horizontal view. Disc is seen protruding into the canal slightly to the left of the midline (arrow).

An example of an MRI of a herniated lumbar intervertebral disc is shown in Figure 3–3. One thing that's good to keep in mind as you and your doctor evaluate your imaging studies is the fact that thirty percent of disc herniations, although present, are not the cause of pain. Therefore you want to be certain that in addition to the imaging evidence of a disc herniation you have the other clinical characteristics of a herniated disc. Certainly before considering surgery or other invasive procedures you want to have the appropriate indications. These are presented in detail in Chapter VII: "To Operate or Not to Operate."

Prior to the more general availability of MRI, CT scans and myelograms were used to confirm the diagnosis of herniated discs. These are still used on occasion when complicated or unusual clinical problems are being evaluated. The CT scan can sometimes present a false positive disc herniation. These and all clinical evaluation items/studies should be combined with the patient's history, physical exam, and personality evaluation for the most accurate diagnosis and treatment plan.

Myelography is sometimes used alone or in conjunction with a CT scan to evaluate a complicated disc problem. In this test, a needle is inserted into the sheath around the nerve, in the spinal canal. A dye that will show on an X ray is then injected. Don't cringe yet. While you may have heard a lot of scary stories, some patients don't find myelography particularly painful. However, in addition to being most likely painful, this procedure is associated with risks such as infection and headaches. Therefore, don't jump into myelography unless you and your doctor have decided to go ahead with surgery if the test is positive. Fortunately for you, CAT scans (computerized axial tomography) are currently supplanting myelograms for diagnosing herniated discs.

Electrodiagnostic studies, electromyography (EMG), and nerve conduction tests are helpful. In the EMG, very fine needles placed in the muscles record their electrical activity. Certain abnormal readings suggest nerve irritation or damage that may be caused by a herniated disc. Nerve conduction studies measure the speed with which the nerves carry out various functions. A slowing of conduction rate may indicate nerve damage from an impinging disc. But myelography gives the best picture of a herniated disc.

How do you avoid a herniated disc in the first place? There are many exotic and elaborate answers to this question, but the scientific evidence supports this answer: Simply nurture your general health, don't smoke, don't drive or ride around in motor vehicles for more than two hours per day, and avoid back stresses, like lifting in awkward positions, that can provoke disc herniation. Certain sports (see Chapter IX) are probably hard on the spine, lowering your threshold for disc herniation. If you already have a herniated disc, see Chapters V and VI on how to treat it, and if all conservative treatments fail, surgery may be necessary (Chapter VII).

ARTHRITIC DISEASE OF THE SPINE

Any type of arthritis that attacks the joints elsewhere in your body can also lodge in your spine. Whenever we have inflammation of the joints, we have arthritis. The inflammation almost always brings pain, and is associated with engorgement of tissues and high concentrations of inflammatory cells such as white blood cells. Arthritis can settle anywhere on the spectrum from very subtle—say, frequent "bursitis" or occasional aches and pains in the joints—to the crippling, deforming disease we hear about on telethons.

The intervertebral joints in your spine are synovial joints, as you learned in Chapter II, and this synovial lining is sensitive to a number of chemical, immunologic, and other disease processes. Would that the Creator had never wrought a synovial tissue, since it plays such a large role in causing pain in our joints. Of course, having no synovial tissue would aggravate the energy crisis. Without the lubricating fluid it produces, we'd have to oil our joints, and change the oil, too, no doubt!

Several arthritic diseases are thought to be based on some kind of allergic or autoimmune response, in which the body's immune system attacks its own tissue. The fibrous tissue called *collagen* that makes up a large part of your bone, cartilage, and ligaments is affected in the so-called collagen diseases—of which rheumatoid arthritis, degenerative arthritis, and ankylosing spondylitis will concern us here. Other systemic collagen diseases, for the record, include lupus erythematosis, periarteritis nodosa, and scleroderma, but we won't discuss them in this book. So back to the back.

Laboratory tests are usually necessary to reveal the immunologic factors involved in the collagen diseases. Then, too, the general manifestation of the disease, including associated skin problems and other disorders, can help a careful internist, orthopedist, rheumatologist, or dermatologist tell you what you've got. Sometimes it's no easy matter to determine which of these diseases is hurting your spine.

Spondylitis (Degenerative Arthritis)

Normal wear and tear in the spine can cause pain and inflammation. Technically this is called *degenerative arthritis.* But that sounds so unsavory that we can instead use the term *spondylitis* (Greek for "inflammation of the vertebra"). Don't let these terms depress you. The normal use of the spine results in certain alterations in the cartilage around the bony tissues, and sometimes painful joints. We're speaking primarily of the intervertebral joints, though the joints between the vertebral bodies can also act up. Consult Chapter II on back anatomy if you need to. While this wear and tear afflicts nearly all spines as they age, only some people appear to have pain associated with the changes.

How can you tell if you're suffering from spondylitis? When wear changes show up on the X ray and nothing else is found to account for your pain, spondylitis is usually implicated. What does the X ray reveal specifically? Osteophytes, or spurs, possibly, as well as minor deformities of the vertebral bodies (see Figure 3–1).

You can ask yourself, is your pain worse after inactivity, say, when you get up in the morning? Does it gradually subside as you move around? Does your back ache more when the weather is cold or damp or the barometric pressure changes? (By the way, now you know why Grandpa could predict the weather by the state of his joints.) Is there a limit to full motion, and pain at the outer edges of motion? Do bending, lifting, prolonged sitting, twisting, or riding in cars or planes hurt your spine? If the answer to many of these questions is yes, you may be a spondylitis sufferer.

Don't despair. The good news is that regular, gentle exercise, good muscle tone, and normal weight maintenance can keep wear changes from causing back pain. And when your back *does* hurt, aspirin and other anti-inflammatory drugs such as Voltaren (diclotenac sodium), Indocin, Motrin (ibuprofen), and Naprosyn are helpful. Occasionally a brace may be recommended. On the rare occasion when the wear changes are confined to one area, foster abnormal motion, and are clearly the source of a patient's backache, a spinal fusion can be considered.

Ankylosing Spondylitis

Spondylitis, as we've said, means inflammation of the spine, and ankylosing means stiffening. Put them together and you have stiffening of an inflamed, painful spine, the hallmark of this disorder. This is the disease, by the way, that *Saturday Review* editor Norman Cousins reportedly cured in an unorthodox fashion: with "laughter therapy." In a book called *Anatomy of an Illness,* he recalls how he checked into a hotel room and watched many solid hours of videotapes of "Candid Camera" and other shows, then emerged with a reanimated will to live and a more comfortable spine. Mr. Cousins may have felt better because he stimulated his body's production of natural painkillers, endorphins (see Chapter IV). A positive attitude is crucial to healing, of course, but in this chapter we'll discuss more conventional treatment.

This very painful form of arthritis commonly afflicts males in their twenties and thirties. As the spine stiffens, the connection between the ribs and the thoracic (middle) spine sometimes becomes so rigid that the patient can barely expand his chest. With a stiff neck and upper spine, he may walk around in a slightly crouched position; in severe cases, major deformity may result.

In the earliest stages, though, these changes may not be so clear-cut. When ankylosing spondylitis starts as low back pain, it will actually turn up in the neighborhood of the sacroiliac joint. That's between the lower back and the pelvic bone, remember? The pain may even be referred to the hip and thigh, confusing the diagnosis with intervertebral disc disease. The case history usually comprises pain in the major joints of the spine and perhaps transient pain in other joints, such as the shoulder, hip, knee, ankle, elbow, or wrist. Characteristically, however, ankylosing spondylitis will eventually settle in the spine.

If your doctor suspects you have ankylosing spondylitis, he or she will perform a few lab tests. The rate at which your red blood cells settle to the bottom of the tube generally increases, and this measurement, called sedimentation, or "sed" rate, is one clue of active disease. Another special test, called HLA-B27, which measures certain immunologic factors, supports the diagnosis.

Unfortunately, we doctors know of no way to prevent this ailment. But once the diagnosis is made, it's very important to perform regular exercises, though severe pain may make it difficult indeed. You should also wear a brace, if necessary, to forestall major deformity. When the deformity is severe and incapacitating, the patient may choose to have his bony spine, *not* the cord, cut through and straightened surgically. Since it's a rather awesome operation, it should be done by an experienced surgeon in a hospital with a reliable spine service. Even so, since one out of every ten or twenty patients dies or suffers major complications, you should contemplate surgery only when you simply cannot tolerate a life limited to seeing only the ground a few feet ahead and never the horizon. Refer to Chapter VII for further discussion.

Rheumatoid Arthritis

This is the bogeyman, the form of arthritis that is most often synonymous with "crippling arthritis" and gives the disease its bleak reputation. While it usually afflicts the knee, hip, hand, and wrist joints more than the back, it can also hit the lumbar spine. For some reason, it's more common in women than in men. The disease inflicts joint deformity, usually making it easy to diagnose. Confirmation comes from laboratory tests that detect the "rheumatoid factor" in the blood. Actually, rheumatoid arthritis isn't just a disease of the joints; it can perform its dirty work on almost any system of the body.

Nobody knows what causes arthritis, but doctors suspect an autoimmune response is to blame. That is, your immune system forms antibodies against its own tissue as if it were a foreign invader; you might think of it as the body turning around and attacking itself.

Aspirin can generally control the inflammatory response. Stronger anti-inflammatory medicines such as cortisone, which can have severe side effects, and nonsteroidal anti-inflammatory drugs are often used to treat rheumatoid arthritis. Gold injections also may improve the quality of life. Sadly, at the present time there's no cure for this unpleasant affliction. Gentle, active exercise and appropriate braces can help prevent progressive deformity, however. Hopelessly destroyed hip and knee joints can be replaced surgically with good success.

SPONDYLOLISTHESIS

This tongue twister (dare even your orthopedist to say it fast!) comes from the Greek for "slipping vertebrae." In this condition, a defect in the bony back part of one vertebra allows the front parts of the vertebra to move forward, out of alignment with the rest of your spine. Picture a child stacking blocks. If the second block from the bottom, say, slides forward, three or more blocks on top of it will tilt, too, right? And that's essentially what happens in spondylolisthesis. When one vertebra slips forward, several vertebrae above it tend to pitch forward as well (Figure 3–4).

This defect, in addition to being common in Eskimos, is seen frequently in several groups of athletes. The players at risk are gymnasts, interior linemen (in American football), sumo wrestlers, weight lifters, and javelin throwers. These sports all require lots of flexion-extension activity or heavy lifting, moving from a flexed to extended position. The defect is created by a type of fatigue break in the bone. This break occurs as a result of many repeated forces on a bone (accumulated impact loading), none of which individually would be strong enough to break it. This is analogous to the march fracture seen in the metatarsal (fore foot bone) of the military recruit who has not done much walking before basic training. No one blow breaks his bone, but the long marches eventually do. A bone scan (page 77) is useful in diagnosing this "overuse" condition.

Here's an interesting bit of low back trivia. Now that you're in "the club" these little anecdotes have a place in your conversations with fellow "low backers." If you study contortionists you'll discover that they can be divided into two groups, those who contort by bending forward (flexing), called Klischnigg contortionists, and those who contort by bending backward (extending), known as Caoutche contortionists. The defect of spondylolisthesis is only seen in the latter group—the extenders—or those who go into great lordosis bending backward. So in order to cause the fatigue failure of the portion of your spine shown in Figure 3–4 you've got to bend backward with force, the way the gymnasts and the Caoutche contortionists do.

The result? Generally, severe low back pain, pain in the hips and thighs, and—when there's nerve root irritation—sciatica, usually in both limbs. Younger people may suffer from spasm or tightness of the hamstring muscles in the back of the thighs, producing stooped posture, an odd gait, and considerable pain. The defect in the back of the vertebra doesn't itself cause pain unless it's the result of a fracture. But it does expose you to some risk of developing the slippage we just discussed. The slippage can be seen on an X ray.

Spine pain due to spondylolisthesis that doesn't respond to conservative therapies like painkillers and braces can usually be alleviated by surgery. You and your doctor may elect a spinal fusion (*arthrodesis*) of the lower part of the spine to the sacrum. If there's a neurological deficit from an irritated sciatic nerve, it may be necessary to remove a portion of the vertebra to relieve the irritation from the root of the nerve.

DEGENERATIVE SPONDYLOLISTHESIS

This diagnosis is similar to the previously described spondylolisthesis, except that the forward slipping shown in Figure 3–4, occurs for a different reason. It happens not because of a defect in the bone but rather because of a deformation, moulding, or yielding of the bone around the joints as a result of wear changes. This condition occurs four times more frequently in people who have diabetes than in those who don't. The reason may be related to relatively weaker ligaments in the diabetics, which could be due to deficiency in the production of collagen, the major component of ligaments.

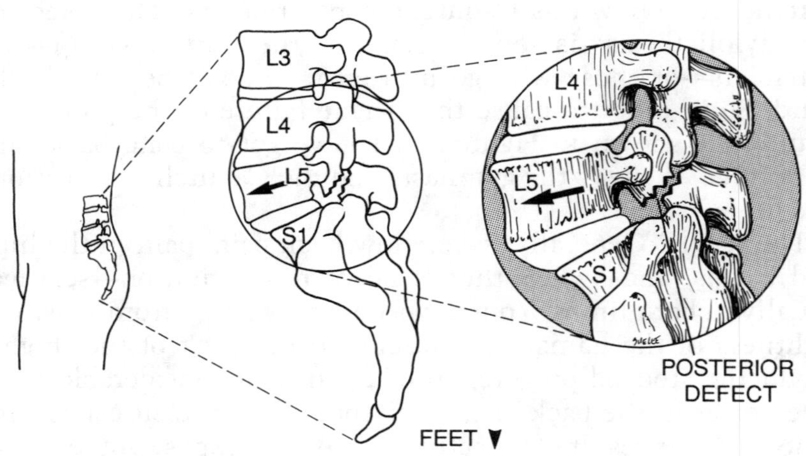

FIGURE 3–4 This is the picture of a *spondylolisthesis* as a result of a defect in the posterior bony part of the vertebral L5. The L5 vertebra has slipped forward (see arrow) in relation to S1. This slip is called spondylolisthesis. This problem is found in a variety of different patients for different reasons. The vertebrae shown are the lumbar 3, 4, 5, and the first sacral vertebra. The spondylolisthesis is at L5/S1. That is where it most commonly occurs; it does sometimes occur at L4/L5. I will discuss spondylolisthesis frequently in the book, so I hope that it has been explained clearly here.

SPINAL STENOSIS

This means that the spinal canal is narrowed or compromised, leaving inadequate room for the nerves (see Figure 3–5). The causes of stenosis vary. Actually, a herniated disc is a type of spinal stenosis, though it isn't called by that name because its clinical picture is different. You see, anything that encroaches on your all-important spinal canal can lead to stenosis. Examples are spur formation around the vertebral bodies; wear changes and distortion around the intervertebral joints, or swelling of the joint's capsule; displacement of the yellow ligament; or thickening of the vertebral body's lamina (thin bony plate). See Figure 3–6. Or, the canal may simply be constricted by congenital malformation. You might wish to refer back to our anatomy lesson in Chapter II to recall what all these mysterious parts of you are.

People over fifty are the most common stenosis victims. Symptoms include substantial back pain with variable leg pain and weakness associated with walking. But the nerve deficit symptoms—weakness, pain, pins and needles, coldness, or loss of sensation in the limbs—have a more generalized and irregular pattern than in disc herniation. Do you have pain after walking, and does it diminish when you walk uphill and worsen when you go downhill? When you stop and rest, does the pain stay with you? Do squatting or sitting, leaning forward and bending your back, help with the pain? Have you noticed that you're relatively more comfortable pushing a grocery shopping cart? This position tends to open up the canal space. A study of figure 3–6 will help you to understand this point better. Do coughing, sneezing, or straining at the stool aggravate your discomfort? These afflictions hint that you may have stenosis. Unlike disc disease and other kinds of backache with an intermittent course, spinal stenosis generally gets progressively more painful.

How does your doctor know if you have stenosis? Your history, physical findings, and X rays can usually uncover the disease. Sometimes myelography or a CAT scan or MRI can help evaluate the exact state of your spinal canal.

I must acknowledge that physicians, being neither omniscient

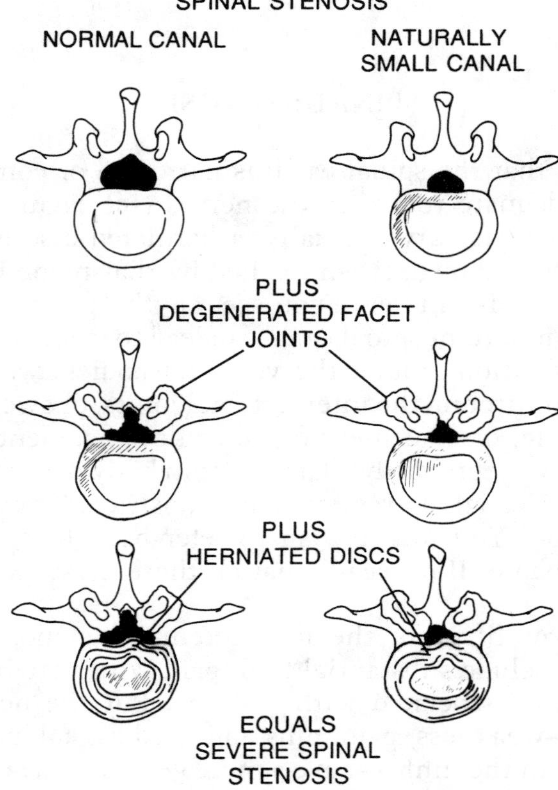

FIGURE 3–5 This figure shows an axial cross-sectional view of a number of spines, emphasizing the shape and size of the spinal canal. Spinal stenosis is a disease in which the spinal canal is encroached upon in various ways. The space available for the cauda equina or the nerves as they pass along the canal becomes inadequate. The top two pictures show a normal canal on the left, and on the right a canal that is compromised as a result of individual development (congenitally small).

The next set of pictures show how degenerative changes of the facet joints and the vertebral bodies can compromise the space available, particularly in the canal on the right that was already small due to individual development (congenitally small).

The next two pictures show that a bulging or herniated disc further compromises the space available in both circumstances. These pictures explain the essence of the disease known as *spinal stenosis.* (Reproduced with permission from White, A.A., and Panjabi, M.M.: *Clinical Biomechanics of the Spine,* J.B. Lippincott, 1990, second edition.)

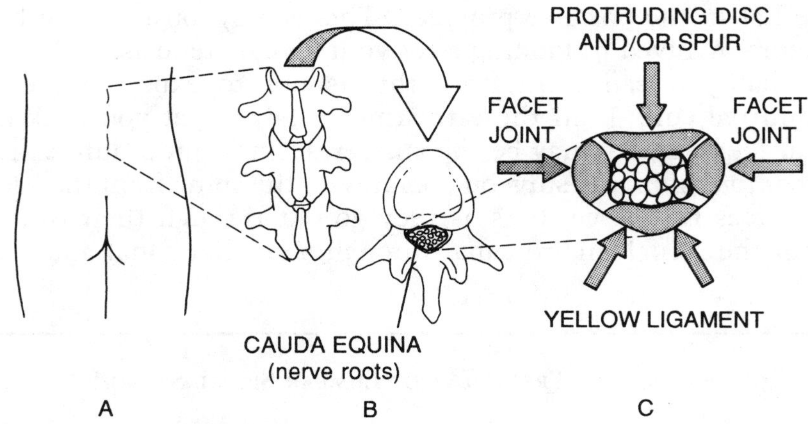

FIGURE 3–6 A) Posterior view of back of patient who has lumbar spinal stenosis.

B) View of L3, L4, and L5 lumbar vertebrae, those most commonly involved in lumbar spinal stenosis. Vertebrae are rotated ninety degrees to allow us to look down the spinal canal where we see the cauda equina, which is a collection of all the nerve roots that run down the canal within the dura. Some of the nerve roots exit at each level to go into the legs. Figure 2–6A shows the cauda equina from the back with the back of the spinal column (spinous processes, laminae, and facet joints) removed along with the dural sheath, which covers the nerve roots.

C) This is a schematic representation of the spinal canal and the *compressed* dural sheath and nerve roots. From the front of the canal the disc and/or a bone ridge (osteophyte) encroaches upon the canal. From the back the yellow ligament, which has lost some or all of its elasticity and become scarred and thickened, protrudes into the canal. From either or both sides a deformed, scarred, and possibly swollen facet joint may encroach upon the space available within the canal. These are the culprits which collectively result in the pain, weakness, and other signs and symptoms of lumbar spinal stenosis.

nor omnipotent, have yet to discover how to prevent spinal stenosis.

Treatment of this disease consists of rest (lying on one's side with hip and knees bent as in Figure 5–12, p. 125, lower illustration), painkillers, and anti-inflammatory drugs, together with support from a flexion corset or brace and gradual, appropriate exercise. You may notice that most of the back problems we're discussing don't get cured miraculously but require patience and tincture of time for recuperation. Please read through the list in the box I've provided. This is a synopsis of the key factors involved in looking after your spinal stenosis.

What you can learn from this is not to expect a quick, definitive cure. If all these treatments fail to get you back on your feet, surgery may be the answer. Using a procedure called *decompression,* the surgeon operates on the spine from the back and frees the nerve roots as they go out through their tunnel from the spinal (main) canal through a smaller canal and into

CONSERVATIVE TREATMENT OF LUMBAR SPINAL STENOSIS*

Medication

- Aspirin and other nonsteroidal anti-inflammatory drugs, Medrol dose pack (prescribed by M.D.)

Orthosis

- Effective thoraco-lumbar spinal brace, which keeps the spine in some flexion

Exercise

- Stationary bicycling—lean forward slightly

Behavior Modification

- Do—use pushcart when shopping, leaning forward on cart. This allows more pain-free walking.
- Do—stop, sit, lean forward gently. This relieves pain by opening somewhat the spinal canal.
- Do—take side-lying position (see figure 5–12, page 125). This too relieves pain by opening up the spinal canal.
- Don't—involve yourself in prolonged standing, heavy lifting, or any extension of the spine; i.e., tennis serve, swimming the breaststroke or butterfly, kneeling in a church pew.
- Don't—sleep flat on your back without having pillows under your knees.

* These recommendations for patients with spinal stenosis problems are to be used in conjunction with a thorough clinical evaluation and patient monitoring.

the legs. The operation is a little bit like what the artist did for us in Figures 2–6A and B. The bony parts forming the back of the spinal canal—including the spinous process, lamina, and yellow ligament—must be removed to make room for the nerves. In some cases, spine fusion is also necessary.

A few other diseases can cause spinal stenosis. Among them are *Paget's disease,* a disease of unknown origin that causes abnormal growth and distortion of a number of different bones; and *fluoridosis,* due to excessive fluoride, which can thicken bone and can contribute to stenosis when there's a preexistent narrowing of the canal. In some cases, scarring and other postsurgical problems like overgrowth of a fusion can lead to stenosis, too.

SCOLIOSIS

You may know this in the vernacular as curvature of the spine (see Figure 3–7). Not all scoliotic spines are painful, but some are. Pain on the inner side of the curve is believed to be due to

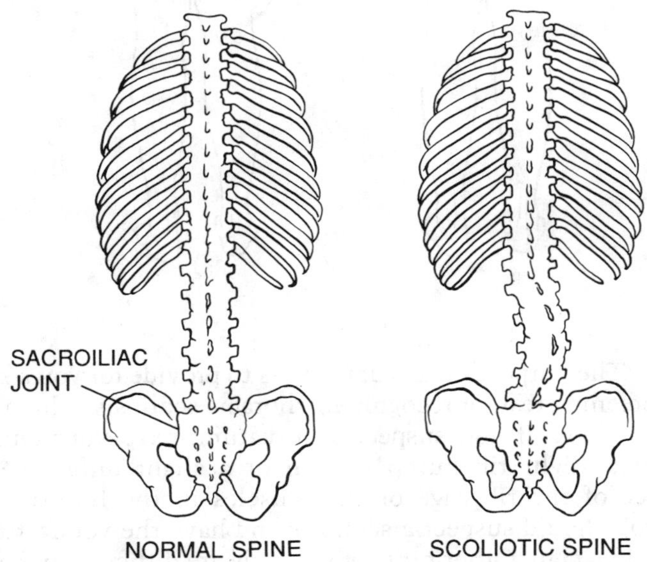

FIGURE 3–7 This figure depicts the major curvature or deformity in a scoliotic spine. This curvature is mainly in the lumbar region. It occurs most often in the thoracic spine. The curvatures associated with low back pain are in the lumbar region.

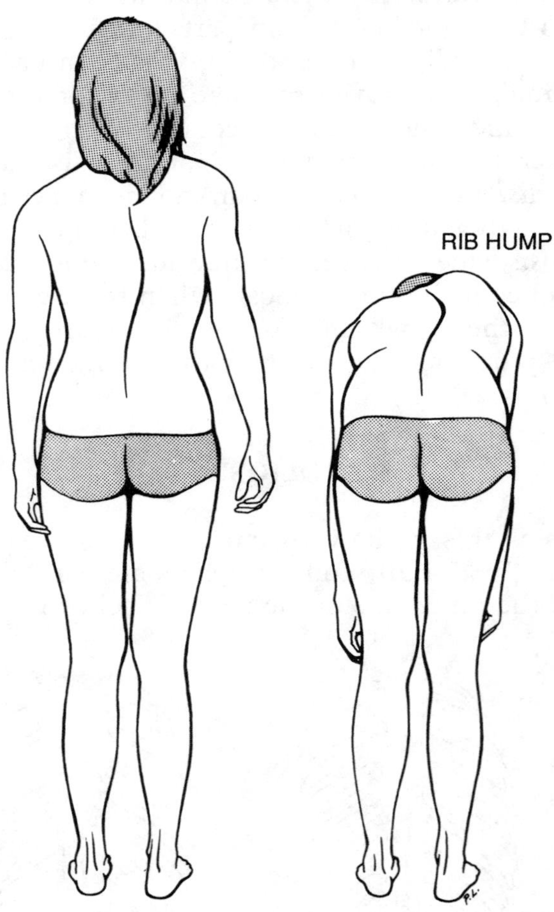

FIGURE 3–8 The purpose of this drawing is to provide for you a brief but reliable screening test for recognizing thoracic scoliosis, which is more common in girls. If you suspect a curvature, have your child bend forward. If a slight rib hump is seen or a slight difference in the prominence of the rib cage or the muscles in the lumbar spine is evident, you should suspect a scoliosis and have the youngster examined by a physician. Other hints of scoliosis are difficulty in balancing or adjusting a skirt at the waistline or difficulty with the hemline. It is important to recognize scoliosis early, because it can be treated more effectively at that stage.

degenerative or arthritic changes, and the outside of the curve may hurt, too. Standing, bending, or doing heavy work usually makes the back hurt more. But pain isn't the only problem. Sometimes severe scoliosis can progress to deformity, and the patient's abnormal posture may even interfere with the working of the heart and lungs.

It's vital to be on the lookout for scoliosis in young people, especially teenage girls. Many communities have formal scoliosis screening programs—an important innovation, since early treatment with a brace can avoid surgery later. But you can do your own at-home screening, too. Does your child's hemline hang differently on one side of her body? Is there a discrepancy in the height of the shoulders, or the protuberance of the breasts or rib cage? Does she have a slight rib hump? Have your child bend over as shown in Figure 3–8. If the answer to any of these questions is yes, take her, or in some cases, *him*—for boys aren't immune—to a qualified orthopedist.

Treatment? A brace and/or a good exercise program may prevent progression or may even correct scoliosis, but a spinal fusion may be necessary in more serious cases.

OSTEOPOROSIS

Here we move from adolescence to a later stage of life. Osteoporosis is probably the world's most common bone disease, for it is almost universal in older women, due to postmenopausal hormonal changes and decrease in activity. Fifty percent of women over forty-five have some X-ray evidence of osteoporosis, and by age seventy-five that proportion soars to ninety percent. As the median age of the U.S. population shifts upward, osteoporosis will probably become epidemic.

Bone is made up of large protein molecules, known as collagen, and a mineral structure built of a calcium-phosphorus complex. The latter is what gives bone its hardness. Aging and mainly hormonal changes accentuated by nutritional problems and inactivity cause bone to lose a great deal of its calcium, so that it weakens. The vertebrae may then suffer small, imperceptible fractures, or large, more obvious breaks, either of which can be excruciating. Note that if this severe pain is associated with a fever, there could be an infection in the vertebrae along with the osteoporosis.

As the bone weakens, such minor-seeming activities as carrying a grandchild, (mis)stepping off a curb, or lifting a stuck window can fracture the back. Some home preventatives include nonslip stick-on tiles in the shower or bathtub, and the addition of a railing to bathtubs, stairs, and other potentially dangerous parts of the house. Also, loose rugs can be removed, or the free edges tacked to the floor. At Boston's Beth Israel Hospital Department of Orthopaedic Surgery, work is in progress to develop a protective device to prevent hip fracture, should the osteoporotic patient take a fall.

Though there's no guaranteed safeguard against osteoporosis, a good diet, plenty of activity (including free-weight training), and sunlight appear to be beneficial. Recent studies show that athletic training programs (low-impact aerobics, swimming, and weight lifting) increase bone density in the young and the elderly. Premenopausal women are encouraged to be active athletically so as to "store up" extra bone mass. Consequently, when they reach postmenopausal status and begin to gradually lose bone mass, they will have some protective reserve. This is the "warehousing concept," or preventative medicine as regards postmenopausal osteoporosis.

This discussion has focused primarily on females. However, let's include elderly males and make a few points here. The points are: regular exercise, regular exercise, regular exercise. Studies show that this tends to help maintain bone mass in postmenopausal females, and definitely improves overall health for males and females. Some physicians recommend estrogen-replacement therapy for postmenopausal women. The attendant risks of uterine cancer with its use can be reduced if progesterone is also utilized. The decision to use postmenopausal hormonal treatment should be made with a physician who will then prescribe and supervise the therapy. Other factors and agents that help to prevent osteoporosis are: fluoride, calcium, calcitonin, androgens, and diphosphanates. Again, you need a physician's advice in determining your treatment.

Whenever possible, the osteoporosis patient shouldn't be confined to bed. Why? Staying active, perhaps with the aid of a painkiller, not only seems to head off further osteoporotic weakening, but also protects against blood clots and lung complications, which often go hand in hand with too much time in bed.

INFECTIONS

Vertebral Infections (Osteomyelitis)

Did you know that bacterial infections can lodge virtually anywhere in your body? Obviously, a penetrating wound or an open fracture that exposes the bone can lead to an infected spine. We know that after surgery one or two out of every hundred patients get an infection in the operated area. Other possible sources of vertebral infections may surprise you: A simple boil on the skin may spread bacteria throughout the bloodstream, and so can, believe it or not, chronically infected teeth or gums. Drug addicts or anyone else who uses unsterile needles may also come down with a vertebral infection. Don't lose sleep over these very rare complications—we're simply presenting the *whole* truth in this book.

Infections of the bladder and kidneys can spread to the spine, because the large network of veins draining these areas is in intimate contact with your vertebral circulation. Finally, diabetics tend to have a lowered resistance to infection in many parts of the body, including the back.

Diagnosis of the particular bacteria that are invading your spine requires either a needle biopsy or an open surgical biopsy of the vertebral body, done under general anesthesia. With the patient asleep or under local anesthesia, a needle is skillfully inserted in the region of suspected infection and a sample is taken. An X ray guides the doctor. Once the specific bacteria are determined, the infection is treated with the appropriate antibiotics. Sometimes, too, surgical decompression, or *debridement* (thorough wound cleansing, removing all pus, dead bone, and foreign particles), is necessary. The more the infection has spread, the more extensive the surgery. That's why infection is important to mention here, even though it's not a very common source of back pain. It is easily overlooked, and that, as we've seen, becomes dangerous.

Discitis

Sometimes one, or occasionally two, discs of the lumbar spine become inflamed and extremely painful, a condition known as discitis. People of all ages get it, though it's much more common in young people under twenty, and its cause remains puzzling. A viral or bacterial infection could be the villain, or discitis may simply be a baffling hypersensitivity or inflammatory response.

In any case, discitis will usually show up on an X ray in the form of a narrowed disc space or *sclerosis,* a local increase in bone density that shows up on a conventional X ray as a white spot. Treatment is a matter of rest, maybe even immobilization with a body cast, and careful observation as the disease runs its course. Discitis can last several weeks to several months, depending on its cause. Steroids, like cortisone, have been used with varying success. Antibiotics are effective if a bacterial infection is the cause.

FIBROSITIS/FIBROMYALGIA/MYOFASCIAL PAIN

For practical clinical purposes, and for the purposes of this presentation, we can lump these three diagnoses together. These three diagnoses are controversial and largely unproven, nevertheless there is a considerable quantity of published papers describing various clinical aspects of these conditions.

Fibrositis means inflammation of the fibrous tissue. Fibrous tissue is the usually thin, strong, low-friction material that separates muscles from each other and from other tissues. Myalgia is muscle pain. Fibromyalgia is pain in the fibrous tissue (fascia) and the muscle. Myofascial pain is pain in the same tissues, but listed in reverse order. That is, myo (muscle) and fascial (fascia). Now wasn't that fun? If you want to memorize the four preceding sentences you can successfully pass yourself off as an "expert" on the condition.

Here are several serious comments about this clinical issue: The problem is more likely to be found in females between twenty and fifty years of age. There is back pain associated with unresolved emotional concerns, sleep disturbances, and immune disorders (sensitivity reactions). At present, the cause of this condition is unknown. There are thought to be changes in the normal physiology of nerve function and changes in the muscles. The beginning of the problem may be an injury, followed initially by back pain in the upper, outer part of the buttocks and pain in the legs. The big feature of this condition is the existence of "trigger points." These are points in the body that are very tender and when touched may elicit what was vaguer, regional pain. Patients are thought to be helped by injecting "trigger points," applying anesthetic spray, massages, or manipulation. Studies show that this group of patients is probably different from those with the common nonspecific low back pain condition. There's much to be learned about this, for while some competent physicians think that this is a definite, distinct, diagnosable, and treatable disease, others are highly skeptical. If you're curious about what my patients are told, here it is: "Don't spend much time or money on the fibrositis, fibromyalgia, and myofascial pain syndromes unless you're absolutely certain that it's worth it!" Time and research will tell us if this is another fad or a substantive recognition of a fully characterizable disease entity. It usually improves once a patient is reassured that it is *not* a serious, permanent, crippling condition.

TUMORS: BENIGN AND MALIGNANT

The first, most noteworthy, message here is that tumors of the spine are *extremely* rare. Probably fewer than one in ten thousand backache patients has cancer in the spine, so why should you be part of this tiny minority? Don't let your mind wander to malignancy whenever your back hurts—just make sure to have a thorough medical evaluation if you've been laid up for over three or four weeks.

But since this is a complete guide to backache, we shouldn't exclude tumors, which, as you probably know, are new growths of abnormal tissue. They come in two basic varieties: benign, or noncancerous, and malignant, or cancerous. If left untreated, a malignant tumor can grow large and/or spread to other locations, and in some situations cause very serious illness or death. Benign tumors grow more slowly and usually are not crippling or fatal.

A tumor can involve or arise from any of the spine's structures: the bone, ligaments, nerves, muscles, or synovial tissue.

Symptoms are variable, but unlike the pain of a disc problem, for instance, which may come and go, tumor pain is generally continuous. And, especially in the case of malignancy, it gets steadily worse, unrelieved by bed rest or respite from activity.

Primary tumors are those that originate in the spine, while *metastatic tumors* come from a primary malignancy elsewhere in the body that has spread and seeded in the spine, commonly the bone. Breast, thyroid, intestinal, and kidney tumors not infrequently send metastases to the spine. Lymphoma-like tumors—that is, tumors of the lymph system—and a disease called myeloma, or cancer of the bone marrow, can also migrate to or originate in the spine, causing pain. But, a note of reassurance: It's quite uncommon for metastatic tumors to show up first in the spine; more often the initial symptoms point to the site of origin. So while metastatic tumors of the spine are slightly more common than primary ones, it's still improbable that your backache is an undiagnosed cancer.

The diagnosis is ultimately made with X rays, and often myelography, an MRI, CT scan, or bone scan. Angiography, injection of a special radiopaque dye into the blood vessels for viewing purposes, may also be done. If a tumor does show up, of course, your doctor must find out whether it's benign or malignant. This is accomplished with a biopsy, which may be either a needle biopsy or a surgical incision to biopsy or remove the tumor. After several days, usually, microscopic evaluation of the tissue sample will give the answer.

Whenever possible, a primary tumor is removed along with a margin of normal tissue to ensure that all the malignancy is caught. This can be a challenging surgical procedure, so make sure you're in experienced hands. A metastatic tumor may also be treated surgically, especially if it turns out to be a solitary secondary tumor. But if the tumor has already spread to several other sites, total tumor removal becomes less pressing. Radiation therapy and chemotherapy (anticancer drugs) can help vanquish both primary and secondary tumors. Metastatic tumors from the breast, for instance, typically respond well to radiation.

Then comes the important necessity of carefully planned surgical reconstruction of the spine. During and after surgery, the spinal cord and nerve roots must be protected, and some method of replacing the excised structures devised. That's because some of the support structure for the spine may be removed in order to get the tumor out, and so human bone—either the patient's own or bank bone—or a kind of acrylic must supplant the missing parts. Obviously, if you have a spine tumor, you'll want to seek an experienced, knowledgeable surgeon and cancer specialist, at a large regional hospital or medical center. A medical team of experts is necessary for these complex medical problems.

Meanwhile, please be assured that most of the other conditions we list in this chapter are much more likely back-pain culprits than cancer.

BACK INJURIES

Of course, your spine is far from invulnerable. As you move about, jog, or lift bureaus, office typewriters, or toddlers, you run the risk of pulled muscles, sprains, hurt ligaments, or fractures of the spine.

Muscle and Ligament Injuries

The back's muscles and any of the ligaments you learned about in Chapter II, like similar tissues in the rest of your body, can be injured or irritated (Figure 3–9). What does you in may be a sudden movement in the heat of a tennis match or a game of touch football, or a fall, twist, or sudden muscle contraction to avoid a fall. To us orthopedists, life sometimes looks like an obstacle course full of potential pitfalls for the back. The pitfalls can result in a strain or sprain to the ligaments, pulled muscle, muscle strain, or charley horse. All of which can make you mighty uncomfortable.

Sudden pain usually follows a clear-cut injury, though there may be a delay of hours or even a day or two. Specific movements tend to aggravate the pain, and muscle injury may bring with it a palpable muscle spasm. Muscle spasms can also happen *without* muscle injury, as a reflex phenomenon from irritated deeper structures, including torn ligaments, infections, tumors, or chronic disc irritation or herniation. The way you move, your posture, and other tests permit your doctor to separate a primary muscle spasm from that caused by some underlying disease.

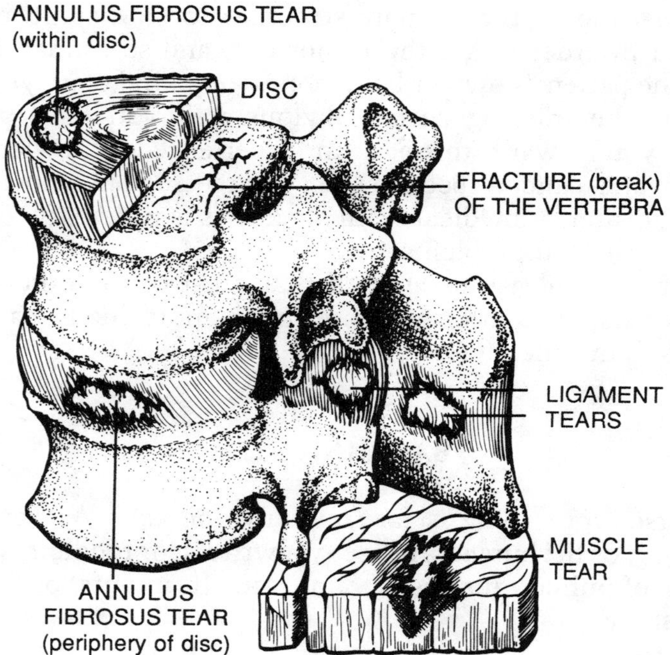

FIGURE 3–9 This picture is to remind us all of the various structures in the spine that can be impaired by injury. These structures, when injured, may cause acute low back pain problems. We recall from Figure 2–5 that there are plenty of nerves around to supply most of these structures; when they are damaged we can expect to have some real pain problems. (Reproduced with permission from White, A.A., and Panjabi, M.M.: *Clinical Biomechanics of the Spine,* J.B. Lippincott, 1990, second edition.)

How do you prevent muscle and ligament injury? Warm-up and stretching exercises before sports or heavy labor are critical, as is proper training in lifting. (Chapters V and IX give more detailed advice.) Treatment most often consists of rest, ice (for the first forty-eight hours), heat, massage, warm showers or baths, and aspirin to combat both pain and inflammation. After a time, as your backache subsides, you can gradually resume activity.

Take solace in the thought that muscle and ligament injuries are *not* often the prelude to a life flat on your back; the odds are excellent that you'll recover fully and spontaneously in about two weeks or less.

Vertebral End Plate Fractures

When you study back anatomy you can see that the vertebral body sports a bony plate at both top and bottom. If you wish, you can visualize the vertebral bodies as a stack of tin cans separated by jelly doughnuts, the discs. In this scheme of things, the cylinder of the can is the vertebral body and the covers at either end are the vertebral end plates. When the end plate cracks or fractures, severe low back pain can ensue (see Figure 3–9).

Usually it all starts with an injury followed by an abrupt spell of low back pain. At first the pain is severe, then gradually subsides after two or three weeks, though some residual discomfort may haunt you for three or four weeks more. There isn't any leg pain unless there happens also to be a disc herniation with nerve root irritation.

Lab tests tend to show a totally normal picture. Special X-ray techniques like a bone scan or a *laminogram,* the first of which allows the doctor to see the bone in slices, the second, accentuates a recent break; both can make the diagnosis.

Safety practices are the only prevention program. Treatment? Bed rest in the early phases, then as your symptoms permit, progressive activity and muscle rehabilitation exercises. When muscle rehabilitation seems unlikely or very difficult, a reinforced corset or lumbar brace may help. Undiagnosed vertebral end plate fractures are fairly rare, but since they can cause perplexing pain, exposure to special X rays may be warranted. Of course, if you suffer from osteoporosis, infections, or tumors, a very slight injury can crack the end plates. Sometimes, too, the end plates become gradually deformed and parts of the disc protrude up into the vertebral body. This condition, called Schmorl's Node, shows up on an X ray and isn't generally thought of as a cause of back pain.

Other Spine Fractures

Unlike end plate fractures, other spine fractures readily reveal themselves on an X ray. Only when the fracture isn't obvious, or your doctor wants to know whether it's a new fracture or an old one, a bone scan may be ordered—breaks more than three to four months old are pretty quiescent on a bone scan.

The same important precautions we keep harping on will help you prevent spine fractures. Treatment may dictate bed rest and the use of a plaster cast or some kind of brace. In severe cases, surgery may be necessary to relieve the pressure on the nerves or to realign the spine with special stainless-steel rods, plates, and screws, or wires with rods. These spine-implant devices help align the vertebrae and protect them from further injury. Physical therapy is the usual sequel.

Once healed, the formerly fractured back generally goes on to function magnificently and painlessly, even when its owner plays rowdy sports or does heavy chores. Isn't this perplexing when you ponder the case of a patient with no X-ray evidence of fracture who nonetheless complains of incapacitating backaches? All I can answer is that pain is subjective, and we doctors still have something to learn about the psychological and even economic factors that affect back pain.

PREGNANCY

Before I'm attacked by healthy, optimistic mothers-to-be, let me say that pregnancy is *not* a disease. Also, it's important to state that even when patients have a back condition and ask about getting pregnant, I almost never advise against it. Never say never, but never do I prescribe medications and never do I recommend elective surgery for back pain in pregnant patients. Read on. There are ways that you, your child-to-be, and your back can cope rather well through this uniquely glorious process.

Blessed event as it may be, pregnancy does cause some mechanical derangement of the spine, as the pregnant woman's increased bulk shifts her center of gravity forward. To maintain equilibrium, as we've said before, the lumbar spine must carry heavier than normal stresses, so pain or actual damage can result (see Figure 2–9 and Chapter V). If that weren't annoying enough, the pregnant state also releases a hormone, relaxin, to loosen the pelvic ligaments. Mother Nature has her excellent intentions, of course—a flexible pelvis permits the baby's head to travel through the birth canal—but unfortunately, this hormone alters the mechanics of the sacroiliac and other joints. Even a normal spine, not to mention one already prone to problems, can suffer, and some of the symptoms can even become chronic, outlasting

CHECKLIST FOR PREGNANT WOMEN

- Understand why you're having trouble (more weight, more leverage, loose joints)
- Learn and practice the ergonomic principles for back care during and after pregnancy
- Do your regular exercises and abdominal strengthening and other exercises prescribed by your obstetrician or midwife
- Get a corset support if you can't find relief
- Virtually all the basics in this book apply to you except that you cannot take medication or have surgery for your backache
- Be patient—you'll do just fine

the pregnancy. Add to this the fact that a pregnant woman no longer has good control of her abdominal muscles, the back's hardworking colleagues, and you get the picture.

We've been asked some key questions about back pain and pregnancy. Here are the answers. The questions will be obvious to us. The position of comfort while pregnant is side-lying, whether relaxing or making love (Figure 8–2, page 225). Sit in the reclined position for relaxation. Generally your muscle strengthening, relaxing, and breathing exercises are best done on your back. If you find positions for anything comfortable yet different from my recommendations, by all means go with what feels best for your back.

Pregnant women with low back pain should be carefully checked for other disease processes, though, naturally, X rays are forbidden during the first three to four months. Then an exercise program for expectant mothers, good body mechanics (see Chapter V), and enough rest to cut down on spine stress make up the pregnant woman's prevention program. A corset like the one shown in Figure 3–10 can help with severe pain. Heat, massage, and tender loving care from family and an understanding mate can't be overprescribed. Conscientious regular exercise (walking, biking, or swimming) to maintain erector spinae and general muscle tone is probably the best thing a pregnant woman can do to prevent back pain.

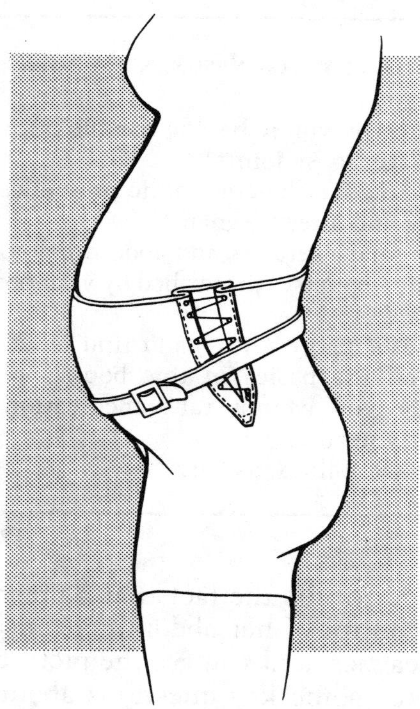

FIGURE 3–10 This is a special corset for back pain in pregnancy. If we refer to Figure 2–9, we can observe how, like the obese man, the pregnant woman has the center of gravity shifted forward. The idea of this brace is to provide some additional support to help the hard-working muscles, and also shift the center of gravity backward so that the erector spinae don't have to work so hard and the forces on the spine are not as great. When the corset can achieve this, the mother-to-be is more comfortable and has less back pain.

OTHER DISEASES THAT HURT YOUR BACK

Sometimes when your back cries for help it's a symptom of a medical problem as remote as the kidneys, intestines, or heart. So here we list some of the systemic diseases that can have repercussions on your spine—though the spine, in this case, isn't the culprit.

Visceral Diseases

Some diseases of the abdomen and pelvic region can show up as spine pain, and these we'll itemize here. One caveat, though: Beware of a psychological phenomenon known as Medical Student's Disease. As medical students peruse their textbooks, they may bcome stricken with a record number of strange symptoms, which tend to cluster around whatever ailments they are currently studying. Of course, male students rarely suffer from ovarian cancer symptoms, nor do female students come down with all the signs of prostatitis, but otherwise virtually any symptom in the internal medicine book may wend its way into the student's consciousness—and "body." Don't you fall prey to this syndrome. One "cure" is to consider whether the aches and pains you're feeling are related to those you just read about here. If they weren't around before, their sudden appearance may suggest sophomoritis, the Medical Student's Disease. Another alternative, when you get weary of your current "disease," is to select a set of symptoms that seem more interesting and less inconvenient and read about them for a while.

By the way, the healthy, robust secretary with whom I work mentioned that whenever she typed parts of this book she got a slight backache. Presumably, you, the reader, already have a real backache and needn't worry about a hypochondriacal one. But I don't want you to "come down with" any of the visceral diseases sometimes associated with backache. If you happen to be a backache-free reader, forewarned is forearmed!

Now let's proceed.

Usually, pain caused by abdominal disease is independent of the kinds of activities that stimulate true spine pain. And neither rest nor the maneuvers that relieve pain from the spine do much to alleviate visceral backache. But because it can be hard to tell whether back pain is coming from your back or from deeper inside the body, it's important to have any persistent backache carefully and thoroughly checked.

Roughly one in ten adults suffers from *ulcers,* which don't *usually* cause low back pain. Yet an ulcer may occasionally reveal its presence as a deep pain in the upper lumbar spine area, either at the midline or on either side. If your ache is due to ulcer, you can expect it to be irritated by chili, curried chicken, Southern barbecue, spaghetti, and pizza, and soothed by milk, cream, ice cream, and antacids. Ulcer pain tends to surface two or two and a half hours after eating. If the pain were caused by a tumor, it probably wouldn't have these clear-cut eating-related and other temporal patterns. Coughing, running, bending, lifting, and other actions that exacerbate other sorts of backache have little bearing on ulcer pain.

Diseases of the large intestine, such as inflammation, ulceration, or tumors, can sometimes lead to complaints of lower back pain. Again, this kind of pain tends to be deep, severe, and unrelated to rest or activity. Sometimes it's affected one way or another by bowel movements. Diseases of the *upper abdominal* structures, like the pancreas and regional lymph nodes, can also cause back pain that may radiate into the hip or thigh as well. Next we must mention the *kidneys* and *bladder* as possible, though improbable, sources of low back pain. Here again, be suspicious of deep pain. Difficulty in urinating or changes in the frequency, color, smell, or amount of the stream, or any discharge from the penis or urethra, are other important symptoms.

In the male, chronic *prostate disease* can cause back discomfort. The prostate gland is a walnut-size, male-only gland at the base of the body. It surrounds the small tube that exits the bladder and goes into the base of the penis. Urinary problems—difficulty in starting or maintaining the stream, for instance—relative sexual impotence, or a penile discharge are clues. Cancer of the prostate or rectum can also produce some of these symptoms. In the female, menstruation can provoke pelvic and back pain. Many back patients suffer most at midcycle or at the time of their periods. Back pain may hint at diseases of the *female sex organs.* Infected fallopian tubes, ovaries, or uterus may be reflected in the lower back. So may endometriosis, a disease in which the endometrial tissue lining the uterus leaks and becomes painful. A prolapsed—or tipped—uterus and tumors of the sex organs can also cause backache. All of these tend to be felt as deep pain, unaffected by physical activity.

Please, dear reader, don't suffer sleepless nights contemplating these remote dangers. If you're in good health and your pains have been with you for only two or three weeks, you've probably no reason to worry.

Back Pain Arising From the Hip

We must also include the possibility that disease of the hip is affecting your back. Arthritis, infections, or a tumor of the hip area could be to blame. And a rare disease called *avascular necrosis,* in which the ball of the femur (thighbone) loses its blood supply, can mimic back problems. Hip diseases usually cause pain in the groin and can be recognized during a thorough physical exam.

Vascular Disease

You probably never suspected, did you, how many parts of your body can affect your back! But bear with me; we're almost to the end of our list.

To all the other obscure and not-so-obscure diseases you've already waded through we must now add disease of the blood vessels. Blockage of either the aorta or the iliac vessels that travel into the hips and legs can produce back pain. Most of the time, what is occluding these vessels is fatty deposits called atherosclerotic plaques.

Vascular patients generally have back and leg pain that gets worse with walking—the faster or the farther they walk, the more pronounced the pain. The pain generally subsides if walking stops and the patient stands and rests. These aches aren't exacerbated by coughing, sneezing, bending, prolonged sitting, and so on. A deep muscular pain in the leg or—more likely—a "pins-and-needles" sensation, like that of a limb that "falls asleep," may be the predominant symptom.

The diagnosis is made on the basis of a medical history, which may include sexual impotence in the male. Pulse may be sluggish at the foot or ankle, behind the knee, or sometimes at the femoral artery in the groin. Ultimately, arteriography—a test in which a radiopaque dye, injected into the arteries, reveals their conditions—confirms vascular disease. Treatment depends on the severity of the disease. The regimen may include a strict diet, regular exercise, and vasodilator drugs to improve circulation. Or, in more serious cases, bypass surgery may be performed.

LEG-LENGTH INEQUALITY

This one is tough to pin down because of the great difficulty of making accurate measurements. Nevertheless, I for one have resisted the idea that leg-length differences may be a cause or a source of persistent aggravation of low back pain. Those who believe differing leg lengths cause pain have varying opinions on how big a discrepancy in length causes pain. Some say very little—less than 1 cm. Others say there would have to be at least a 2 cm. difference. If a patient with back pain and leg pain on the same side as the long leg consistently measures a 2–2.5 cm. (¾–1 inch) difference, we think that there's no risk in trying a shoe lift of 1–2 cm. (½–¾ inch) on the short leg.

"IT'S ALL IN YOUR MIND"

You may not realize just how intimately your body and mind affect each other. We'll scrutinize the emotional underside of back pain in more detail in Chapter IV. But for the moment, let's just say that separating bodily aches from the more ethereal aches of the soul is a less straightforward matter than you might think. Every physical pain impinges on your mind, and psychological pain, in turn, sends messages to every corner of your body. And so, to complete our roundup of the causes of backache, we can't neglect the following.

Depression

It's not that rare for severely depressed patients to focus on the lower back as the source of their pain. These patients are neither "faking" nor carping, for their hurt *feels* absolutely real, though no organic cause may be found.

If you have a thorough physical and your doctor suggests your backache may have its roots in your mind, don't feel angry or ashamed. Of course, doctors aren't infallible, and it's possible your doctor has overlooked a hard-to-diagnose physical problem. Of course, even depressed or severely disturbed patients can have real organic diseases. On the other hand, an experienced physician is *usually* capable of recognizing when a back problem is largely due to depression. Certainly before you rush into surgery for a back disease that doesn't really exist, get a second opinion.

Hysteria

Hysteria originally meant "wandering womb" in Greek, for it was thought to be due to an odd displacement of the female organs. Now it's medical parlance, applied to males as well, for a "disease" based more on emotional imbalance than organic disturbance. When it comes to back pain, some patients may be confined to bed in order to retreat from emotional stress, avoid lovemaking, win sympathy from others, or for any number of unconscious reasons.

Though hysterical backache, fortunately, is usually short-lived, it isn't always easy to treat. Tranquilizers and painkillers are all often ineffective and in many situations should not be used. In any case, psychiatrists, social workers, ministers, and others adept at dealing with the mind are more appropriate managers for this "backache" than orthopedists or neurosurgeons.

Remember that hysterical symptoms often look and feel very real while they're around, and the afflicted is not a mere malingerer or complainer.

Camptocormia

While you're not likely to be suffering from this dramatic hysterical disorder, it belongs in our list of emotional ills. Classic cases of camptocormia have reached epidemic proportions in the military. A typically young, modestly educated soldier comes to the doctor complaining of severe back pain, and his posture may be so tilted as to make the Hunchback of Notre Dame look like a West Point plebe by comparison. The treatment? The doctor may say, "You have a back condition that, though deforming at the moment, will improve. But your condition makes it inappropriate for you to remain in the military, so we'll let you go home as soon as your spine straightens up a little." The patient usually straightens up completely within a week or two.

Compare this situation with that of a worker who drudges at an ill-paid, boring, unsatisfying job and comes down with a back injury that can earn him workman's compensation for life. In such cases, even the backache sufferer himself may be confused about how much of the pain is in his back and how much in his head. More about all this in Chapter IV.

Malingering

In a sense, all malingering is a form of "compensationitis," though the disability payments may be in the form of exemption from the draft, escape from burdensome responsibilities, or extraordinary attention from doctors or family members. It is generally distinguishable from an unconscious behavior pattern—say, hysterical paralysis—though the differences can be murky, and the degree of sophistication with which patients present their symptoms varies all over the board. More about malingering later.

THE BACKACHE WITH NO NAME

Medical books call it "idiopathic back pain," but don't let the lofty term impress you—it's really medical jargon for "who knows?" It might seem a bit ironic to end our comprehensive chapter on the causes of back pain on a note of bewilderment, but the fact is that some backaches never do yield a clear-cut cause.

Eloquent testimony to the pervasiveness of "idiopathic back pain" is the fact that, in December of 1980, a workshop on this subject was organized by the National Institutes of Health, the American Academy of Orthopaedic Surgeons, and the Orthopaedic Research Society. Epidemiologists, psychologists, psychiatrists, anatomists, bioengineers, neuroscientists, orthopaedic surgeons, rheumatologists, sports medicine and occupational medicine experts, and anesthesiologists all convened to plan a multidisciplinary attack on this mystery. The focused research program that resulted will help us to discover the precise cause of your aching back in the future.

A workshop was convened in 1989 by the same organization, as a follow-up to the 1980 workshop. This second meeting is published by the American Academy of Orthopaedic Surgeons in the book *New Perspectives on Low Back Pain.* The full citation is listed in the bibliography at the back of this book. That publication is produced for the biomedical scientist, but it can be useful to anyone interested in the state-of-the-art, best scientific information. (See Bibliography, Chapter 3.)

Chapter IV

Pain and the Mind

"Man is chastened with pain upon his bed and with continual strife in his bones, so that his life loathes bread, and his appetite dainty food."

—Job 33:19–20

It seems like a downer to start our chapter with one of the bleakest Biblical tales. But the seeming senselessness of Job's woes brings us to a central problem of pain. Job was a pious man who feared, respected, and followed God. Still he suffered plague, blight, and boils and couldn't understand why. After many well-meaning but not-too-helpful suggestions from friends and neighbors, Job finally got a message from God that said, in effect, "Keep the faith, baby." This answer may be as good as any to the "why?" of pain. Sometimes this is simply our lot. If you can keep the faith, be patient, and remember that back pain, however dreadful, never killed anybody, you're well-equipped to move ahead. With this as a positive attitude, you're definitely ahead of the game.

Why do some people suffer and not others? Why, as any backache victim will wonder, am *I* afflicted? Is there something I can do about it, or am I doomed to be a passive victim? There is plenty that you can do to help yourself, and you are by no means a doomed victim. Read on.

In the Brain

Pain isn't as simple as it may seem. First of all, your pain isn't actually "in" your lower back; in a very real sense, it's in your brain. This gives us a clue about how to deal with it.

Two true stories, back to back, will serve us here.

The first takes place in 1967, in the one-story frame building housing the orthopaedic wards at Fort Ord Army Hospital. Here injured Vietnam veterans are being treated in a large open ward.

A twenty-three-year-old recruit, shot in the right hand in combat six months earlier, lies in one of the beds. Right after his injury his wound had been thoroughly debrided (washed with sterile water and all the dead, damaged, and dirty tissue cut away), but he'd gone on to develop an infection. That infection had been successfully treated in the Philippines.

Like many of his fellow Vietnam vets, however, the young man became depressed, frustrated, and hostile. An aspiring electrician, he worried that his maimed hand might interfere with his career. He became more and more uncooperative and combative, and his hand also went through some strange changes. The hand and arm started to swell. The skin got very slick and discolored, fluctuating between extreme wetness and extreme dryness. Most of all, his arm became so sensitive to pain that merely the movement of air in the region triggered sheer agony. Traffic in his room had to be kept in "slow motion" to minimize air turbulence.

All this, despite the fact that his infection had obviously cleared up! Why? The young man was suffering from something doctors call "causalgia," or "reflex sympathetic dystrophy," which often follows major or minor injuries. It's a clear-cut example of how emotional distress greatly exaggerates an initial organic problem, heightening pain sensitivity out of all proportion. Its treatment consists of psychiatric help, a supportive environment, and frequent novocaine blocks of one of the sympathetic nerve centers in the neck region. In this case, when I left the hospital, the young man was moving his arm with little pain, on the road to recovery.

Now let's journey to the other end of the spectrum. Again our story takes us to Vietnam.

The colonel, who had been evacuated forty-five minutes

earlier from the battlefield (the medical evacuation system in Vietnam was the best in history), was alert and talkative and didn't complain of pain. At first, a doctor would have thought him normal but for the fact that he was a little excited. A quick glance at his feet, however, revealed that the left one was hanging from the leg by a couple of tendons and muscle fibers. The exposed bone was packed with more mud than I'd seen in six months of treating some pretty severe injuries. A few days later, when the colonel was medically stabilized, he was able to relate what happened. His tale was confirmed by several of his men.

While on a search-and-destroy mission the soldiers had been cleverly ambushed, and the colonel saw several of his men wounded. As the ambusher started to retreat, the colonel caught sight of him. His anger and frustration gave way to elation and he set off in pursuit of the enemy. Then the colonel stepped on a medium-sized land mine, which blew his foot off. But undaunted or unaware, he continued the chase for three or four minutes. Though his men noticed he was running with a limp, it wasn't until he had collapsed from shock and loss of blood that they caught up with him and discovered the cause: an almost completely severed and dangling foot. This seasoned colonel didn't deny his pain, but said that in the heat of the moment it had felt more like a sprained ankle.

Here are two dramatic examples of how pain is filtered through the mind. In one case, the patient's negative emotions intensified his pain; in the other, the peculiar *élan* of the battlefield dimmed what should have been agony. It turns out that these perplexing "psychological" phenomena may be partly physiological, rooted in some tricks of human biochemistry, as we'll see.

You don't have to be a recuperating soldier, of course, to witness the subjectivity of pain. There may even be cultural differences in pain reaction. Scandinavians, New England Yankees, and the Irish are supposed to behave stoically in the face of pain, while people from Jewish, Italian, and other Mediterranean cultures are traditionally much more vociferous in their complaints of pain, often curbing their activities in response. Then there's the stereotype of Asian reticence about expressing pain. Granted, these are generalizations that may or may not apply to individuals.

There may also be sexual differences that affect how much pain a person feels. In our culture, for instance, it is less acceptable for men to cry than it is for women, perhaps making it harder for men to deal with pain. Also, when men become dependent because of back disability and pain, it may cause them a great deal more tension, anxiety, frustration, hostility, and guilt than it does women in our society.

The point is this: Your psychic structure at any given time—including your own personal philosophy, religion, or cultural conditioning—can elevate or lower your pain threshold. Obviously, medicine lacks a "painometer" to objectively measure pain intensity. We have to take the patient's word for how much he suffers.

Now, *why* do we have pain in the first place? First, pain is a mechanism to alert us to injury so we react appropriately. We move our hand instantly away from a hot stove. When we severely sprain an ankle or break a leg, we don't usually walk on it. Pain can also be a signal that something more subtle is wrong. We may find that a long drive in the car without rest stops makes our backs ache, or that certain foods cause ulcers and burn holes in our stomachs.

Another, more philosophical theory of pain is that it puts pleasure in perspective. Without pain, the philosophers ask, to what can we compare pleasure? Plato, in his allegory of the cave, felt that one couldn't appreciate light until he/she had experienced darkness. To this idea, I've always objected that I'd willingly accept the challenge of appreciating intense pleasure without any reference to pain whatsoever!

The Gate Control Theory of Pain

What happens to us physiologically when we feel pain? If you touch a hot stove, for example, the nerves in your skin are vigorously stimulated, and they send high-magnitude impulses along the nerve fibers into the spinal cord. Then they cross from one side of the spinal cord to the other, and ascend into the midbrain, in the center of your brain. Here, in a part of the brain called the *thalamus,* pain transmission seems to stop. The interaction between the thalamus and the convoluted outer cortex, the "thinking" part of your brain, is still quite mysterious. What is the connection between the transmission of nerve

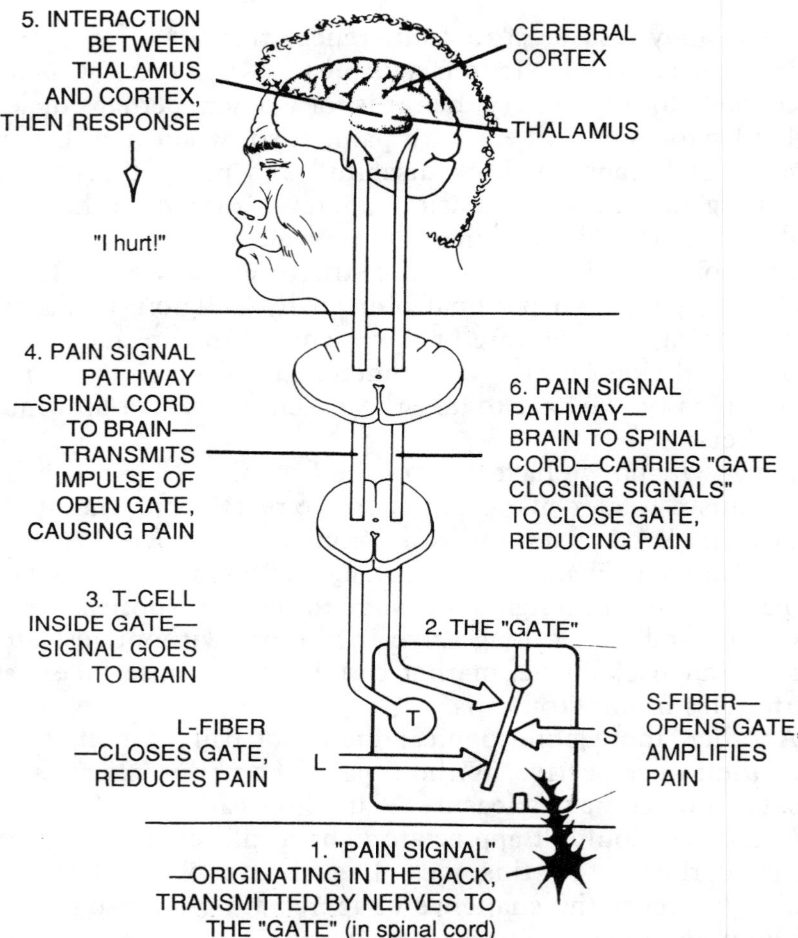

Figure 4–1A and 1B This somewhat complex diagram explains a great deal about pain. You can benefit from this book without tackling this illustration, but I urge you to study it, because it will help considerably your understanding of pain. Let's give it a try. 1A illustrates the theory and 1B the theoretical mechanisms through which a broad variety of clinical phenomena may occur. Let's begin with 1A. First, at the bottom of the figure we see that there is a pain signal or stimulus that originates somewhere in your back (1) and is transmitted by the nerves to the "gate" (2), which opens, triggering the T-cells (3) that send the pain signal up the spinal cord (4) to the thalamus. There is an interaction between the thalamus and the cortex of the brain and the pain signal is felt by you and you respond, "I HURT!" (5). The brain can produce signals that travel down the spinal cord to close the gate (6). The structure of the nervous system is such that even without such

CORTICAL AND THALAMIC INFLUENCES
BLOCKING OR OPENING GATE

BLOCKING GATE
pain medications
tranquilizers
placebos
meditation
euphoria
endorphins

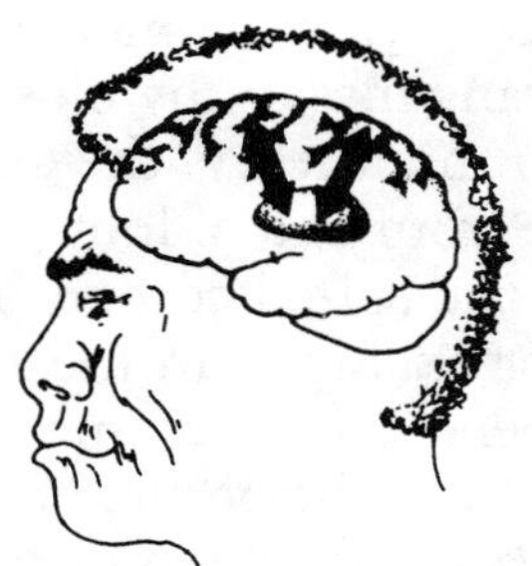

OPENING GATE
anxiety, depression
sadomasochism
memory of pain
life-situation crisis
chronic pain

OPENING
OR BLOCKING
cultural factors
personal philosophy
feeling about work
feeling about sports
monetary factors

"I hurt! I'm OK!" depends on interactions
between cortex and thalamus

CORD LEVEL
BLOCKING
dorsal column
stimulator
tractotomy
endorphins

PERIPHERAL
BLOCKING STIMULI
acupuncture
electrical stimulation (TENS)
heat, cold, massage
traction, manipulation
salves and ointments

THE "GATE"

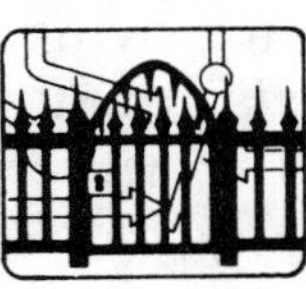

BLOCKING,
ELIMINATING
OR CORRECTING
SOURCE
facet neurectomy
discectomy
spine fusion
chymopapain
anti-inflammatory drugs

signals from the back or the brain, other fibers, the S-fibers and the L-fibers, can affect the intensity of the pain—the S-fibers tending to open the gate wider, amplifying the pain signal, the L-fibers tending to close the gate, reducing the pain signal. Thus, sometimes pain signals aren't transmitted to the brain, or are transmitted only weakly (remember our colonel in Vietnam). Another thing to bear in mind is that the spinal cord and midbrain can produce endorphins, chemicals that reduce pain either by acting on the "gate" or the brain, and sometimes both.

In 1B, we find suggestions as to how pain may be stimulated or suppressed by events taking place in the brain. We also see how peripheral events can cause or suppress pain. The endorphins may work at both sites. May I suggest that you look this figure over again after you've finished this chapter. You'll see a lot more in it.

fibers in the thalamus and your ultimate "ouch!" or some less reserved exclamation initiated in the outer cortex of the brain?

Now we come to the gate control theory of pain (see Figure 4–1). It suggests that a "gate" somewhere in the spinal cord slows or stops pain transmission by closing and increases it by opening. According to this theory, the "closed gate" and "open gate" signals emanate from one of four places: the brain's outer cortex, the midbrain, the spinal cord, or nerve fibers peripheral to the spinal cord—for example, in the skin and joints of back and limbs. As it happens, small-diameter fibers called *S-fibers,* which carry impulses from the peripheral nerves into the spinal cord, do "open the gate," freely transmitting pain messages. Conversely, large-diameter fibers, the *L-fibers,* "close the gate." Other fibers, thought to send messages from the midbrain down into the lower parts of the central nervous system, also close the gate.

Let's look at the "ouch" of low back pain. Nerves run throughout your lumbar spine, so virtually any of them can transmit pain. If arthritis of the facet joints is the pain source, the nerves that carry the "ouch" from the joint into the spinal cord can be destroyed in a procedure called a *neurectomy.* The result? No nerves, no pain. Another way to close the pain gate is with a spinal fusion, which gets rid of the "ouch" by basically eliminating the joint and removing the possibility of motion.

If the intervertebral disc is at fault, and you remove the disc, the mechanism irritating the nerve is gone. A wide variety of surgical procedures similarly block pain transmission somewhere between the original "ouch" source and the brain. The closer these procedures come to the brain, the more radical they are. We just mentioned neurectomy, in which a nerve is effectively cut just before it enters the spinal cord. Moving higher up the nervous system, a *tractotomy* cuts the nerve within the cord itself. There also have been operations in which certain nerve tracts *within the brain* have actually been severed.

But there are other, nonsurgical ways to close your pain gates. The L-fibers, the gate-closing nerves, can be stimulated instead. How? Acupuncture, transcutaneous electrical nerve stimulation (TENS), heat and ice massage, and regular massage all probably send stimuli to the cord and midbrain via the peripheral nerves, telling the midbrain to fire the L-fibers that close the pain gates. So may traction, manipulation, and mildly irritating or soothing salves and ointments. You may remember the dorsal column stimulator that was popular in the sixties. In this technique, an electrode implanted in the dura covering the spinal cord sent electrical signals to "close the gate." The common denominator of all these methods is that they interrupt pain messages between the back and the brain.

And let's not forget drugs. Where do they work in the central nervous system to block pain messages? The answer, of course, is in the brain itself. Tranquilizers and muscle relaxants, for example, probably interfere with communication between the cortex, your "thinking cap," and the deeper thalamus. Actually, you don't even have to take a drug to change the way the cortex and thalamus commune. Transcendental meditation, hypnosis, and other relaxation techniques appear to work at this site, as does the famous "placebo effect." The placebo effect dictates that one in every three people will have real pain relief from a fake "painkiller." All that is necessary is that they *think* it's a real pain pill, though it may be a simple sugar capsule.

Again, you see how the psyche operates in pain perception, perhaps even changing the way parts of our brain and nervous system "listen" to one another and send nerve signals. On the darker side, anxiety, depression, and other negative emotions intensify pain, either lowering the threshold for pain sensitivity or altering the brain's interpretation of it. The reason chronic pain is such a tough nut to crack is that the memory of pain tends to lower your pain threshold, resulting in a more intense response. And for good or ill, life crises—like divorce, the death of a loved one, a job change, or even a promotion or high honor—change pain perception. Even finances obtrude. A person with modest savings who is about to retire may find it difficult to return to work with a disabled back. But another person, who must attend a rigorous business meeting to close a multimillion-dollar deal, is likely to be more successful at closing the "ouch" gate. Take a few minutes to study Figure 4–1B. Then think of ways that you can control your own pain gate. Drugs are best considered only as temporary short-term gatekeepers.

Natural Painkillers

Now, in the 1990s, we can add one more piece to the pain puzzle. A few years ago, scientists were startled to discover that our bodies produce their own painkillers, called *endorphins,* the natural version of morphine. Different mechanisms can stimulate the brain to produce endorphins. In fact, the once-puzzling pain relief afforded by acupuncture, meditation, and the placebo effect seems to be due to these chemicals, which attach to receptors, or target sites, within the brain and spinal cord and dull pain. There's good reason to believe that emotional and cultural factors also influence the amount of endorphins you produce. Even natural childbirth, wherein training, relaxation, and concentration can make the brain block or reinterpret pain, may depend on endorphins. The "jogger's high" and the strange analgesia of the colonel with the severed foot owe something to these morphinelike chemicals.

Much of what we've just discussed in terms of gate control can be explained as follows: Whatever "closed the gate" stimulated the body's natural painkillers. Bear this phenomenon in mind when we talk about how to treat your own back pain.

The Relaxation Response

I assume that you are sitting or reclining as you read this book. Take a moment now and really get comfortable. Now breathe in a relaxed, ordinary way and mentally repeat the word *one, one, one. . . .* If other thoughts intrude, gently ignore them, continuing to think *one, one. . . .* Go on repeating *one,* softly pushing all thoughts out of your mind. Concentrate and continue this for four or five minutes. You may close your eyes if you wish, and continue for another five minutes. But don't go to sleep. . . . You have just experienced what my friend and colleague Dr. Herb Benson, of Boston, calls "the relaxation response."

According to Dr. Benson, the relaxation response is at the core of the prayer practices of many of the world's religions. Its elements include a relaxed position, concentration on breathing, and the repetition of a particular statement, prayer, or syllable, while keeping extraneous thought out of the mind and staying awake. If you've tried transcendental meditation or another meditative practice, you'll recognize this exercise as virtually identical, except that repetition of the word *one* replaces the mantra or prayer.

While some of the profound effects of the relaxation response remain rather mysterious, it's obvious to doctors and laymen alike that it reduces stress. Thus, it can make pain patients a great deal more comfortable. Here again, the brain and spinal cord may be secreting their own internal opiates, the endorphins, when you put yourself in a relaxed state.

Biofeedback is a close cousin of the relaxation response. Usually, an electronic sensor is set up to pick up the electrical responses from a muscle that contracts in association with tension. The patient learns to relax him/herself and the muscle as a voluntary controlled response. This process, if effective, then reduces the pain experience.

Mind as Ally—or Enemy?

Are you wondering why we're spending so much time on parts of you remote from your aching back? Does our discussion of "pain gates" and internal opiates strike you as obscure? Well, in the next chapter we'll give you very precise instructions for dealing with the physical side of back pain: how to prevent it, how to heal it. This chapter is devoted to your *emotional* care.

Now you've learned how your body and mind work together when it comes to pain. Pain will be around to challenge mankind for a long time, unfortunately. You can get considerable help from the outside—from doctors, family, friends, and relatives—but you'll ultimately need a strong dose of your own thought control and optimism to overcome your disease. This is no abstraction. If you learn to draw on your mind's latent healing powers, it will make a huge difference to your back.

How can you make your emotions work for you instead of against you?

Get involved in something "outside yourself"—a hobby, helping others, exercise, music, etc. We know that people who have "something better to do" don't suffer as much.

Coloring Your World

Here we'll talk about the virtues of a positive attitude. Don't let the Norman Vincent Peale overtones turn you off. This section may even be the most important part of this book.

As a doctor, I'm struck by the fantastic rehabilitative abilities of certain groups of patients. Again and again I've noticed that amateur and professional athletes, people who own their own businesses, and people in leadership positions—executives, teachers, coaches, school principals, community leaders, and so on—make amazingly fast and thorough recoveries from their back ailments. Why? It's simple: These people possess high motivation and a positive mental attitude. That's not to say that *all* executives embody such praiseworthy traits, or that nonprofessional, nonexecutive people aren't capable of great optimism under stress. The point is not the occupation or the socioeconomic status, but the mind-set.

The message you can take home is this: Make up your mind, here and now, that you want to get well. Cooperate conscientiously with your treatment. If you do, there's little doubt you'll do much better.

Dear reader: These last three sections may contain the most important and helpful message in this book. Read them again . . . and again. Read the whole chapter again if you don't understand or agree with these statements.

Now that I've begun to preach a bit, let me warn you about the other side of the coin. Two frequent tragic figures, in my experience, succumb to the deadly duo of backache and a negative mental state. I've dubbed them the *Poor Soul* and the *Compensation Tragedy,* but in real life there's considerable overlap between the two.

I don't expect to dazzle anyone with any psychiatric elegance here; I simply draw on my own clinical experience with these unfortunate people. Some of you may suspect you fall into one of these categories. If so, I hope you'll feel you're treated fairly in this section, and more important, that you'll find the impetus to recognize yourself and turn your situation around before you reach the point of no return.

The Poor Soul

We've noted that pain is a spectrum running from something primarily organic with a faint psychological overlay, to the primarily psychological with a hint of real disease. The Poor Soul can start anywhere on the spectrum. Wherever he begins, though, he soon becomes rewarded, consciously or not, by persisting in his pain-behavior pattern. How can pain be rewarding? Well, it may mean escape from sexual intimacy—the "Sorry, not tonight, dear" syndrome—or from work responsibilities at home or on the job. It may be a weapon to threaten, punish, blackmail, or manipulate relatives or friends. It may gain the attention or sympathy of someone who otherwise won't give you the time of day. It may serve as a "reason" for not achieving a personal goal in life. "I would have been a great ball player but . . . I injured my back." How many times have we empathetically listened to that or some similar story?

The pain pattern persists at both conscious and unconscious levels, perhaps becoming ever more unconscious. The patient arrives at his doctor's office so depressed, hostile, or guilty, or so determined to maintain his pain behavior, that diagnosis and treatment may be very difficult, if not impossible. And he keeps going back to the doctor to document the disease, maintain sympathy, and alleviate guilt. Sometimes he'll refuse to communicate his symptoms clearly or to follow his doctor's advice. He may even become outright hostile toward physicians and other practitioners.

Sometimes there's a clear-cut diagnosis, followed by transient improvement or actual deterioration. At other times, there's an imprecise diagnosis, and surgery or other invasive tests may be performed. These procedures almost always aggravate the Poor Soul's overall condition. But no matter what happens, the Poor Soul returns for more and more therapy and, appropriately or not, opts for one or more operations. It's a fact of life that if a patient complains of backache long and vigorously enough to enough people, including a number of surgeons, he'll sooner or later end up on the operating table. So the cycle goes. The Poor Soul's reward system may be reinforced or it may break down at any point, due to his own frustration or that of those around him, leaving depression in its wake. This pain pattern can run for two, fifteen, or twenty-five years.

How do you recognize a Poor Soul? Usually, he or she lacks animation and facial expression, rarely makes eye contact, and may hobble, limp, or walk with crutches, cane, or walker in a dramatic fashion. He may be obese or dramatically emaciated. For him, life has no joy. Over the months or years, as his all-consuming pain behavior isolates him from friends and family, his only contact with the world may be the games he plays with health professionals. Games that no one wins.

Why do we take the time to paint the Poor Soul's wan portrait? Merely as a warning. I want to remind you that just as a positive attitude can work miracles, a negative attitude can permit a back problem to dominate and devastate your life. If you think you resemble the Poor Soul in any respect, turn around right now and run as fast as you can in the opposite direction. Start by discussing your problem openly and frankly with your doctor, or anyone else who will listen.

The Compensation Tragedy

If this section prevents just one Compensation Tragedy, it's worth the time and space.

Let's start with the unlikely subject of pirates. Some of the following information comes from a lecture by compensation expert Rodney Beals, M.D., presented at the 1979 American Academy of Orthopaedic Surgeons' course on the spine in Philadelphia.

Pirates had a fairly standard system of operation. Expenses included costs of the ship, provisions, a surgeon, a shipwright, and compensation for disability. After subtracting operating expenses, they divided the profits. The disability costs included scheduled and unscheduled benefits. Examples of *scheduled* compensation are as follows, expressed as pieces of eight:

Right arm	600	Left leg	400
Left arm	500	An eye	100
Right leg	500	Finger	100

Examples of unscheduled compensation are described:

> "Our surgeon [evaluated] the wounded [finding] four crippled and six hurt, to whom we gave six hundred pieces of eight a man and a thousand to those who were crippled, as was our custom."

Some people question whether contemporary compensation laws have evolved much from those developed by the pirates. While workmen's compensation—whereby the employer bears the cost of a job-related disability—serves an obvious purpose, our present system also prolongs disease instead of promoting health. One study of patients hospitalized for back injuries revealed that compensation patients received two hundred percent more physical therapy than noncompensation patients, even though they had thirty-three percent *less* impairment.

New Zealand provides us with an example of how compensation laws can affect patterns of disease. In 1979, what is thought to be the most comprehensive accident compensation laws in the world were passed in that country. These laws provided that a worker injured on the job could stay home and his employer would be required to continue his full pay for *one week*. Once passed, absenteeism rose decidedly. Many workers with minor injuries who would have previously continued work immediately after first-aid treatment instead began going on compensation for *one week*.

And, as you might guess, the number of tests and X rays is directly related to your insurance coverage. The consequences? First, unnecessary X rays mean needless radiation exposure, and tests like myelography pose even more serious risks. And these diagnostic tests can represent "documentation" of a real disease in the patient's mind, when there may be only a minor or nonexistent problem.

The cost to society is only part of the compensation picture. The other, more ominous cost isn't financial. There are data to show that backache patients receiving compensation don't respond as well to treatment as patients cared for under another system. The appeals process, which allows patients to appeal a case after it is closed in hopes of getting a better award, lifts recuperation to another level of complexity.

Sometimes we see patients who have had ten or twenty back operations and are still suffering. They're on full disability, but do you think they are happy? Enough myelograms and surgical procedures can themselves result in an organic basis for pain.

And remember that pain behavior is complex and tricky. Don't naively assume that once your case is settled and you are compensated you can turn off your ailment at will. It might not work. Somewhere along the line the chronic-pain patient loses touch with reality and his whole life revolves around his disability. To compound his misery, even the most compassionate doctor, nurse, or therapist, put off by the patient's hopelessness or hostility, may covertly avoid him.

The lawyer is literally a limited partner in this venture. He or she invests his/her time and energy plus *your* body. Once the settlements are made or not made, the lawyers, insurance adjusters, and others withdraw. You may be left with a less-than-healthy mind and body, weary family and friends, and a growing acquaintance with the druggist.

Never forget that your number one priority is to get back to normal as soon as possible. Endeavors to beat the system subvert that goal, and you risk becoming the pawn of your employer, insurance company, lawyer, doctor, or other practitioner.

The Unbroken Circle: Your Real Backache and Your Spouse

Having just traced a saga of family manipulation and medical-legal tangles, let me now seek to exonerate the patient with real backache. It is one of the most excruciating and disabling illnesses around. The pain is comparable to that of a severe toothache, with some important differences: All a toothache sufferer need do is eat a soft diet and deaden the pain while a backache victim may not be able to walk, run, ride, swim, make love, dance, or move around at all. On top of that, you may not receive much sympathy for a disease that can't be diagnosed or treated with certainty. Backache is chronic and unpredictable, with a typical course of transient improvements and setbacks that can severely tax family members. So let's address the patient's family for a moment. The key words are patience, sympathy, understanding, and practical adjustments. Here are some undesirable scenarios that can occur without the above.

Say the back patient is the wife of a busy professional man who depends on her behind-the-scenes productivity in order to devote *his* full energies to work. Now she's laid up, and he resents the desertion of his able assistant. Many men who gallantly adjust to a wife's acute illness become intolerant of a chronic disability. Even when finances allow some domestic help, the husband may complain of the stranger's way of doing things. Basically, he may assume his wife's problem isn't real. He may even indulge in the paranoid fantasy that she is punishing him with her affliction.

How does he react? He may either discourage her from seeing doctors or push her around from practitioner to practitioner. He may pressure her into inappropriate surgery or oppose a needed operation.

Now let's change the identity of the patient. Let's make him the breadwinner.

At first, his wife may welcome his unaccustomed presence at home, the time for casual discussion, newspaper reading and television watching *a deux,* and so forth. Yet, as his condition becomes chronic, the backache sufferer quickly gets depressed, angry, guilty, or afraid and is no longer such a pleasant companion.

What can you do if you're the spouse of a backache victim? First of all, don't propel your partner around to multiple practitioners, though sometimes a second opinion is desirable. Above all, don't badger him/her into unnecessary surgery; think how you'd feel if the operation backfired and made your spouse worse in some way. Don't deny your partner's pain. Be patient. Though you can't feel a tumor in his/her back, thank heavens, acknowledge that there *is* a disease there. Be sympathetic. Remember your spouse's fine track record: He/she certainly doesn't want to fail you now, but is profoundly disabled. Be understanding.

If you work, consider telling your colleagues or superiors about your home situation, explaining that you may have to be less productive than usual. Perhaps specific adjustments—more assistance on the job, changed deadlines, or new strategies—can remove some of the pressure. Be practical.

You and your spouse might take several one- to two-hour "vacations" from each other during the day. As the pain becomes tolerable, invite some close friends in once or twice a week. Feel free to discuss the disease's course and prognosis, but don't let the conversation revolve completely around your mate's disability. When possible, go out for a walk or a ride. The backache sufferer can lie in a reclining seat or in the backseat of the car, sitting up to see the scenery at intervals. Drive-in movies are great. And now is the time for some loving sexual ingenuity (see Chapter VIII).

As the back ailment becomes chronic, the challenge thickens. Careful communication, understanding, and mutual support are crucial. If your family life becomes severely restricted it may be a good idea to step back and talk to the physician, a social worker, or some other advisor about such possibilities as retraining for an alternative career. Whatever you do, *please* don't fall into the saga of the eternally treated, multiply operated upon, poor soul or miserable compensation patient. Be positive.

Remember to nurture your spirit as well as your back. As we said at the beginning of this chapter, your body has its own internal control mechanisms for pain. You merely need to help it work. If marshaling your own dormant recuperative powers means meditation, positive thinking, acupuncture, biofeedback, psychiatric or psychological help, family counseling, or any combination of the above, do it. Just remember: Relatives, friends, doctors, other medical personnel, and the whole health care system can help, but *you* are the most important ingredient in the successful outcome.

Chapter V

Basic Back Self-Care

A Manual of Prevention and Home Treatment

Ah, you've arrived. This is the core chapter of the book, especially for those of you who are impatient with the arcana of spine ailments and just want to know how to take care of your back. These are the pages that should be read, reread, and assimilated into your life-style.

It contains what I consider the most reliable information, culled from sound scientific research and my own twenty-nine years of experience with patients. You'll be told precisely how to put it into practice. The underlying formula is the maximum comfort and minimum harm to you. The "first physician," Hippocrates, whose two-thousand-year-old oath new doctors still repeat, advised, "*Primum non nocere*," or, "First of all, do no harm." Not a bad place to start. We're all aware that medical and pseudomedical procedures can do harm. When you get to Chapter VII, you'll hear much about possible surgical harm. But, as your own physician, you can also harm yourself if you aren't properly informed. By mastering the ABCs of back care, you'll begin, I hope, to solve some of the problems of your back.

Now, not all of you are alike and of course you don't all have the same disease. Some of our suggestions will work for some readers, some for others. Hang on to those that work well for you; forget about the ones that don't.

Our first section deals with specific prevention tactics, which should become your constant companions over the years. But if you're already lying flat on your back and want to get to the straight talk of healing, read on.

HOW TO PREVENT BACKACHE

Now you're a student at our Low Back School, the goal of which is to nurture your back in your daily life. Presumably, most of you have had some backache, so prevention may seem academic right now. But "it ain't necessarily so." After you recover from this bout, you'll be highly motivated to head off a recurrence. It wouldn't be unusual, either, for you to become a back-care evangelist, lecturing friends, lovers, and family about how to prevent a first attack.

Some of our prevention principles are covered elsewhere, but let's review the basics: rest, proper nutrition, ample exercise, and weight control.

Staying Slim and Working Out

Shedding excess pounds reduces the loads your beleaguered spine must carry around. Unhappily, there is no magic diet. Sorry to break the news so ungently. Albert Einstein said, "Energy is neither created nor destroyed." In your body's terms, the weight you walk around with represents the calories left over when you subtract the calories used up from those consumed. These facts of the physical universe may seem self-evident, but fad diets tend to obscure them. We must admit that although there is lots of data to support the assertion that avoiding obesity is good for you in many ways, the statistics reviewed in Chapter I do not *prove* that if you are overweight, your back is more likely to hurt.

Regular exercise not only burns up your adipose tissue, it also maintains muscle tone, good circulation, and mobility. We've noted in Chapter II that good muscle tone is essential to a robust spine. And when weight is in the form of fat rather than muscle, it tends to be distributed so as to shift your center of gravity forward—hardly a fine state of affairs for your back.

The bottom line is that any physical exercise more strenuous than merely sitting on your derriere has some value, especially if done two or three times a week, at least. Chapter IX, devoted to sports and the back, lists the risk factors of various sports. If you have a serious back problem, of course, you shouldn't take up a high-risk game. Again sticking with the facts, although some studies show that being in shape protects you from backache, there are some that fail to show any benefit.

Good Ergonomics

We learn algebra and history in school; we may even dabble in Greek or ancient Aramaic; but how many of us, unless destined for a career in a white coat, learn even the rudiments of our own anatomy? Few of us get enough health education. How many mothers teach their small children that the way they sit, ride in the car, sleep, and lift things directly affects the spine? But since you're converts to back care, you already know that such factors as a sedentary life, driving long distances, and lifting objects way out in front of you or with a twisting motion threaten your back. Right?

Under the upcoming "Do's and Don't's" section, we'll give ergonomics lessons for a number of occupations, including homemaking.

Back Care on the Job

Industries could help out a lot by redesigning work environments. Better-designed secretarial chairs, desk and worktable arrangements, and motor vehicle seats, for example, would spare many employees' backs. It would be nice, too, if basic back education for high-risk workers and supervised exercise programs became part of the wave of the future. A simple but critical innovation is to minimize the times a worker must lift something off the floor. By starting the hefting from at least two feet *above* the floor level, the employee will avoid dangerous bending.

Our hospital has a safety committee that consulted me about secretarial chairs. One zealous member wanted to change all the institution's chairs to "wipe out backache." Of course, back pain is so multifaceted that better seats alone won't eradicate it as the Salk vaccine might wipe out polio. But why not start by describing the perfect secretary's seat, since it's such an everyday example.

The ideal secretarial seat should be adjustable to the ideal height, permitting you to sit with your feet flat on the floor, your thighs resting comfortably on the seat and your knees bent about ninety degrees. It should support your lumbar spine with a good adjustable backrest, with its most prominent part at the middle of the lower back, right at its point of greatest inward curvature. The backrest should have a rigid spring soft enough to let you lean back ten to twenty degrees but stiff enough to support you in the upright position. It's also nice if the stiffness or resistance of the backrest (its ability to "go back" or change its angle) is adjustable. Swivels and wheels? So much the better, if you must face in several different directions like a Hindu goddess and move small distances. The ideal chair should be upholstered with a material that permits heat transfer and doesn't allow too much body slippage. (Figure 5–1.)

Of course, in the best of all possible worlds, we'd all be sitting in individually molded chairs that precisely fit the contours of our particular backs. But in a world of limited resources, taking a tip from this chapter's recommendations will do. We can at least expect a comfortable chair that supports, and doesn't irritate, our lumbar spine. We'll talk more about seats toward the end of this chapter.

What if your job requires heavy lifting? Well, you can take a hint from weight lifters and use a large belt or small abdominal corset for additional support. This precaution, based on the concept of intra-abdominal pressure described in Chapter II, also has the psychological value of reminding you to think before you lift. Evaluate your work environment.

DO'S AND DON'T'S FOR A HAPPY BACK

Now let's take a stark look at exactly what you do at home and on the job. If you're scrupulous about heeding the following do's and don't's as they apply to you, perhaps your backache will take a long vacation or even divorce you.

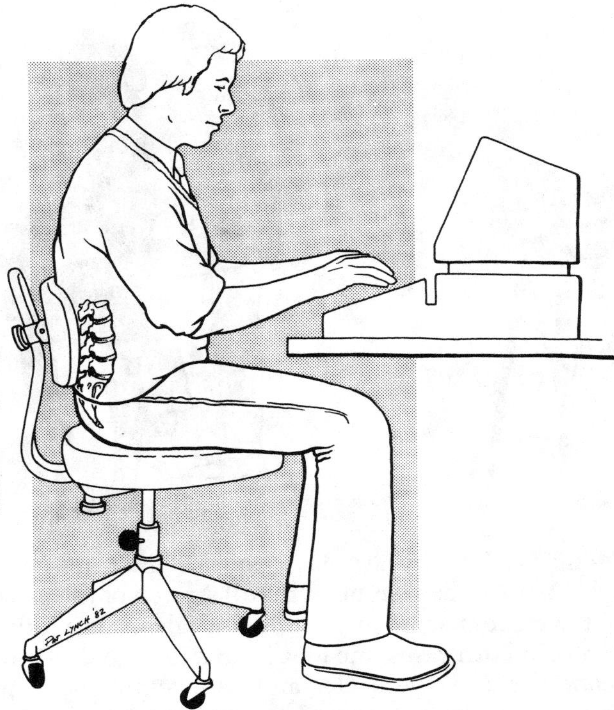

FIGURE 5–1 The ideal secretary's seat. Note the back support just at the level of the lumbar spine. It's flexible so that the secretary can lean back, yet it's supportive. There is good support for the thighs. The feet are flat on the floor, the knees are bent at ninety degrees. The chair can swivel, and it's on rollers. The height of the seat, the level of the back support, and the rigidity of the backrest can all be adjusted to the individual's needs. Small armrests are a nice option.

For Home Workers

DO step on a box while ironing, and station one leg on the base of the cabinet when washing dishes. Remember the bar rail. (Figure 5–2.)

DO use a high—above waist level, at least—table for changing the baby's diapers to avoid undue bending while lifting.

DO carry the baby as close to your body as possible, against your shoulder. (Figure 5–3).

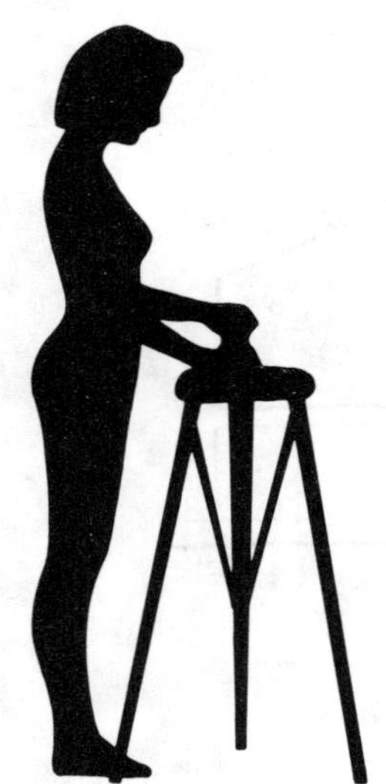

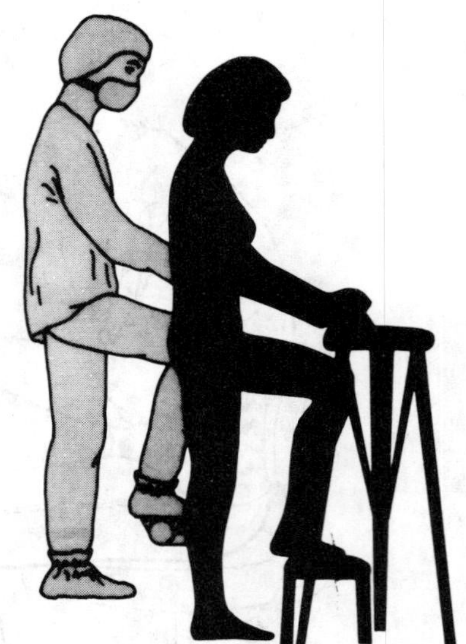

FIGURE 5–2 This is the "why bars have bar rails" picture. On the left we have a swayback (extended) spine with full stretch of the psoas muscle. On the right we see a woman ironing and also one working at the operating table. In both cases one foot is on a footstool (bar rail) to flex the hip, *relax* the psoas muscle, and *relieve* the back pain. This important principle of ergonomics has been recognized by successful drinking establishments for a long time. (Reproduced with permission from White, A.A., and Panjabi, M.M.: *Clinical Biomechanics of the Spine,* J.B. Lippincott, 1990, second edition.)

DO bend your knees and keep objects (or babies) close to you when lifting. Let your legs help you lift (Figure 5–4). Don't lift the way the man does in Figure 5–5.

DO use a long-handled vacuum cleaner and kneel on one knee instead of bending over from the waist. (Figure 5–6.) Use sponge-rubber knee pads. Always use your hands to support yourself when you must bend from the waist. According to my patients, vacuuming is one of the most notorious backache irritants.

DO use shopping carts and helpers as much as possible when loading and unloading groceries.

DO use care in lifting packages out of the car trunk. Position the package close to your body before lifting.

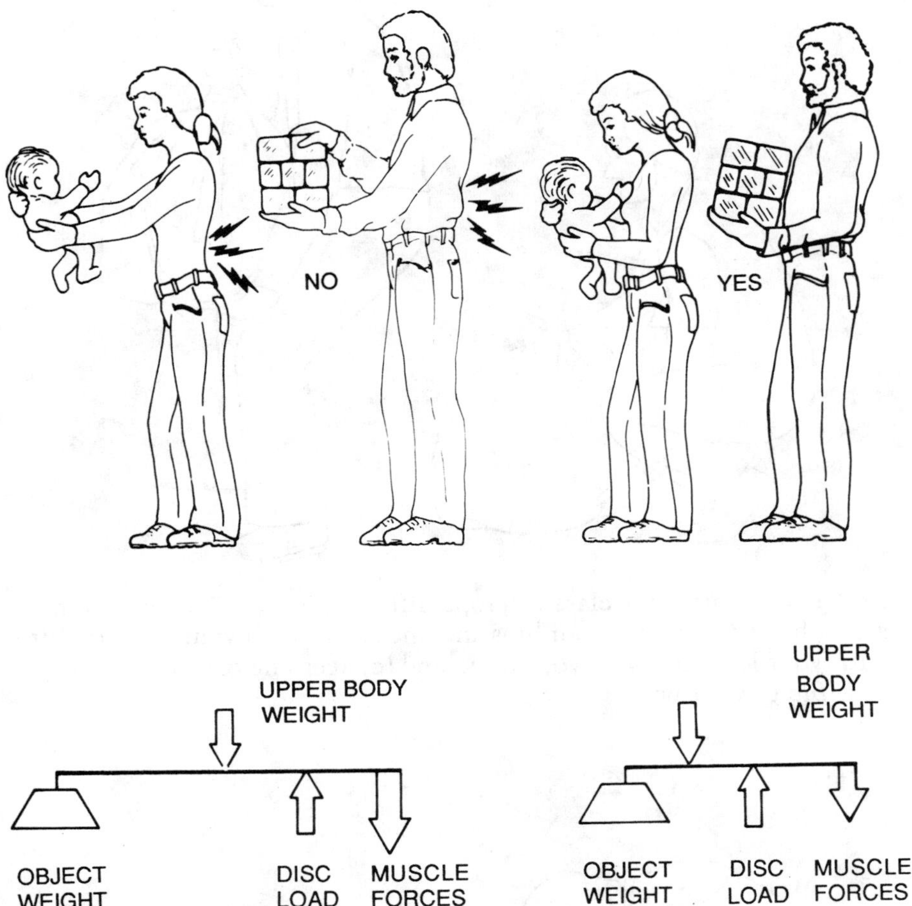

FIGURE 5–3 This picture is worth a moment of your study, as it will enhance your understanding of back mechanics. First, you must simply compare the *NO* picture on the left with the *YES* picture on the right. Even if you aren't interested in *why,* simply remember to lift and carry objects and babies as close as possible to the body. A study of the lever systems shows that the forces on the back (the disc) depend upon (1) the weight of the object lifted, (2) the weight of the upper body, (3) muscle forces, and (4) lever arms. The *NO* picture creates large lever arms, requiring large muscle forces. The result is considerable force on the back (the disc). In the *YES* picture the lever is shorter and the muscle and back (disc) forces are reduced. (Reproduced with permission from White, A.A., and Panjabi, M.M.: *Clinical Biomechanics of the Spine,* J.B. Lippincott, 1990, second edition.)

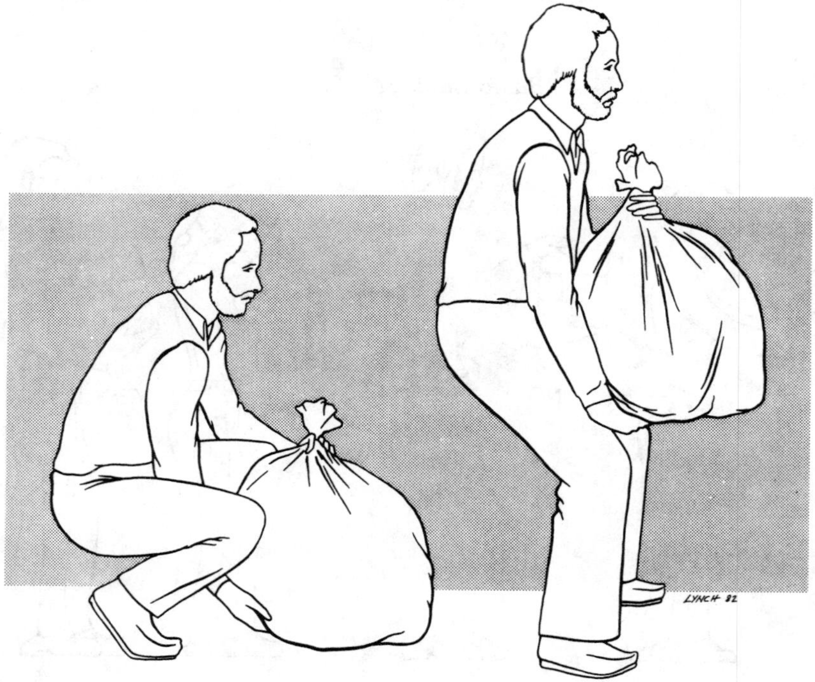

FIGURE 5–4 This is the classic "proper lifting" picture. The main points are (a) bend down with your hips and knees, *not* with your back, (b) lift with your legs, *not* with your back, and (c) keep the object *as close as possible* to your body.

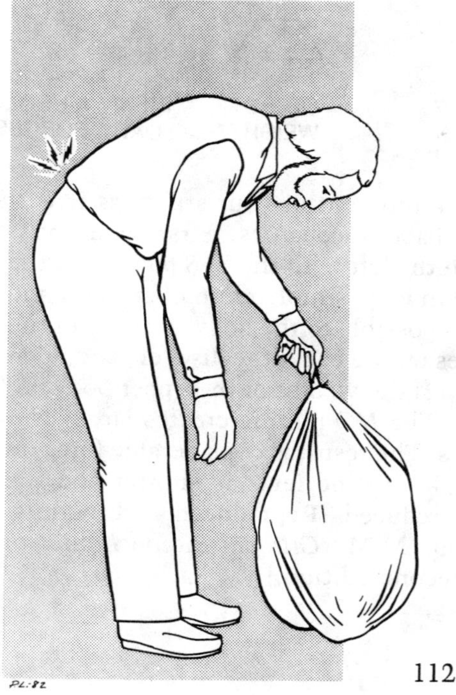

FIGURE 5–5 This is the classic "wrong way" to lift!

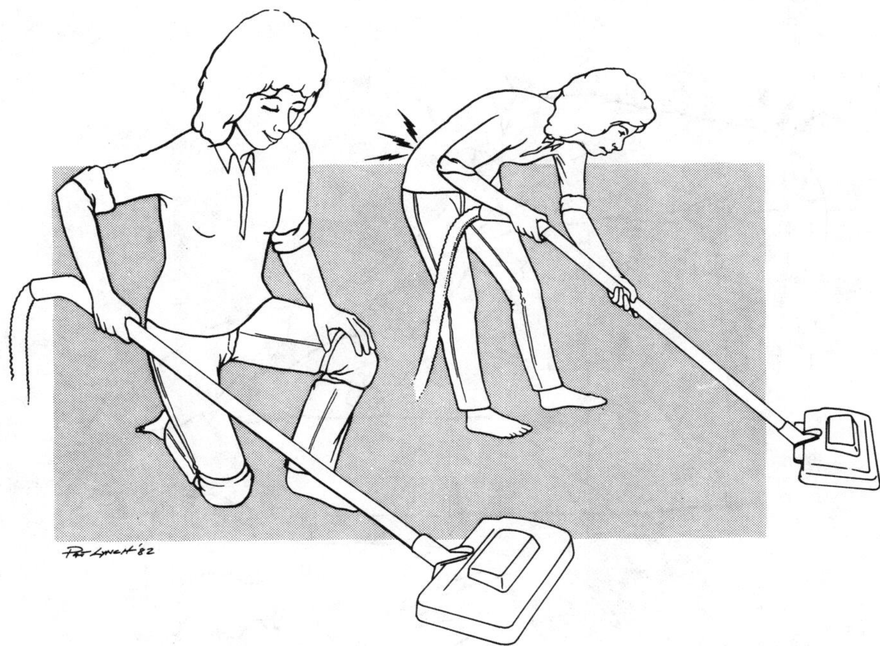

FIGURE 5–6 This is to protect home workers with backache from what is probably their most threatening task. With a fresh new backache this job simply ought to be avoided. Otherwise it should be performed *not* in the usual manner of bending at the waist. It should be done down on *one* knee. If your knees are sensitive, get some sponge-rubber knee pads from any sports shop—a worthwhile investment.

DO kneel down for gardening and break it up into five- to ten-minute intervals. Don't bend at the waist.

DON'T vacuum for long periods at a stretch. Break the job up into five- to ten-minute periods, with several hours or days in between. If you have back pain, have someone else do the vacuuming.

DON'T bend over to make a bed. When you can, kneel on the bed with one knee. Brace yourself with your arm to take pressure off your back. Another useful technique is to kneel on the floor at each side of the bed to straighten or tuck in sheets. (Figure 5–7.)

DON'T try to open a stuck window if it's too tight; get help.

DON'T jerk-lift anything, stuck windows included.

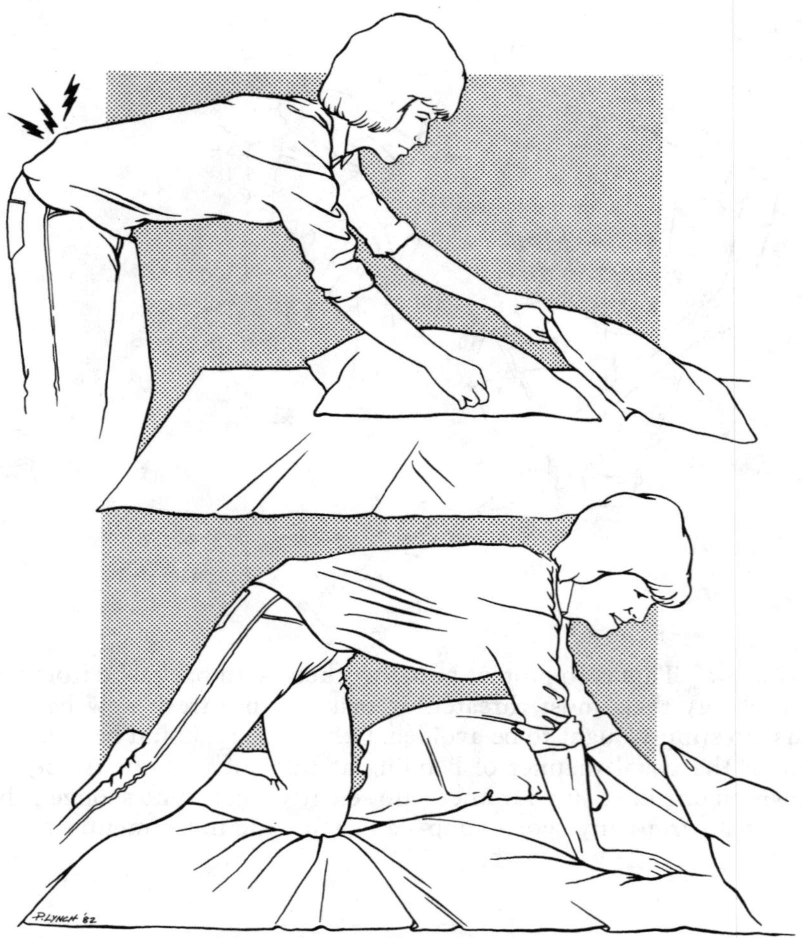

FIGURE 5–7 The home worker can avoid a lot of back pain irritation by simply supporting the upper part of the body on the hands and knees when making the bed. It's better to have both sides of the bed away from the wall so you don't have to reach as far across the bed.

For Executives

DO get an appropriate chair.
DO get enough exercise to counter your sedentary work.
DO get up and move about from time to time when you dictate or talk on the phone.

DO break up car and plane trips. Get out of the car and walk a bit at intervals; walk about the airplane cabin every hour or so.

DO travel first class when feasible, as the extra room is easier on the back.

DO consider using light luggage and briefcases with shoulder straps. This can be a lifesaver on a business trip.

DO balance the luggage you carry on either side of your body. If your load must be one-sided, alternate it. Keep luggage to a minimum.

DO use a collapsible luggage carrier with wheels whenever possible.

DO consider changing your job organization, location, and so on to meet your back's special considerations. It need not compromise, and may actually enhance, your effectiveness.

DON'T overload your briefcase.

DON'T drive long distances without rest stops.

DON'T go all out on the baseball diamond, or in any athletic field of endeavor, when you've been sedentary and out of condition. Work up to it gradually.

DON'T play golf unless you're aware of the risks and are willing to accept them. (Unless you are one of the lucky low back golfers who can get away with playing golf. See Chapter IX.)

DON'T have surgery just to get back to work two or three weeks sooner. Give bed rest and nonoperative treatment a good chance to cure you.

DON'T hesitate to get up and move around the board conference room after prolonged sitting. At least four out of five present will understand.

For Secretaries

DO obtain a comfortable, appropriate seat. (Figure 5–1.)

DO move about to decrease your sedentary time.

DO consider a chest- or waist-high working surface as a part-time alternative to sitting.

DO walk about sometimes when you're on the phone.

DO occasionally hand-deliver correspondence—using the stairs frequently—instead of sending it by messenger. The exercise will be good for you.

DON'T arrange your desk so you're frequently twisting from one position to another.

DON'T bend over files for extended periods.

DON'T, if you happen to wear high heels more than 4.5 cm. (1¾ inch), walk around in them all day. Keep a spare, low-heeled pair in your drawer.

For Hospital Workers

DO wait for help in lifting patients. Yes, everyone's busy, but they'll be even busier if you're *home* with a bad back.

DO use transfer boards when possible to transfer patients from bed to stretcher, and so on. If it's not an emergency, it's worth the time.

DO put your foot on the bottom of the operating table or hospital bed (like a bar rail) to relax your psoas muscle while attending to an operation or caring for a patient at bedside. (Figure 5–2.)

DO sit down to make a difficult vein puncture or a blood pressure reading rather than bending over the patient and struggling for several minutes.

DO have an appropriate chair to read and study in.

DO remember that *pushing* a hospital bed or stretcher is better than *pulling* it as far as your back's concerned.

DO transfer your weight from one foot to the other when standing for long periods of time (more than several minutes).

DO raise the patient's bed to a comfortable level—waist level—when working with him/her.

DON'T assume *you* have cancer. We medical people always assume the worst when we get sick.

DON'T assume that, unless you keep working when you should be resting your bad back, all your patients will die. Someone else will take good care of them for you.

DON'T fail to be as careful and conservative with yourself as you would be with a patient.

DON'T lift improperly because you think nothing can happen to *you.*

DON'T climb up on a patient's bed with your knees and try to lift him.

For Flight Attendants

DO pay special care to your lifting techniques.

DO maintain good overall muscle tone, especially in your abdomen and legs.

DO use wheels and carts to help transport your luggage. Maybe other travelers will learn from you.

DO get help from colleagues for difficult lifting.

DO look around you and suggest changes in work requirements and cabin design that could unstress your back.

DO push rather than pull serving carts up and down the aisles.

DO keep your back straight and bend from the knees, and keep the object close to your body, when lifting liquor kits and other heavy objects.

DO take time and care in stowing and retrieving things from under seats. Always get as close as possible to the object and avoid jerking motions.

DO always bend from the knees and keep your back straight when removing and passing trays. If your back is bothering you, just pass the first tray to the aisle-seat passenger. Then, while leaning one arm on the back of the seat in front, pass the tray with the other. This will avoid the stressful position of bending at the waist and holding something way out in front of you.

DO, when carrying trays, pile them one on top of another when possible. Carry no more than three at a time, close to the body, with your elbows straight.

DON'T try to lift heavy objects into the overhead compartments.

DON'T make long reaches with a food tray—delivering a tray over two passengers to the one in the window seat, for instance. Chapter II explains why this maneuver is dangerous. Passengers: When sitting in that window seat gazing at the moon, give the attendants a break and help pass the tray.

DON'T reach above your head or out from your body to lift even moderately heavy objects.

For Pilots and Cockpit Crew

DO get up and walk through the cabin a few times. The kids will love it, and it will be great for your back.

DON'T sit the whole time.

For Heavy Laborers

DO look for ways to reduce the injury potential in your workplace. The ideal is for everything that needs to be lifted to be two feet off the floor.

DO put a priority on good abdominal, leg, and general muscle tone. A recent study of Los Angeles firefighters showed that good conditioning *prevented* back injuries.

DO ask for assistance from coworkers in heavy-lifting situations.

DO consider wearing a small back support or a large belt if you're doing lots of lifting. Though it remains unproven, this idea is theoretically sound.

DO use all available lifting aids whenever possible.

DON'T push yourself, doing too much too soon during your convalescence from a back problem—but DO get back into the work environment and routine as soon as you can.

For Everybody

DO be patient—*you will* get better.

DO what you can to control stress, depression, and anxiety in your life.

DO be thoughtful of your back when making love.

DO get adequate exercise, especially strengthening your abdomen.

DO change position often, if you're sitting a lot. Sit on one hip for a while, then the other, then both. Then slouch a bit, before sitting erect for a while.

DO rest your arms on armrests when available, or on your lap when they're not.

DO try to use a chair that supports your lower back and has the potential to recline to about a 120-degree angle. Its seat should be wide enough for you to move around in it, and it should have armrests.

DO put a blanket or towel behind your lower spine while driving, and two pillows under your passenger-side arm as an armrest if there is not one in the auto. Rest your other forearm on the armrest built into the driver-side door. If none is present, improvise one there too.

DO obtain and use a cruise control in appropriate conditions when driving an automobile. This gives you more freedom to move about, shift your weight, and change the position of your back.

DO use a footstool or foot rail when standing for long periods—when ironing, at a bar, and so on. Now you know why bars have bar rails.

DO get a long shoehorn if bending forward to put on your shoes aggravates your pain.

DO try to balance the load you're carrying on each side.

DO perform exercises that strengthen your stomach muscles. Stomach-tensing (isometric abdominal) exercises are better than sit-ups if you already have a bad back. Also, it is a very good idea to strengthen the back muscles. See pages 133–37 on exercises. Just two small precautionary notes: 1) don't become a fanatic about them, and 2) don't take your conscience on any long guilt trips about doing them.

DO exercise when you sit for prolonged periods in planes, trains, buses, and cars. See Figures 5–8 and 5–9 for your "Olympic class" seat exercises.

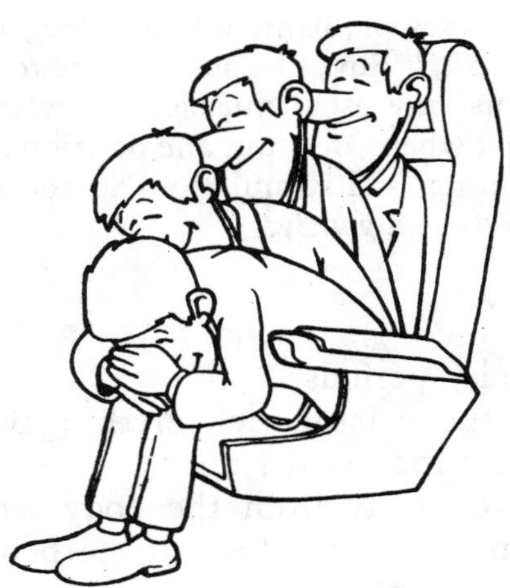

FIGURE 5–8 Draw the stomach fully in. Bend forward at the waist until the chest touches the thighs, then *gently* take the upper torso back to the upright position. Use your hands to help push yourself up. Do this twenty or thirty times about every two sitting hours. This is not for those of you with a sharp new back pain. It's good for all the rest of us. Remember this rule, however: If it hurts, don't do it. The advantage of this exercise is to stimulate circulation and prevent stiffening. (Figure reproduced with permission from the *SAS In-the-Chair Exercise Book*, Bantam Books, Inc., 1979.)

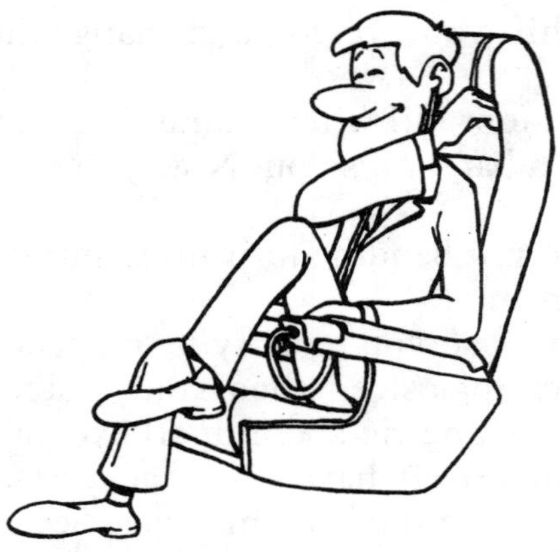

FIGURE 5–9 Lift the left and right knees alternately toward the opposite elbow. Reach a bit toward the opposite knee with the elbow. This is good for circulation, and it imparts a very slight and well-controlled axial rotation to the lumbar spine. This prevents the stiffness in the knee joints and spine that can occur with prolonged sitting. These exercises should be repeated fifteen times in each direction for every two hours of sitting time. (Figure reproduced with permission from the *SAS In-the-Chair Exercise Book,* Bantam Books, Inc., 1979.) The more inquisitive reader may ask, "Why is he advising me to bend forward as in Figure 5–8, and to use my psoas muscle and twist a bit in Figure 5–9?" The reason is that when you sit in *one* position a *long time* your spine needs a bit of motion and stimulation. So you should do these two exercises, but *slowly* and *gently.*

DON'T sit for extended periods.

DON'T bend over at the waist to pick anything up—or for more than a few seconds for any reason.

DON'T hold packages away from the body with your arms extended. Keeping the load close to the body reduces the burden on the lower spine.

DON'T do any vigorous back activity first thing in the morning, when your discs are more injury-prone because they have absorbed some extra fluids while you were lying down sleeping.

DON'T jog on very hard surfaces, especially if you're overweight and lack good jogging shoes. The combo of hard surface, poor footwear, and a bulky, awkward body can upset an already sensitive spine.

DON'T do exercises that involve twisting and turning. Remember what we said of twist-induced back pain during the Chubby Checker heyday?

DON'T work standing on a hard surface if you can avoid it. If you can't, invest in some thick crepe or soft rubber soles and heels to absorb some of the impact.

DON'T become an unhappy compensation cripple.

DON'T carry your wallet in your back pocket if you have back pain and sciatica, as the wallet presses on the sciatic nerve when you sit or drive, aggravating your condition. This is an example of what we call in medicine a "pearl of wisdom," and I learned it from a truck-driver patient of mine with sciatica! It certainly makes medical sense, since we doctors press on the sciatic nerve, just as a back wallet does, when we test for sciatica.

DON'T give up! It takes time. Follow this book and *you will* get better.

Summary of Preventative Measures

- Stay "in shape" (workout)
- Learn and practice good ergonomics both on and off the job
- Learn these do's and don't's and practice them, as they relate to you

HOW TO TREAT YOUR OWN BACKACHE

Okay, you just did something to your back. You hit a beautiful topspin serve. You lifted a tire out of the trunk of your car and twisted around to put it on the ground. Or perhaps you simply bent over from your chair to pick up a paper clip.

In any case, the pain hit. Maybe it was a mild stitch at first, but over the next few hours it turned into a full-blown backache. You may have pain in one or both legs, in the hip or thigh area, or radiating all the way down to your heel, even your toes.

What do you do now?

You can manage this yourself, as long as you haven't had trouble urinating or distinct weakness in your legs. If you *have* had such problems, get to a doctor straightaway.

Why am I making such a big deal out of this rather mundane bodily function? Because if you've got backache, and suddenly either can't urinate or hold your urine, you may have a very large herniated disc that has popped out of place. If it's displaced enough, it can hamper the nerves controlling your bladder, bowels, and legs. This situation requries immediate medical attention.

Otherwise . . . here it comes: "Take some aspirin, go to bed, and call me in the morning." Don't toss this book into the trash compactor yet. For reasons we'll elucidate in a moment, bed rest and two aspirin every four hours as tolerated is the very best prescription at this point.

Best Bed Tactics

What's the optimum lying-in-bed position for your sore back? Either on your back with your hips and knees bent (as in Figure 5–10) or on your side, again with hips and knees bent. Try it, you'll like it; it relaxes the key muscles and takes the burden off your spine. But if you find a more comfortable position, enjoy it, and if you'll drop me a postcard describing it, I'll share it with others. You can try putting two or three pillows under your knees, or hanging your legs over the edge of the couch. Some-

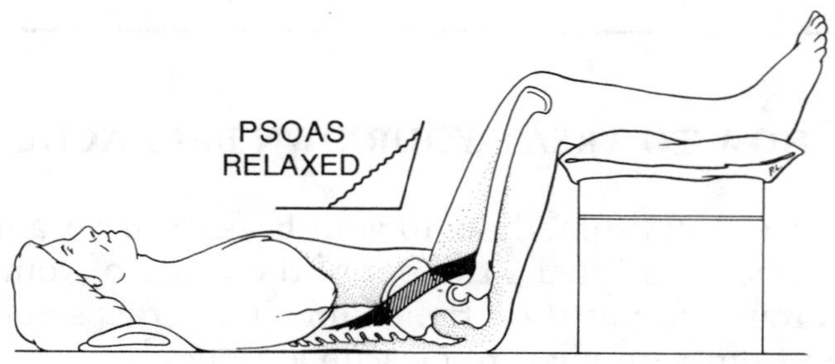

FIGURE 5–10 This shows an effective method for relaxing the psoas muscle and easing the stress on the low back. With the hips flexed and the weight relieved by being on the back, the spine is least likely to be irritated. Alternative and equally effective positions are shown in Figure 8–2A and B.

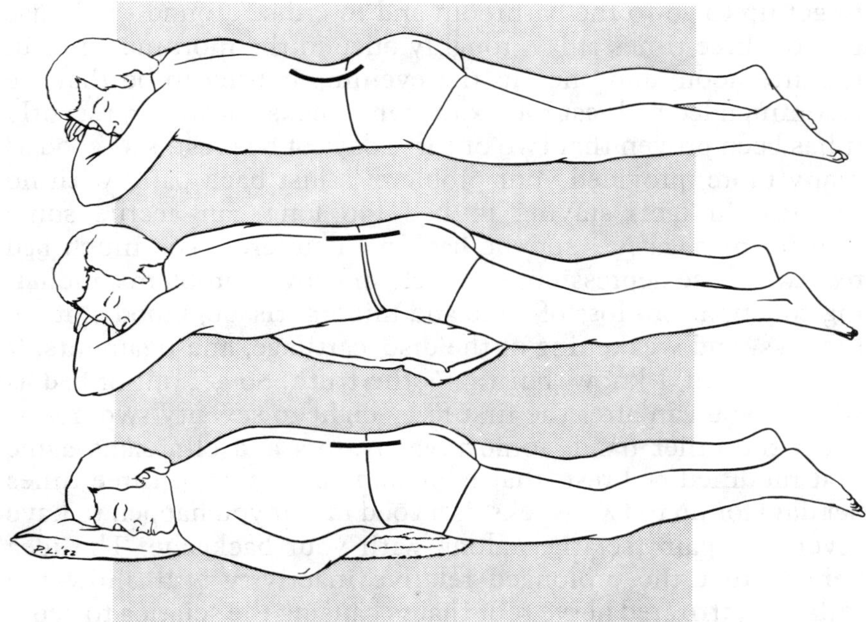

FIGURE 5–11 The "sleeping on the stomach" problem. The top illustration depicts the swayback or slightly extended spine. Figure 8–1 shows us why that's a problem. Thus, the backache patient should avoid sleeping on the stomach. However, for variety, or if you simply *"must"* sleep on your stomach, try the tricks shown in the lower two illustrations. You can straighten out that spine a bit with a pillow or a towel and/or by sleeping with your forearms underneath your pelvic bone.

times placing four or five blankets on the floor provides a firm surface that you'll prefer to sleep on for several days. A position that's *not* apt to please your back is lying on your stomach, which causes irritating lordosis (swayback). Some patients tell me, "I'm in a real bind, because I prefer to sleep on my stomach, but my back really wipes me out when I do." If this distress applies to you, try this. Sleep on your stomach, but with your arms or a rolled towel supporting your hips, as shown in Figure 5–11. This position supports the spine and may relieve just enough swayback to permit you to sleep on your abdomen. Try it!

At first, you should stay in bed for two or three days. Feel free to get up to go to the bathroom and to cruise around the house two or three times a day, roughly once in the morning, once in the afternoon, and once in the evening. It used to be that we recommended bed rest for six to eight weeks. However, recently it has been proven that two or three days of bed rest is as good as many more, provided your problem is just back pain, with no sciatica. In fact, staying in bed too long can accrue some significant negatives for the back pain sufferer. Too much bed rest can cause depression; stomach and bowel problems, including constipation; loss of bone and mineral tissue; blood clots in the legs; and weakening of the disc, cartilage, and ligaments. It sounds awful, I know, but that's the truth. So get out of bed as soon as you can after the first forty-eight to seventy-two hours.

On the other hand, some investigators and clinicians agree that modified bed rest (that is up and about two or three times per day) for up to two weeks, is a good idea if you happen to have severe leg pain (sciatica) along with your backache. The idea here is that the prolonged relative inactivity will allow the inflamed, irritated nerve root that is causing the sciatica to "cool down."

Mealtimes may be problematic, as sitting up will probably irritate your back. You *can* stay in a near-reclining position and eat from some type of tray, but make sure you're not twisting your spine to eat from a tray at your side; you'd be better off eating at the table or standing at a counter and returning promptly to bed.

Making Light of Bedrest

The banality "Forewarned is forearmed" applies here. If your back forces you to bed for a period, watch out for unwanted pounds. Inactivity plus the likelihood of boredom-inspired munching will make you less svelte than formerly. We've noted that weight stresses the lumbar spine. Don't fall into the vicious cycle of back pain leading to inactivity, leading to weight gain, leading to more back irritation, leading to more immobility, and so on. It may hurt, my friend, but now is the time for a little willpower on top of all your other trials. If you diet, however, follow a sensible low-calorie regimen, not a fly-by-night miracle diet. Take a generic multivitamin pill once a day.

Getting In and Out of Bed

Getting in and out of bed with a backache is a sophisticated art. Consult the diagrams in Figure 5–12.

To get out of bed, first lie on your side, facing the side of the bed from which you plan to arise. Then work your way over to the edge of the bed. Now, without twisting or bending your back—keeping it straight—let your lower (bedside) arm push you slowly up to the sitting position. At the same time, move your legs over so they can fall to the floor. This motion is similar to that of a woman, heavy with child, getting out of bed. Follow

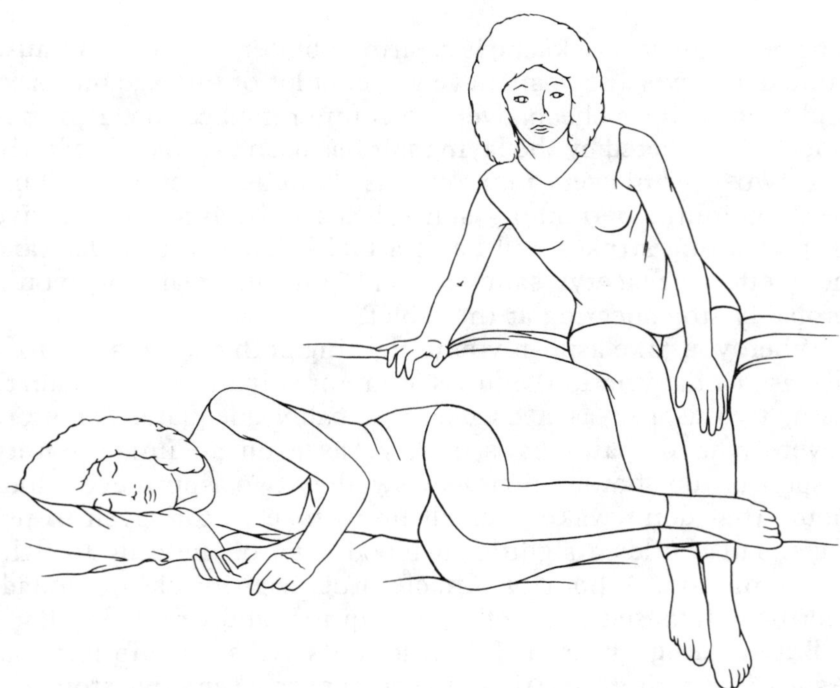

FIGURE 5–12 Here we see the side-lying position, with hips and knees flexed for a relaxed, pain-free back. This is also the position one should move to before getting in and out of bed. The text describes this maneuver in detail on this page and the next. This figure also shows the use of the arm to push up when getting out of bed or to let yourself down with when getting into bed.

that example, if you've ever seen it. If you do this maneuver carefully, you'll spare yourself some pain.

Getting back into bed, do the reverse. First, sit on the bed, resting your pillow-side arm on the bed. Gradually bring your legs up as you slowly let your body down by shifting your weight from your palm to your forearm, then to your elbow, your shoulder, your neck, until you're fully reclined. Now move to your favorite position.

If your back is very painful, have someone help you by slowly lifting your legs as you let your body down.

Aspirin and Other Friends

The best drug for backache is aspirin or buffered aspirin. Because comedians over the years have gotten a lot of mileage out of it, and because it's a cheap, over-the-counter medication, aspirin is not well respected by the layman. It has been estimated that 650 mg (two aspirin) every four hours is about as effective as 50 mg of Demerol (meperidine). Aspirin has also been found effective in preventing strokes and heart attacks. Once you understand how effective acetyl salicylic acid (aspirin) really is, you'll probably stop sneering at the tablet.

When you take aspirin you're fighting both the cause of your disease (inflammation) and its symptoms (pain). For moderate pain, two aspirin as needed are probably adequate. For more severe pain or pain that's clearly based on an inflammatory response, you should religiously swallow two aspirin every four hours (but don't wake yourself up to take it) for seven to ten days. This builds a significant blood level of the drug to fight inflammation. A homely miracle drug, aspirin: cheap, nonaddicting, purchased without a prescription, and very helpful!

But no drug on earth is without its risks and limitations. Aspirin can irritate gastritis, ulcers, or even a sensitive stomach. If that's the case, try buffered aspirin, or taking aspirin with a small bit of food or in an enteric-coated form (which keeps the aspirin isolated as long as it's in your stomach). It can also be taken rectally.

Aspirin can also cause abnormal bleeding in some circumstances. Check with your physician if you think you're at risk.

If you're one of those who for one reason or another can't

tolerate aspirin, don't despair. There are substitutes. Tylenol (acetaminophen) is a similar nonprescription painkiller. Indomethacin and ibuprofen (Motrin) are nonsteroidal anti-inflammatory drugs. These are now available "over the counter" under the brand name Advil. Thus, you don't need a prescription. These nonsteroidal anti-inflammatory drugs have gastrointestinal side effects, and therefore precautions must be taken. Always take these medications with a small snack. If one bothers your stomach, try a different one. Also, it shouldn't be used by patients with GI-tract difficulties. There is a new drug that can block most if not all the gastrointestinal problems associated with the nonsteroidal anti-inflammatory medications. The generic name is misoprostal and Cytotec is a brand name. A prescription is required. Newer nonsteroidal anti-inflammatory agents like naproxen (*Naprosyn*), sulindac (*Clineral*), and diclofenac sodium (Voltaren), can also be used to alleviate back pain. For women, Motrin is as effective a painkiller as codeine. A physician should prescribe and supervise the use of all prescription medications.

The question of *muscle relaxants* almost invariably comes up. I prefer to make my patients comfortable without resorting to them. Muscle spasms, caused by the disease in the spine, may actually be protective—and when the disease wanes, the spasm should disappear. On the rare occasion when I do prescribe a relaxant, I prefer cyclobenzaprine (*Flexeril*).

If you happen to be taking this drug for low back pain and or sciatica, remember this important point! It is possible that this medication can cause urinary retention; that is, you may have difficulty or be unable to pass your water. You should report this to your doctor immediately or, if you go to an acute-care facility, let someone know the problem may be due to the medication you're taking. The reason for all this emphasis is that someone may fear that your inability to void is due to a huge disc herniation. Loss of ability to urinate based on a huge disc herniation requires surgical removal of the disc, on an urgent basis.

The next chapter, on medical care for the problem back, will attack these pharmacological matters in more detail—including the use of stronger painkillers, narcotic and nonnarcotic. For most backaches, however, aspirin or another nonaddictive medicine is the drug of choice.

Heat, Ice, and Massage

Heat is another ally while you're on your back. An electric heating pad is as good as anything, though some people will prefer moist heat. Moist heating pads are generally available at any large drugstore or home health aid store. So long as it isn't too hot and doesn't damage the skin, any form of heat will do.

What does heat or ice do for you? By soothing your aches, it can help break up the cycle in which muscle spasm causes pain, causing more muscle spasm, causing more pain, and so on. Refer back to the "gate control" theory of pain in Chapter IV. The sensory input from heat or ice application (and massage, too) may somehow block pain transmission, or it may cause local circulatory changes under the skin.

Massage? Clearly, massage, laying-on-of-hands, tender loving care—and any sensual pleasure derived therefrom—are good for the back as well as the soul. Both heat and ice massage probably stimulate endorphin production and the "placebo effect" (see Chapter IV), which can have potent benefits.

While I believe any kind of heat application works equally well, the particular massage technique and the skill of the masseur or masseuse are probably important factors. Oddly enough, ice massage, simply rubbing the back with ice cubes, comforts some sufferers. If it helps, don't worry about *why.* It can't harm you.

The question frequently arises, which is better, heat or cold? First answer: Use whatever feels best to you. Second answer: Generally, in an *acute* strain, or with a muscle-pull injury with spasm, ice is likely to be better in the first forty-eight hours, and heat thereafter.

GETTING WELL

How Long, Oh Lord, How Long?

Observe yourself for signs of progress. Chart your recuperation in terms of what you can do today compared with yesterday or two or three days ago. You'll no doubt find you're improving—gradually—and that there are more and more things you can do without the excruciating pain that heralded your ailment. A little back diary can help you keep track.

We've indicated that the bed rest should be limited to two or three days. If you're not getting worse, and are improving just a little bit, consider taking aspirin and reducing activity (not bed rest) for as long as two or three weeks before consulting a doctor. This assumes you have no problem urinating; if you do, see a doctor at once. If you should get progressively worse for several days even though you're doing all the right things, you may want to see a doctor about adding stronger painkillers to your regimen. Most people, however, will recover on a course of reduced activity, aspirin, *patience,* optimism, and following the advice in this book.

Bye-Bye, Backache Blues

What should you do when you start to feel better? How can you gauge how much activity your back can withstand? As soon as you can move with minimal pain, you can begin to walk around the house a little more. Then, when you've managed at-home maneuvers with little pain for two or three days, you can start pondering a more rigorous exercise program (see pages 133–37) and a return to work. If commuting requires a long drive, have someone else drive at first, and you can lie either on the backseat or in a front reclining seat, if your car has one.

Starting back to work on a half-day basis may be wise. But as long as your back pain doesn't come back to haunt you, you can plunge right into a full schedule. Even with some residual back pain—as long as there's no major setback—you can progress to full-time work over the course of seven days or so. Once you're almost free of pain, you can start the basic sit-up and leg-stretching exercises described on pages 133–36.

If your job involves heavy manual labor, however, your back-to-work scenario is a little different. You'll need a five- to ten-day essentially pain-free interval beforehand, then *light* duty (policies permitting). That means lifting no more than twenty-five pounds and no bending or twisting. If this is a problem because of your actual work situation, or if you have any questions, you should probably consult a physician about what your back is capable of handling.

Despite our keep-a-positive-attitude theme, I must warn you

that sometimes patients who cautiously start back to work have a setback, and their pain comes back full blast. Despair not; you won't be a lifelong cripple. But you must take it from the top, more or less, and start recuperating all over again. You'll work yourself back to health sooner than you think, so try again.

Convalescence: Step by Step

Let's describe the convalescent period—between recovering from acute back pain and returning to the workplace—in a little more detail.

First a sermonette: In the last chapter I warned you against the tribulations of compensationitis, and now I'd like to take on the other end of the spectrum, those people who think the sun will be stuck below the horizon if they don't get back to the office and make it all happen. Don't worry. The work crew / company / hospital / government / store / university / team / family / business will still be there. Of course, you're needed and missed, but don't wreck your back by playing the martyr, the hero/heroine, and "totin' them bales" prematurely. You may be strong as an oak, but yield to back pain like a willow to the wind and you'll bounce back sooner.

What are the risks of too much activity too soon? You may reirritate your spine and cause a setback that will prolong your overall convalescence.

One signpost of recovery is the amount of time spent out of bed and moving about. You should do a bit of sitting, but not too much, as it puts a big load on the spine. When you can sit without back pain for over twenty minutes, you'll know you can gradually increase your activities.

Noting the amount of pain-free time you spend each day is a good gauge of how much you can stay out of bed. Another pretty specific milestone is how much walking you can do. You can gradually extend your distances as your back permits.

Sometimes you can do a little gentle testing of your work conditions. Try desk work when there are other signs of recovery. Various kinds of heavy work can also be performed as a test run.

After you return to work, stop and lie down for a few minutes if your back bothers you. This is crucial advice, as it often prevents a reinjury or setback. Let me repeat it *con brio: If your back hurts, stop and lie down for a few minutes with hips and knees bent!*

Here's a summary of some key back-to-work information as espoused by Professor Alf Nachemson of Sweden.

Back-to-Work Checklist (Reminder)

- Don't lift heavy objects
- Whatever you lift, keep it close to your body
- Have lumbar support and armrests where you sit
- Avoid bending and twisting
- Change positions frequently
- Don't sit in low chairs

EXERCISES

Exercises are important and they *do help!* Once you get back to work, or even a few days before, is the time to start an exercise program. In my opinion, the simple, straightforward exercises below represent the best advice current medical knowledge has to offer you. A word of warning: Don't confuse complexity with efficacy. I suspect some exercise programs may seem more compelling because they're complicated. Don't worry—sometimes simple is beautiful.

Walking, Bicycling, and Swimming

We now recommend what we consider a simple, straightforward, effective exercise program, of which there are several key ingredients. They are: 1) regularity, 2) trunk muscle strengthening and endurance, and 3) palatability, i.e., that the exercises be somewhat interesting and enjoyable. Regularity is important to stimulate endorphin secretions (our own internal pain control substances). There is evidence that good functional (strength and endurance) trunk muscles support the spine and help in rehabilitation and prevention of recurrence. Finally, since we are all endowed with the inalienable right of the pursuit of happiness, among other things, we need to "have fun" doing the exercises. Moreover, if in this process of fighting the backache battle we can become habitual exercisers, this would be a bonus. It takes six weeks to develop a habit (a good or bad one). To develop a healthy exercise habit, tie it to a current habit—for example, your daily dental hygiene. Tell yourself, "I can't brush my teeth until I've done my back exercises." The tandem approach is a successful one. The exercises suggested, and the schedule recommended, are designed to provide aerobic fitness as well.

In our routine program, patients gradually work up to a point where they can walk, bicycle (mobile or stationary), or swim for a half hour to three quarters of an hour at their own pace, three to five times per week. We suggest that one or any combination of the three activities is fabulous! The patient is advised to gradually work up to the half-hour range, and to continue with mild pain as tolerated, but to stop when there is severe pain.

Walking can be done as a slow, relaxed, recreational walk or it can be done with as much vigor as tolerated. A fifteen-minute mile is excellent for aerobic conditioning. Headsets with music, humor, foreign-language lessons, sermons, lectures, letter tapes, or unmentionables are suggested to make it fun.

Bicycling inside or outdoors is generally an exercise well tolerated by those with back pain. As with walking, one can gradually build up to the suggested thirty- to forty-five-minute workout, and go at one's own pace. Supplementary entertainment with audio or, if stationary biking, audiovisual tapes can enhance the fun.

Swimming is often described as the best all-around exercise, as well as the best exercise for patients with low back pain. Swimming tends to require work from all our muscles, provides superb aerobic conditioning, and takes lots of the load off our backs. We ask our patients to use any stroke or any combination of strokes that they enjoy. The butterfly stroke aggravates lots of patients because of the extensive extension (swayback or lordosis) of the back. However, if it *does not* bother you and you like the butterfly—no problem. The guidelines for pain are the same as stated above.

These are our recommendations. Certainly any sport or exercise activity that does not aggravate one's pain can be helpful, as well as invigorating. We usually like to discuss these sports individually with the patient. Our goal, of course, is to help the patient get back to doing whatever it is he/she wants to do.

Jogging or "wogging" (a combination of jogging and walking) can often be participated in successfully without pain, as can golf, tennis, sailing, softball, bowling, and many other activities, although some seem to be more likely than others to cause difficulty. The recommendation is best made after a careful discussion with the patient about a particular sport and the past and current history of tolerance and incidence. There's a lot more about sports and the back in Chapter IX.

You've just been exposed to my first choices of exercise, but following is a discussion of some other reasonable approaches that have been utilized and prescribed for patients with back problems.

Sit-ups

Sit-ups have been considered important, because they strengthen the abdomen and in theory relieve the spine of stress. (Figure 5–13.)

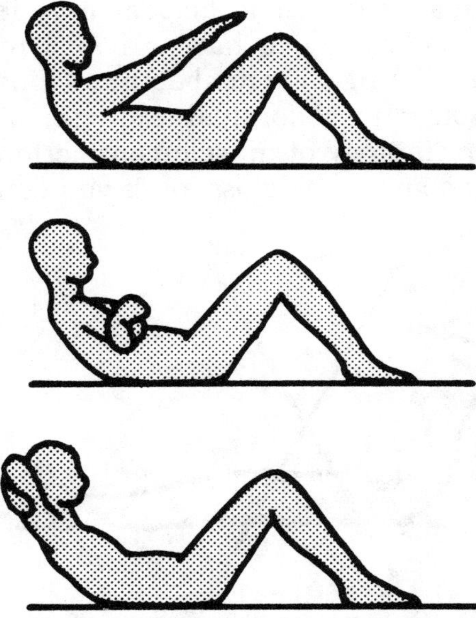

FIGURE 5–13 These exercises are good for strengthening the stomach muscles after you've gotten over the initial sharp back pain. These sit-ups increase in difficulty from top to bottom, because you shift the center of gravity upward by moving the arms closer to the head. The top one is fine and the best for most readers.

Sit-ups should *not* be done with the legs straight, or with the feet or legs hooked under some fixed object (Figure 5–14). Why? Doing them that way makes the psoas ("filet mignon") muscle work too hard, imparting high stress to your spine. And this phenomenon aggravates rather than alleviates any existing backache—and may even be undesirable for someone *without* back pain.

So start the exercise lying flat on your back with your hips and knees bent. In the beginning you won't have much strength, so you need do no more than just reach for your knees by raising your head, shoulder, and upper back off the floor (Figure 5–13). If you can do this twenty to twenty-five times once or twice a day, you'll develop abdominal tone and protect your back. As you gain strength you can increase the difficulty by putting your arms behind your head.

Isometric Abdominal Exercise

Tighten your throat, bowel, and bladder muscles. Then press hard, as if you were trying to have a bowel movement, and concentrate on tightening all your abdominal muscles. This, my friend, is the isometric abdominal exercise. There's a mini course on the terminology of muscle contractions on page 138 and the definitions are in the glossary. If you don't particularly

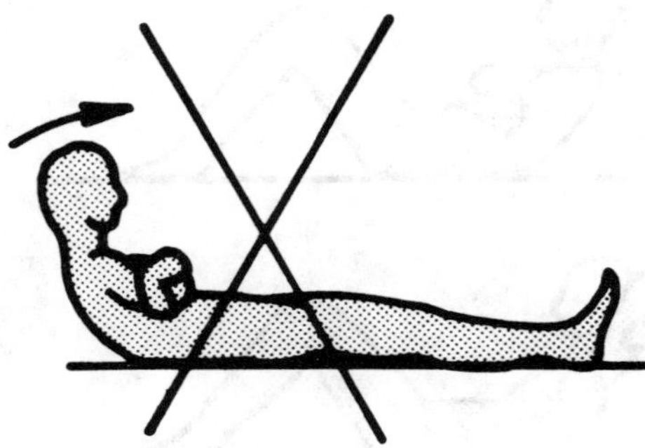

FIGURE 5–14 This is no good for the back, even if you don't have backache. It is the best way to strain the spine, because when you do sit-ups this way, or with something holding your feet down, you use the psoas muscle and stress your back. This obviously is what you do when you lean over the side to balance a sailing craft. See Sailing, Chapter IX.

enjoy studying these terms don't worry, you *can* take good care of your back without memorizing their definitions. The beauty of these exercises is that you can do them riding in a car, standing, listening on the phone, or whenever. Their purpose is to tone up your abdomen, and you should do fifteen or twenty of them three or four times a day. I think that this is the best exercise of all, especially if you are only going to do one exercise. If you have heart disease, it should not be done without consulting your doctor.

BACK MUSCLE EXERCISES

Some clinical studies and a number of therapists have emphasized strengthening the back muscles, mainly the erector spinae group. There are two ways to achieve this. One is to simply lie face down and raise the head and upper chest off the surface. The other is illustrated in Figure 5–15. Start down on "all fours," then lift one arm and the opposite leg to a position parallel to the floor, hold a second and then place them back down on the floor. Then do the same with the opposite arm and leg. This is not easy because it requires good balance and strength. If you can work up to ten or fifteen repetitions for each arm and leg daily, you will have significantly strengthened your back muscles.

Knee-to-Chest Exercises

Take a look at Figure 5–16. Lying on your back with your hips and knees slightly flexed, take one leg and pull it up to your

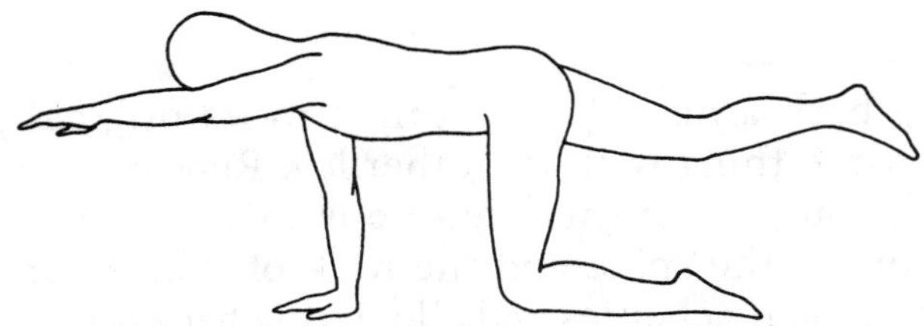

FIGURE 5–15 An excellent though not easy exercise to strengthen the back muscles. (Reproduced with permission from White, A.A., and Panjabi, M.M.: *Clinical Biomechanics of the Spine,* J.B. Lippincott, 1990, second edition.)

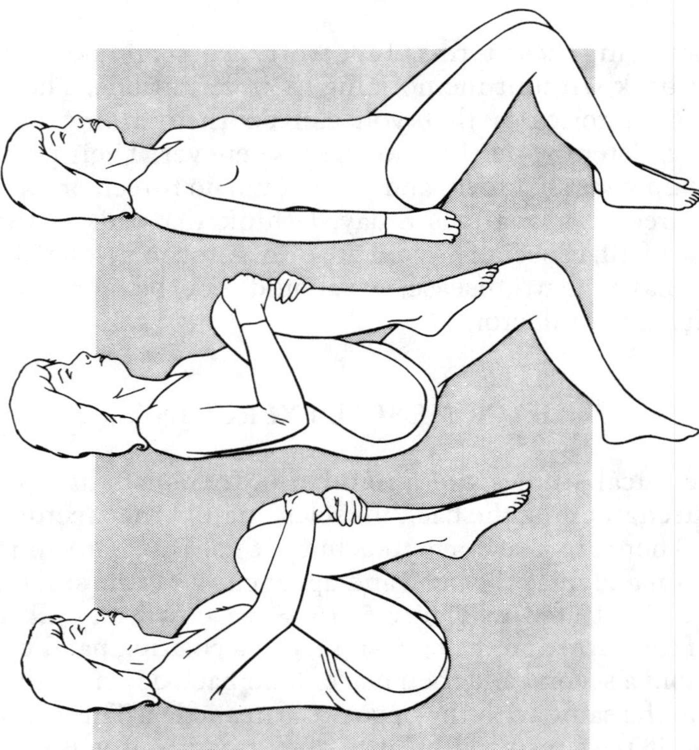

FIGURE 5–16 This figure demonstrates the single and double knee-to-chest exercise. The top picture shows the starting position; relaxed, flat on the back, with hips flexed and feet flat on the floor. Next, pull the right knee to the chest. Complete the last few inches by pulling with the arms. Then let go, relax, and repeat with the left knee. The double knee-to-chest exercise is done as shown in the bottom drawing. If you are one of the few patients who experiences additional pain following these knee-to-chest exercises, don't continue them.

chest, using both arms. Then return it to its original position and do the same thing with the other leg. Repeat ten times for each leg. The purpose of this exercise is to stretch the muscles and ligaments in the spine and the back of the hip, improving posture and spine mechanics and alleviating back stresses. It can also be done by bringing both knees up simultaneously, also repeated ten times.

Twice a day is best, but even a consistent once-a-day habit should benefit you greatly.

However, be advised that some of you, especially if you're afflicted with sciatica, may find this exercise irritating. If so, *don't do it.* This rule applies to any activity that makes your back hurt more, for the old "work through the pain" concept is a fallacious one.

The Pelvic Tilt

If you're a dancer or a lover, or both, it may inspire you to learn that this movement is essentially the "front bump" in dancing and the pelvic motion basic to lovemaking.

Back up against the wall or lie on the floor. Now put your hand behind your lower back, feeling the arch there and noting that the back isn't touching the wall (or floor) at that point. Then try to flatten the back to eliminate the gap. When you've done this you've done the pelvic tilt. Do fifteen to twenty of these every day and that should suffice.

This exercise strengthens the front spine structures and stretches the back ones. And it moves the lumbar spine from a lordotic (swayback) position to a straighter position that's better for your back. (Figure 5–17.)

SOME THINGS YOU NEED TO KNOW ABOUT MUSCLES, EXERCISE, AND LOW BACK PAIN

There are three important, practical questions to be discussed concerning low back pain. First, how important is trunk muscle function in the evaluation, treatment, rehabilitation, and prevention of low back pain? Second, assuming that strong erector spinae muscles are important, what is the best way to strengthen them? Third, if one decides to strengthen these back muscles, what is the importance of various types of exercise machines that are available for monitoring the muscle activity?

If you have back pain rehabilitation in the 1990s, you're very likely to be faced with some of the following terminology, so before I discuss muscle strengthening allow me to share with you a brief glossary of muscle contraction terminology. Your therapist or physician may on occasion use one or more of these terms.

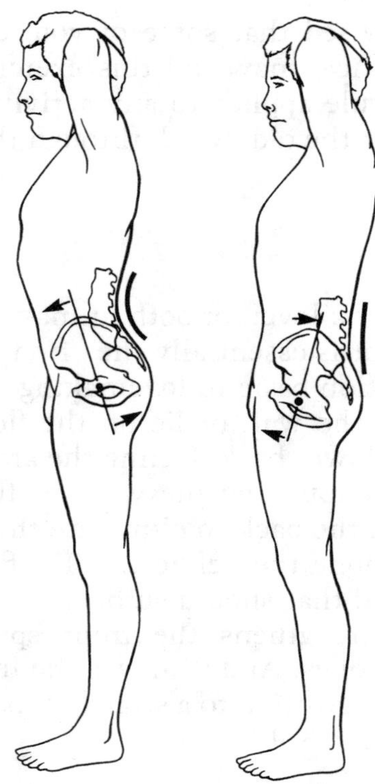

FIGURE 5–17 The "pelvic tilt" exercise can be difficult to explain, but between the text and the good work of Pat Lynch, our dedicated illustrator, we think we've explained it. On the *left* we see the position of the low back and pelvis in the swayback or extended position. I describe elsewhere (Figure 8–1) the theoretical negatives of this position. The pelvic tilt shown on the *right* rotates the pelvis and straightens out the spine, which accentuates the positives and eliminates the negatives. The forces are better distributed with the pelvic tilt as shown.

On the left is the relaxed swayback position. On the right, the arrows show the forces that must be exerted by muscles to rotate it to the proper position. The text tells you how to get your pelvis in this more healthy position. Now you must get in the habit of keeping it there.

Isometric Contraction—there's *tension* in the muscle (it contracts), but it *does not* change its *length.* Consequently, nothing moves. I discussed this type of contraction when we reviewed "isometric abdominal" exercises.

Isotonic Contraction—there's *tension* in the muscle (contraction again), but this time, it *does* change its *length*. As a matter of fact, it shortens and something moves. Take a sip of coffee. When you lift the cup you contract and shorten your biceps muscles, and the coffee, with its familiar, stimulating aroma, moves to your welcoming lips. That is isotonic contraction.

Eccentric Contraction—there's *tension* in the muscle (you got it: contraction), it changes *length*, but this time it doesn't shorten, it *lengthens!* Right! It's just the opposite of isotonic contraction. Would *lengthening contraction* be a more explicit term? Some people think so. You be the judge. Here's an example of eccentric contraction. You have a sip of coffee and put your cup back on the table. The weight of the cup and its contents is resisted by the biceps muscle involved in an eccentric contraction. The muscle lengthens as it contracts to assure a gradual safe descent of the cup of coffee to the table.

Isokinetic Contraction—there's *tension* in the muscle (right, it contracts: the common denominator). However, this time there's a smart and powerful machine that can be set to select and control the speed at which you can move your arm, leg, or trunk. The rate of muscle shortening can be held constant. Machines that do this eliminate certain variables and make possible a more standardized analysis of muscle strength and fatigue.

Isointernal Contraction—tension in the muscle and change in length, but this time the smart machine can control and keep constant the load or the force that the muscle must exert.

Testing equipment is available to control resistance and rate and range of movement (acceleration, velocity, and distance). This leaves only the torque as an independent variable, which makes it possible to compare a patient with him/herself and with others in a standard method. The Cybex and Kincom are examples of computerized machines that measure the power, strength, and endurance of various muscle groups.

So to summarize and review, there's tension in the muscle every time—that's contraction. Sometimes the contracting muscle a) keeps the same length, b) shortens, or c) lengthens. Moreover, in the contractions in which there is change of length, there are machines that can select and keep *constant* either a) the speed at which the muscle can change its length or b) the loads that must be overcome as length changes. Are you thoroughly confused? If not, let's move on. If so, let's move on, bcause understanding this muscle physiology is by no means crucial to getting rid of that backache.

Let's continue with some additional background information. Analysis of trunk muscles shows that the extensors (back muscles) are generally stronger than the flexors (abdominal and psoas). My athletic daughters were amused to find out that although men are as a group stronger than women in the absolute sense, on a "pound-for-pound" basis women are stronger. In addition, research shows that women demonstrate greater endurance in their trunk muscles. It seems that we're all destined to show distinct loss of strength in the trunk muscles, beginning around "forty-something."

Most muscle strains and acute soft-tissue injuries of the spine and trunk recover completely in three to six weeks. Although machine-controlled muscle testing provides some quantitative assessment of functional capacity, it can be irritating if started too soon after onset of the acute condition.

As mentioned previously, there is moderate evidence that less than good trunk strength may predispose one to having a backache. Studies show that sit-ups, extension exercises, and electrical stimulation of muscles enhance endurance but not strength. Trunk muscle strength can be improved with a six- to twelve-week exercise program.

In recent years there have been some prominent studies of the use of trunk muscle exercises in the treatment of our fellow humans suffering with low back pain. As we've mentioned before, there are no strong consistent ropes of evidence to support claims for their efficacy. The current literature promotes the idea that trunk-therapeutic (abdominal and/or extension) exercises, in conjunction with back pain school, work hardening programs, are beneficial.

Studies of the electrical response of muscles, as well as mechanical studies of the trunk muscles, show an association of trunk muscle fatigue and low back pain.

Let me now attempt succinct answers to the questions posed at the beginning of this section.

Q. *How important is trunk muscle function in the evaluation, treatment, rehabilitation, and prevention of low back pain?*

A. It is important.

Q. *Why?*

A. Because patients with low back pain have decreased strength, and more of them are likely to have less endurance. In all probability, the development of strong trunk muscles, particularly the erector spinae, is useful in the treatment, rehabilitation, and prevention of low back pain. However, the clinical evidence to prove this is not as strong as we would like it to be.

Q. *Assuming that strong trunk muscles are desirable, what is the best way to strengthen them?*

A. Swimming, stationary bicycling, walking, back extension exercises, and the use of various electronic machines to increase muscle strength.

Q. *How important is it to use various exercise machines for monitoring muscle activity?*

A. The currently available evidence does not prove that they are essential. They are nice to have, and appropriately used they can make a contribution. There is also an unproven but probably psychological advantage in that the patient can "see progress." This, I believe, has motivational value to the patient.

Even though there is no hard scientific proof, the best available prevailing current opinion for the 1990s strongly suggests that exercises do help. So good luck, and get to work!

When NOT to Exercise

Don't exercise right after getting out of bed in the morning. Your discs have taken in fluid while you were lying in bed with no gravitational forces on them. Thus they are tense and more prone to irritation. Wait two hours before doing your exercises.

Don't do any exercise that causes severe pain. Whenever your back gets worse, you should decrease your activity. And don't abandon all hope: It's highly probable you'll gradually recover again without a relapse.

DEVICES FOR DAILY LIVING

Mattress Connoisseurship

The morning can be a stiff and painful time of day for the backache sufferer. So now let's talk about beds.

First, don't be hoodwinked by terms like *orthopaedic* or the root *ortho-* affixed to particular beds or mattresses. Words like *posture, medical, osteopathic, chiropractic,* and so on, while perhaps evocative of white uniforms, don't guarantee better sleep or a disease-free life, either. Your own preference is a good place to start. After all, you spend approximately a third of your life either recreating, procreating, or recuperating there, so one's free choice of a mattress ought to be a birthright.

Let's start with the simplest scenario. If you have a normal back and no acquaintance with backache, then in addition to being an unlikely reader of this tome, you should choose your mattress entirely on the basis of comfort. "Sleeping around" on different mattresses in department or furniture stores is an inevitable part of the selection process. Once you've narrowed your choice to two or three mattresses or beds, explain to the salesperson that you need to try it out for a half hour or so.

All other things being equal, a relatively firm mattress is best. And you can, of course, make up a rather firm bed by laying down a ⅜-inch (1-cm.) plywood board on some cinderblocks or a wood frame and then using a three- to six-inch piece of foam rubber as a mattress. Another alternative is to put a plywood bed board between your innerspring and your mattress.

Now, if you're a backache victim, everyone has probably told you, "Get a hard mattress, as hard as possible." That advice is basically sound. To test out how a firm mattress would treat your back, put six or eight blankets on the floor and sleep there for three to five nights. Feel better? If so, then a very firm mattress should be a good investment.

But, again, individuals are unpredictable. Some of you back-pain sufferers may not sleep comfortably on a hard mattress, and something medium or even soft may suit you better. If you do prefer a softer mattress, and the sleeping-on-the-floor test doesn't do anything for your back, by all means go with the soft mattress.

What about water beds? Trial and error is the best *modus operandi.* If you like it and it doesn't hurt your back, enjoy sleeping on the waves. You might first test one out in a motel. But I don't think there's any back magic to slumbering on H_2O.

Here's some useful specific information about beds that I'm happy to be able to pass on to you. Drs. Garfin and Pye in Southern California completed a very useful study. They compared the effects of four types of beds on patients with long-term low back pain. Allow me to present the four types of beds. Bed #1, a *hard bed* (seven hundred and twenty individually reinforced coils and built-in bed board). Bed #2, a softer bed (a five hundred-coil bed, no bed board). Bed #3, a commercially available water bed (filled to a depth of 25 cm.). Bed #4, a "hybrid" bed (a combination of foam and water). Results—the majority of patients preferred the hard bed and thought their back pain improved more after two weeks on it. The water bed came in second—the second-largest number of patients showed improvement using it.

I haven't meant to be inconsiderate of your spouse—or, as Charles Osgood so glibly puts it, "POSSLQ" (pronounced POSS EL Q" and meaning Persons of Opposite Sex Sharing Living Quarters). In any case, I'd hope that some reasonable compromise could give you both satisfactory sleeping arrangements. You probably can't expect your mate to be happy on the floor for nights on end! One possibility is to soften a very firm mattress on one side with a sponge-rubber covering. Your ingenuity may suggest others.

Corsets

Corsets have been around for centuries, mostly to accentuate the positives and eliminate the negatives in the female form, and occasionally the male. But here our topic is therapeutic corsets.

The rationale for the corset is that if the spine can be immobilized and rested, it will be irritated less and therefore hurt less, thereby unweighting your spine. I suspect, too, that there's an emotional value in making your back feel more secure and supported: If it "feels better" for your back to wear the corset, then enjoy it and don't worry about your muscles wasting away.

Next come more sophisticated spine-immobilizing devices like braces and casts, which ought to be prescribed by a physician. We'll discuss brace and cast technology in the next chapter.

A Guide to Seats

Well, you've gotten out of bed, you've dressed, with or without a corset, and now you're about to drive or ride to work. During many parts of your day you're going to be in a seat. What is the ideal seat?

That depends, in part, on what you're sitting down to do. So we'll break this down into categories. Much of the following information is based on experiments that measured intervertebral disc pressures as well as the sitters' subjective comfort ratings.

It appears that the more a seat is reclined, up to a hundred and twenty degrees, the more comfortable it is. A distinct lumbar support is better than an indistinct or absent one. Armrests decrease the forces on the low back. Plenty of space on the seat platform is desirable, because it supports the thighs and allows for comfortable shifts of position. Readers who have compared long airplane trips in first class with those in economy class will attest to this criterion.

Another factor is the position of the entire seat in relation to the floor. That is, if the angle between the seat's back and bottom is ninety degrees in the erect position, and the entire seat is tilted twenty degrees in relation to the *floor,* the forces on the spine are reduced, even though the angle between back and seat hasn't changed. This concept (shown in Figure 5–18) may seem abstract, but it can, in fact, be used by a weary driver with a multiply adjustable power seat.

Avoid low chairs.

Car Seats

Individual taste surfaces here, for we know that some people will ride in a terribly uncomfortable seat if the car satisfies the ego. But if you drive a great deal and back comfort overshadows ego gratification, select a comfortable car seat. Why not rent several cars and find one or two with comfortable seats, driving

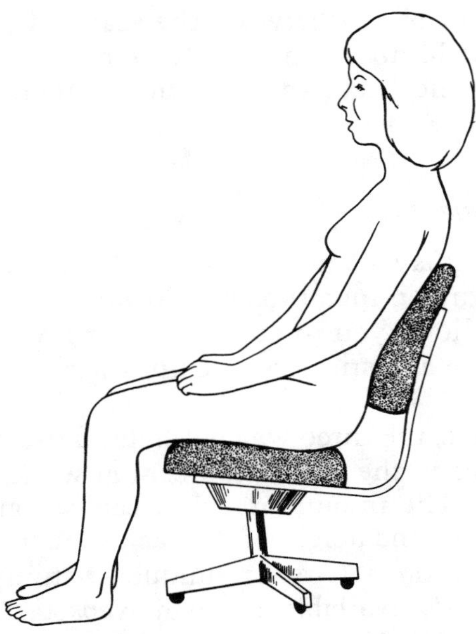

FIGURE 5–18 This shows the principle of fully tilting a chair to the horizontal to unweight the spine and relax the back muscles. By *tilting* the bottom or seat part of the chair, it is possible to decrease considerably the stresses on the spine. This type of chair can be returned to the upright position and locked for working.

them enough to be certain before you make a purchase? You can also get information from friends in your search for the "ideal seat."

It's well known that the Volvo Corporation has spent a good deal on human spine research, using the information to design its seats. And the multiply adjustable power seat system, which allows the driver more changes of position, also has its virtues.

Here are a few car-seat-enhancing tips: If there isn't an armrest on either side, improvise. A pillow will serve, either next to the door or on the middle part of the seat. Long trips make an armrest particularly desirable. If you're driving, relax your arms by hanging them steadily on the steering wheel, which unweights the spine and relaxes the shoulders. Recline in the seat as much as you can and still see the road; you may want to alternate this position with one in which the seat is more erect and pulled close to the steering wheel. You can use a towel, small blanket, or pillow between the seat and your lower back for that crucial lumbar support. Remember to place it at the curved part of the back, the way the secretaries' seat fits in Figure 5–1.

Seat Accoutrements

A few devices may come in handy. An air pillow, a small eighteen-by-eighteen-inch rubber pillow with a detachable hand bulb inflator, allows you to pump up your low-back support to the desired bulge and stiffness. It comes with straps that attach to any car seat.

Another device, the three-way portable adjustable orthopaedic seat, can be used in the car, at home, or at work. It boasts some real advantages: The amount of recline can be controlled, as well as the prominence and height of the back support. Therefore, the seat can be fashioned to your unique anatomy and comfort requirements. (It's available through *Nepsco, Inc., 53 Jeffery Avenue, Holliston, Massachusetts 01746,* for about seventy dollars.)

Let's mention a few more car-seat helpers. One is a seat-within-a-seat, usually just a bottom and a back, either or both of which may have cushioned wire coils or springs. There are also wedges that fit right into the angle where the seat back meets the base in an attempt to offer lumbar support. But these tend to be too low. Such devices can be found at a large auto-supply or "truck stop" store. But try the towel or pillow trick first. If it helps, go to an air pillow or an adjustable orthopaedic seat.

Seats and Standing Desks at Work

Now that you've made it to work, you'll probably have to spend several hours on your derriere—which puts more force on your spine than standing does. If you enjoy the luxury of an executive chair, have it fit the criteria of the ideal seat. Consider having all the seats under your domain come as close as possible to the ideal traits while remaining functional. While you're at it, why not arrange for all the future seats purchased by the company to pamper your employees' backs?

Secretarial seats with lumbar supports, armrests, and a reclining option are available. In some cases, of course, armrests aren't practical. Draftsmen and other desk workers can have appropriately designed chairs that don't interfere with their work. Improvisation can improve your work seat, as it did your car seat, if this year's budget doesn't allow for buying more chairs.

For several years patients have asked me about furniture that substitutes as a chair in which people can kneel and work, read, etc. The weight is carried partially by the rump, but a significant portion of it is carried by the shins and lower leg. Well, happily, now I can give an answer. Balans chairs (Figure 5–19), as they are called, were studied and found to be less comfortable than more conventional chairs and using them caused increased muscle activity in the neck and back. This implies more stress or strain occurs in the position in which this device is used. Nevertheless, some patients like them. My advice is if you like it and are comfortable in it, use it. However, there is no evidence that it's

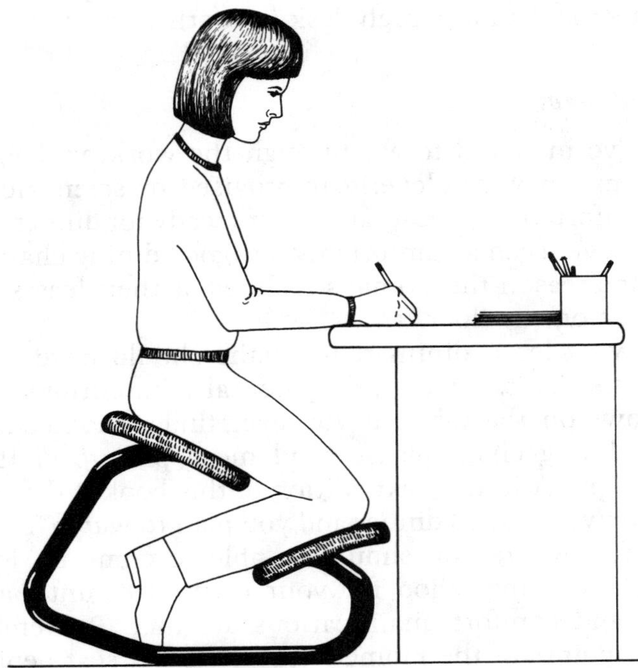

FIGURE 5–19 This is the Balans "chair." Weight is carried on the rump and the shins. While these are marketed as "more comfortable" chairs, clinical studies suggest that they are not. However, if you try it and like it—that's all that matters.

going to be helpful or therapeutic for a bad back. The price of a Balans chair ranges from two hundred to over three hundred dollars.

Don't forget that just about everything you can do sitting can also be done standing up. It may be worth it to build waist- or chest-high platforms (with bar rails) as alternative workbenches. It isn't written in stone that a typewriter won't work if its operator is on his/her feet. You can even read—this book, for instance—standing at a high desk. In fact, I've found a number of my patients who would usually be doing a great deal of sitting have been helped tremendously by standing desks, and I think it's a very important point to consider. Depending on your individual preference and comfort, a standing desk will be the height of your waist, at minimum, and your nipples, at maximum. It should incline up and away from you. (If you're unable to locate one, or have one built, try contacting *Peabody Office Furniture Corp., 234 Congress St., Boston.*) A high stool with a back and a foot rail at a high desk is another option.

Home and Hearth

Now you've managed to get through the working day; you've driven home in your cleverly improvised or scientifically designed comfortable car seat; and you're ready for dinner. Unhappily, I've never seen a comfortably designed dining chair, which may be one reason the Romans reclined at their feasts and the Japanese sit on the floor.

At the very least, dining-table chairs should have armrests, and if yours don't, forget early parental admonitions and rest your elbows on the table. If you ever find a biomechanically designed dining chair, please send me a picture of it, and I promise to put it in the next edition of this book if there is one.

Now you've finished dinner and you plan to watch TV or read a bit. Here's where you should be able to come up with the perfect seat. Simply shop for your own "10" until all your aesthetic and comfort qualifications are met. Remember the four basic points of the biomechanically ideal seat depicted in Figure 5–20. Take seriously the careful search for a truly comfortable chair that has the biomechanical characteristics described here for you. This can be an important lifetime investment of time and money.

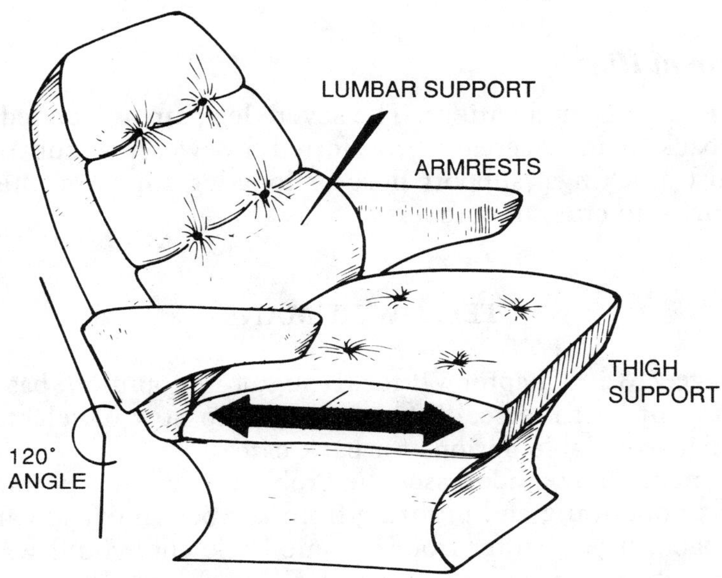

FIGURE 5–20 This figure depicts the important elements of the biomechanically ideal seat, your ideal chair for maximum low back comfort. Features include (1) significant lumbar support, (2) the ability to recline at least a hundred and twenty degrees, (3) armrests, (4) ample thigh support and room to change position. As long as you have these four basic elements, you can do anything you like with design, upholstery, and the like, and have the best seat for relaxing your back. (Reproduced with permission from White, A.A., and Panjabi, M.M.: *Clinical Biomechanics of the Spine,* J.B. Lippincott, 1990, second edition.)

Vibrating Chairs, Beds, Massagers

Massagers, which come with some mattresses and reclining chairs, can certainly soothe the back and relax tense muscles. A simple hand-held vibrator—its honeymoon-catalog aura aside—can also ease the painful parts of your back. The cheapest one that is safe and feels good is probably the best buy. Though these devices, of course, don't cure any basic problem, they can put you in a relaxed state, the virtues of which are laid out in Chapter IV. Whether the laying on of human hands or the application of an electrical masseur works best is purely a matter of individual taste and availability.

A Helpful Hint

This is a tip from a patient. The severe leg pain associated with low back pain is greatly comforted by wearing substantial support stockings (support hose or long-leg supports). Just for comfort—no cure, of course.

FELLOW HUMANS

See page 213 in Chapter VII for listing of my opinion, based on the current best medical information, as to how to select from the major available options for back care.

Our next chapter addresses the Problem Back. It is a practical guide to obtaining and profiting from the best medical care for your back. If you suffer from chronic backache, you'll want to turn the page for an inventory of all nonsurgical treatments, from acupuncture and spinal manipulation to traction and trigger point injections.

Reflecting on the references to "epidemics" in Chapter I and home remedies in this chapter, it seems to me I have painted a pretty dismal picture of everything you must do to avoid backache. It goes something like this: Don't work too much; don't sit too much; don't make love too much. Don't lift too much; don't drive too much; don't smoke; don't play golf. Don't get promoted or divorced; redesign all your furniture; don't put on weight; and, of course, don't "stress yourself."

In real life, though, just two or three minor adjustments, like a new mattress, a moderate exercise program, and breaking up long car trips, may do wonders in keeping your backache at bay. Now, if you *don't* have chronic or intractable pain, this is the ideal time to save your back. I believe that this chapter should be read and reread from time to time until it becomes second nature to you. Also, remember that most people get rid of their back pain in two to three weeks. May the Force be with you!

Chapter VI

The Problem Back

Nonsurgical Treatments

BACKACHE, ESPECIALLY the chronic or recurrent kind, isn't an easy companion to live with. Back care is a field full of confusion, contradictory opinions, unanswered questions, myriad therapies—orthodox and not-so-orthodox—and, yes, some dubious practitioners. (Figure 6–1.) Is it any wonder that you sometimes feel like a wanderer in a medical and quasi-medical labyrinth? Alas, there *are* no foolproof cures. When we fully understand spine disease, we'll let you know. However, we *do know* that if you follow the guidelines presented for you here and you do your best to be patient, you will gradually improve.

What this book can do for you, is to serve as a survival manual. We'll guide you through the intricacies of doctors' offices—and acupuncture clinics. Not all back care is administered by M.D.'s. This chapter will acquaint you with just about all the known nonsurgical back treatments, noting everything we presently know about their value or lack of it. It will help you pick your way through the B.S.

When to Get Help

In the last chapter we told you how to treat your backache at home. But sometimes you should take your back to a good doctor. Here is a list, in order of urgency, of all the circumstances that warrant medical intervention.

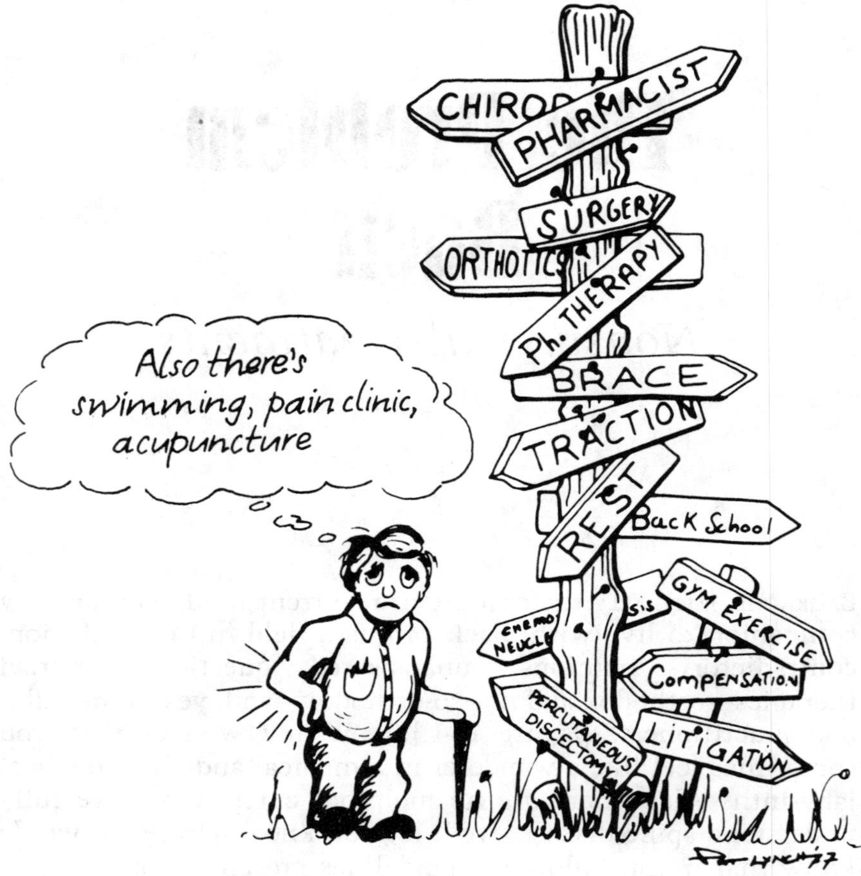

FIGURE 6–1 Dear Reader, I know some of you must feel like the fellow in the cartoon. He obviously doesn't think his situation so funny, and you may not either. There are lots of options for treating your back and it's normal to be a bit confused at some point. We recognize that there are plenty of directions you can take. We've provided information here and in the next chapter to help you in deciding which road is *best for you.* (Reproduced with permission from White, A.A., and Panjabi, M.M.: *Clinical Biomechanics of the Spine,* J.B. Lippincott, 1990, second edition.)

CHECKLIST FOR WHEN TO CALL THE DOCTOR

1. You are having trouble urinating, especially getting the stream flowing.
2. You have weakness in one or both legs that is getting worse.

3. Your severe back pain is preceded or accompanied by involuntary weight loss or pain elsewhere in the body.
4. Your severe back and leg pain is accompanied by a fever that isn't an obvious cold.
5. Your pain is very intense and getting worse no matter what you do.
6. You've got backache and/or leg pain associated with pain or swelling in other joints: fingers, wrists, elbows, hips, knees, or ankles, for instance.
7. You've had moderately severe back pain for an extended period (three to four weeks). Or you've had several episodes of severe backache and want to find out what's going on.
8. Your back and/or leg pain is constant, severe, and doesn't improve with three to five days' bed rest, and two or three weeks of home and/or self care.
9. You've done the best you can and you just can't stand it anymore.

These are all excellent reasons to see a doctor. I suggest you consult a good general practitioner, board-certified family practitioner, internist, rheumatologist, orthopaedic surgeon, or neurosurgeon. On page 184, I've provided some tips intended to help you select the best doctor for your back.

Most backaches can be well managed by your primary-care physician; however, there may be situations in which you want to see a specialist even though surgery may *not* be in the offing. This is the case when there's long-term back pain without sciatica or neurological problems, such as weakness or numbness.

Getting Along With Your Doctor

This book is intended as a handbook of practical survival, as well as a reliable source of information. So we must point out some of the pitfalls in your path, one of which is possible prejudice on the part of fellow humans. If you happen to be African-American, female, obviously poor, Jewish, Catholic, Irish, Italian, Chicano, or whatever, you may be treated prejudicially. We in the medical profession would like to think that all of us are without prejudice, but unfortunately, that just is not the case. If a doctor or some other professional treats you disdainfully for no reason, be suspicious. Consider changing doctors.

Ask around; find a doctor who has taken good care of a friend or a member of your own family. If you have a friend with a good doctor, let your friend tell his doctor about you and your problem. Then tell the doctor that you sought him/her out because of a friend's recommendation. He/she will appreciate the compliment.

Medical schools teach us to "humanize" our patients. This is important. What it means is that in addition to evaluating and treating a patient we must somehow communicate with him/her as a human being. There are infinite possibilities: How's your golf? Your wife? Your kids? Did you see the game last night? Let me suggest that you the patient also humanize your doctor.

Working With Your Doctor

You've found a doctor you like. How do you get the most out of your relationship with him/her? The trick is *not* to take the attitude that says, "Okay, I hurt; now, I'll bet you can't make me stop hurting." The trick is to take the attitude that says, "I have this disease—Doc, let's you and I work together to lick it." If you and your doctor can develop that type of relationship, you're way ahead of the game!

First, ask enough questions to satisfy yourself that you understand what your back is doing. Hearing the doctor intone the diagnosis is great, but make sure you *understand* it, too. How serious is it? What is the prognosis? Remember that many back conditions don't have a precise diagnosis. That's okay, provided your doctor has noted your history and thoroughly examined you. You should be examined for tumors, infections, and any other specific, treatable disease such as ankylosing spondylitis, which requires special management. Ask whether other tests are necessary either to confirm the diagnosis or to search further for causes.

Once you grasp the diagnosis and the ins and outs of the disease process, you and your doctor can confer about your treatment. Ask for the rationale, benefits, and risks of a recommended treatment. You should know both its pitfalls and its prospects for success.

If everything makes sense to you, follow your doctor's pro-

gram conscientiously. I italicize the advice because the treatment can't work if you don't do it. You'll never know if it *could* have worked if you don't give it an honest try. This is referred to as "patient compliance," and *your* compliance in the care of *your* back is essential for a successful outcome. When you go back to your doctor and he assumes you've tried Treatment A, and it didn't work, he'll suggest Treatment B. Generally, as you progress from A to B to C, the risks, as well as the possible benefits, escalate. This rule is almost as inevitable as the investment "laws" dictating that risks increase in proportion to profits. If you bury your money under the mattress, you probably won't lose it, but you won't earn any interest, either. If, on the other hand, you put it into venture capital, you may get a twenty, thirty, or fifty percent return, but you risk losing your entire "bundle."

If what your doctor is telling you does not make sense and he/she is unable or unwilling to explain things so that they do make sense, then you deserve at least another opinion, if not another doctor. You are an important human being with an important problem. You deserve to know and you deserve to understand.

Listen to Your Body

Seeing a doctor doesn't absolve you of responsibility; you're still your own best physician, in that only you dwell inside *your* body.

Pay attention to what circumstances and activities seem to provoke back pain. You can do this in your head; if you're either compulsive or forgetful, jot down your observations in a little notebook. Do stress, changes in the weather, certain sports, certain chairs/beds/cars, some sexual positions, airplane trips, a hobby or work activity seem to trigger a backache? Next ask yourself what makes your back feel better. Some of the preceding activities might end up on the *good* list. What about aspirin, a glass of wine or a cocktail, or a certain sport like swimming? This information will help you avoid pain and enjoy comfort. When you turn up distinct trends or correlations, tell your doctor; they could help determine your diagnosis as well as influence treatment.

Use your own mind, psyche, ego, faith, intellect, will, or whatever you call the spirit inside you. If you've mastered Chapter IV, you know that a positive attitude is a potent force in your treatment program. Something you already possess—a philosophy of life or health, a religious or secular commitment—or something new can help sustain you. Perhaps it's some form of autopsychology, the "relaxation response," biofeedback, meditation, self-hypnosis, or anything else that bolsters your will to recover. Maybe your doctor, minister, friends, or family can be of help. Utilize all the resources that are available to you. Take control of your backache situation.

The Placebo and the Natural Course of the Disease

Let's revisit our old friend the placebo. We've already introduced you to the placebo response, but further acquaintance seems fitting here.

There's a copious list of backache treatments, generating two chapters, one for nonsurgical and another for surgical procedures. Why? Because fifty to seventy percent of adults at some time in their lives will suffer an attack of low back pain. A rarer disease generates fewer opportunities to try out different treatments, and still fewer opportunities for them to catch on.

A major factor in any treatment's success is the placebo phenomenon, which is really built into the human psyche. When you're treated for any painful disease, a successful outcome boils down to changing your behavior from an "I hurt" mode to "I feel better; I no longer hurt." A worthless sugar pill touted as an effective medication will switch one out of every three people from "I hurt" to "I'm better." All in their minds? Not exactly. There are situations in which real, measurable changes have followed placebo treatment.

What does all this have to do with the treatment of backache? First, when we talk about any treatment's success rate, bear in mind that thirty-three percent of patients can be cured by *belief* in the treatment alone, the placebo effect. Furthermore, when it comes to backache, recall that by waiting and doing nothing, seventy percent of you will be well in three weeks, ninety percent in two months. That's written into the natural course of the disease. Now we begin to understand that any treatment, whether traditional or exotic, acclaimed for healing seventy percent of all seekers isn't necessarily the greatest boon to mankind. When we factor in the placebo effect and nature's own healing hand, the proportion of success directly attributable to the treatment drops dramatically. This is not to deprecate the placebo effect. In fact, as we discuss specific treatments, we'll applaud the harnessing of your own faith and self-healing powers. Moreover, placebo treatment may also induce the body to secrete its own morphinelike drug, endorphins.

The Parable of Frog Surgery

There's a familiar tale in medical circles about placebo surgery.

Once upon a time, a patient complained of severe stomach pain, which he described as though it were "a frog jumping around there." Every possible test—X rays, a barium enema, gallbladder studies, and numerous lab tests—turned up nothing. The patient consulted a psychiatrist, who listened carefully to the description of the ailment and concluded that the patient was emotionally disturbed. Yet months of intense psychotherapy didn't alter the man's complaint.

In desperation, the man's physicians, psychiatrists, and surgeons, after long and intensive discussion, finally decided to relieve him of his suffering with placebo surgery. They made an incision, opened the patient up, sewed him up again, and reported they'd found a large frog in his stomach. They even produced a frog they'd preserved in a jar of formaldehyde. After a few days, the once-frog-plagued patient was pain-free and living a normal life.

After several weeks, however, the man felt fresh discomfort in his stomach, and its nature was such as to convince him it was exactly the same pain. When he consulted his doctors, they pointed out they had already removed the frog from his stomach. The patient was pensive for a moment. Then he said, "I think I know what happened, gentlemen. You've done an excellent job of removing the frog. But it's clear that you left the eggs behind and now there's another frog."

This story points to some of the vicissitudes of the mind and the pitfalls of placebo treatments.

A COMPLETE LIST OF NONSURGICAL BACK TREATMENTS

Now back to where we left off in Chapter V, which focused on the "do it yourself" mode of treatment. Some of this section will also be "do it yourself," but much of the treatment here is for the longer-term back problem and is likely to be utilized by a physician or therapist, since in this chapter I focus on chronic, severe backache. Many of Chapter V's lessons will also apply to those of you who have been seeing a doctor longer and are contemplating some more sophisticated remedies. So bear with a bit of recapitulation.

Bed Rest and Painkillers

Bed rest minimizes the mechanical irritation of your spine and reduces local inflammation. Since local inflammation in the back's anatomic structures—like the facet joints and surrounding nerves—probably produces much of your back pain, resting in the proper position (see Chapter V) allows nature to heal most patients in two or three weeks, even though I recommend that you limit your actual bed rest to two or three days.

We also told you of the wonders of good old aspirin and itemized a few other drugs, both prescription and nonprescription, that may be useful. But what if your backache is really excruciating and the remedies have not worked?

When your pain is very severe and unrelieved by two aspirin every four hours, your physician may sometimes prescribe a narcotic analgesic. Usually this means codeine or Demerol, in addition to an anti-inflammatory drug. Narcotics can relieve the agony of the acute phase but shouldn't be relied upon for long-term treatment. They're addictive and you soon build up a tolerance to them. The exception to the rule is a very serious, specifically diagnosed chronic pain problem, such as inoperable cancer.

What about muscle relaxants? Usually your muscle spasm will subside on its own as the pain and inflammation wane. I repeat that I'm not an enthusiast of these drugs, which alter your central nervous system and mental processes and have not been proven to specifically relax muscles. However, on the rare occasion when a severe muscle spasm is unresponsive to rest or anti-inflammatory and other drugs, I sometimes prescribe cyclobenzaprine (Flexeril) or diazepam (Valium). As with anything else, I try to use the lowest effective dosage, prescribing medication at the earliest possible time in my patient's best interest.

Heat and Massage

We talked about the soothing virtues of these age-old remedies in Chapter V. Their success rate is on a par with other nonsurgical treatments and, delightfully, it's very hard to harm yourself with either. Skin burns can occur in connection with heat application. Massage poses occasional social complications. But otherwise, I'd say massage and heat application constitute a riskless therapy that satisfies the patient's need to be treated. Who can argue against something that can make people feel better, even though it may contain no special elixir?

Braces

In the last chapter we said that a corset can serve as a stand-in for firm abdominal muscles. The next, more sophisticated level of abdominal support is the lumbar or lumbosacral brace. It extends from the pelvis up to the middle of the rib cage. These braces come with a variety of rigid components running down and across the body. Several common back braces are shown in Figure 6–2. Some actually go down to the trochanter, the prominent bone on the side of the hip. Being held in a tight clasp, the wearer is reminded to restrain his motion.

Why a brace? Besides giving abdominal support, the brace, with its rigid parts, further immobilizes the spine. But by supporting the trunk muscles, some studies suggest, the brace may usurp their functions, leaving them to fade away, as inactive muscles are wont to do. Paradoxically, another experiment showed that when a patient walks in a rigid spinal brace his erector spinae muscles are actually *more* active (as measured by their electrical response).

If you decide that maximum bracing is the treatment for you, two specific braces represent the optimum state of the art, the Boston Brace and the Raney Flexion Jacket. Both are rigorously

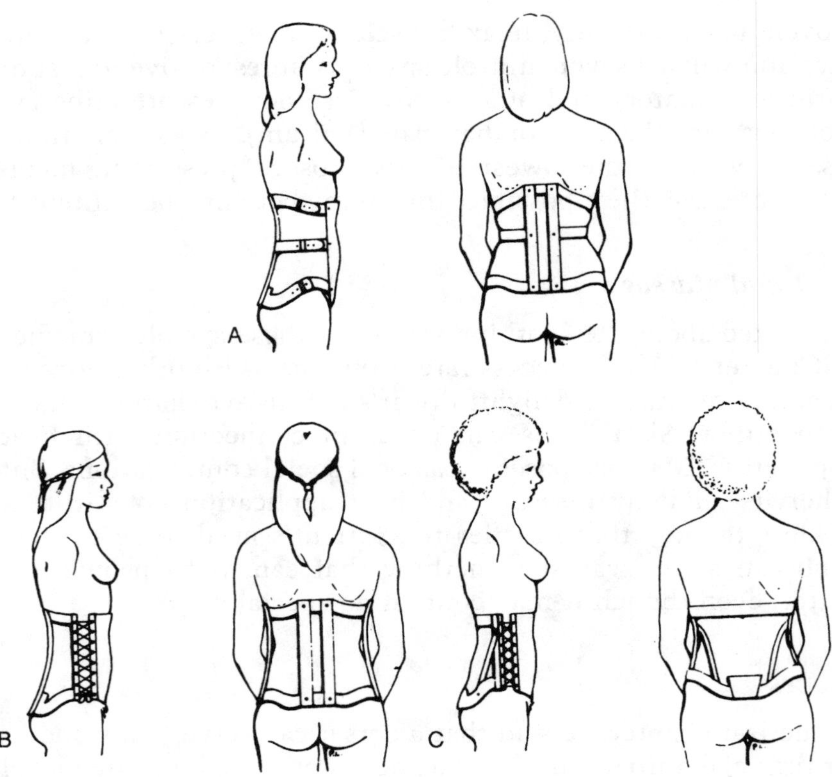

FIGURE 6–2 Here are several braces that you may consider for low back pain. All of them can be effective. Several others are described in the text. A) is the Mac Ausland or chairback brace, B) is the Knight brace, and C) is the Williams brace. Note that all three of these have a good abdominal support. This is a key factor in their efficacy. (Reproduced with permission from White, A.A., and Panjabi, M.M.: *Clinical Biomechanics of the Spine,* J.B. Lippincott, 1990, second edition.)

designed for effective abdominal compression and for a slightly flexed lumbar spine. Lumbar flexion decreases the backward bulging of the disc and reduces some of the forces on the lumbar spine's posterior elements. But these braces are not cheap. And like drugs and surgery, they should be prescribed only after a thorough clinical exam and an adequate trial of less expensive therapy.

Plaster Casts

The plaster cast differs from corsets and braces only in its greater rigidity. It can be made to fit your individual contours as well as the average brace, but, of course, you don't have the option of conveniently taking it off. Because a cast is temporary and cheaper than any other bracing device, it's often used on a trial basis to predict how you'd fare with a brace. It can also test to some extent the efficacy of a proposed spinal fusion.

Though no definitive clinical studies have tested corsets, braces, and casts, there's no question they sometimes make patients feel better and are reasonable alternatives to more drastic therapies. Their risks come mainly in the form of nuisances. Braces may irritate the skin or bony prominences or make your back more painful. More ominously, a too-tight cast, or even a slightly snug one, can occasionally result in "cast syndrome." This is a serious problem that results in vomiting and/or severe abdominal pain as one of your major abdominal arteries squeezes against the upper intestines. If you come down with these symptoms, see a doctor immediately to head off major gastrointestinal upset or disease.

Traction

In a nutshell, traction pulls the upper and lower parts of your body in opposite directions to ease your low back and/or leg pain. It can be done either continuously for several hours, or intermittently—pull, release, pull—for seconds or minutes. There have been several clinical studies on various traction techniques. Sorry, folks, but the results indicate that traction really doesn't seem to work. So let's move on.

Spinal Manipulation

Yeah, I know you've been waiting to hear what I have to say about chiropractors. Well, here it is. What I am going to say about chiropractors is very little. This book is about low back pain, how to treat it, how to survive it and live with it, not about political, socioeconomic, or other aspects of various forms of practitioners in this world. I have already emphasized for you the medical implications of backache, have given you my best opinions as to how you ought to behave vis-à-vis when and how and what type of medical attention to seek for your backache. So. Let's go ahead to the issue of spinal-manipulative therapy. I suspect that even this disclaimer won't defuse controversy or misunderstanding, and no doubt chiropractic critics and devotees alike will be pleased and offended in turn by what I write here. My goal is simply to present the facts as objectively as possible and let you form your own conclusions.

Whole books have been devoted to the numerous, complex maneuvers involved in spinal manipulation (see Bibliography). Yet, whatever external technique is applied, the possible movements of the vertebrae themselves are limited by nature. You can carry out whatever bodily contortion you like, but your vertebrae can move only in certain possible ways. All of the possible movements are indicated by the arrows provided in Figure 6–3.

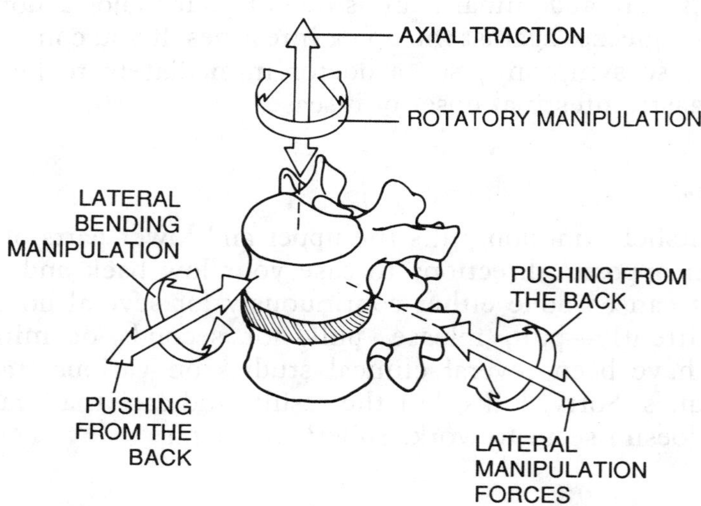

FIGURE 6–3 This is to show all the possible ways that we can cause a vertebra in the spine to move. These various movements can be achieved through spinal manipulation, traction, or exercise. No matter what you do to the spine, here are all the motions you can possibly achieve. (Reproduced with permission from White, A.A., and Panjabi, M.M.: *Clinical Biomechanics of the Spine,* J.B. Lippincott, 1990, second edition.)

Now let's try to be a little more scientific and objective. In 1975 the National Institute of Neurological Diseases and Stroke (one of the National Institutes of Health) sponsored a workshop on the "Research Status of Spinal-Manipulative Therapy." (See Bibliography.) Here is a quotation from the summary of that workshop, which drew a number of osteopaths, physicians, chiropractors, and scientists.

> The concept of chiropractic subluxation [that is, nonobservable partial dislocation in the normal position of two adjacent vertebrae] remains a hypothesis yet to be evaluated experimentally. We believe this has been one of the frustrating aspects . . . When one is correcting a "subluxation" that cannot be perceived by independent scientific observers, it is difficult to convince those observers that the treatment is effective . . .

In other words, the question of spinal manipulation's efficacy remains in limbo, since independent clinical and scientific observers remain skeptical of its unverified premises. Yet spinal manipulation is one of the most popular backache treatment methods, and it deserves a detailed, fair look here.

It's cogent to bring to your attention another document, in case you'd like to study this topic in more depth. The publication is "Position Paper on Chiropractic"; the full reference is in the Bibliography. It contains an updated, thoughtful, and comprehensive review of manipulative therapy and its individual as well as societal implications.

Common Manipulation Techniques. Since manipulation techniques would fill a large tome, we'll confine ourselves to the best-known ones. The simplest manipulation consists of pressure applied directly to the spinous processes of a given vertebra. This can be done by pressing a finger into the vertebra or with the palm or the ball of the hand. There is also a limited maneuver that can be performed on the front of the neck or, in a very relaxed patient, on the front part of the lumbar spine. Again, the finger is usually supplanted by another part of the hand. Most manipulations are done *indirectly,* by twisting the head, shoulders, and hips, displacing the spine with a twisting motion, as shown in Figure 6–4. A more direct manipulation is shown in Figure 6–5.

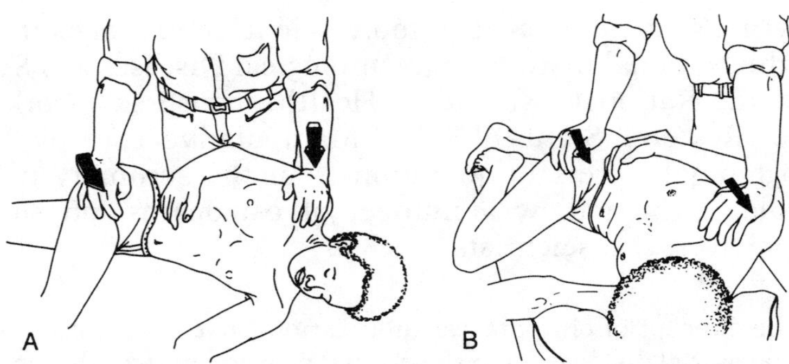

FIGURE 6–4 This particular technique of spinal manipulation is probably the one most often employed by medical scientists. A) This shows the technique from the frontal view. The major force is from the therapist pushing the pelvis forward with his right hand, while with the left hand there is a moderate thrust in the opposite direction. B) This is an axial view, which shows how the two motions impart an element of twist to the lower portion of the spine. (Reproduced with permission from White, A.A., and Panjabi, M.M.: *Clinical Biomechanics of the Spine,* J.B. Lippincott, 1990, second edition.)

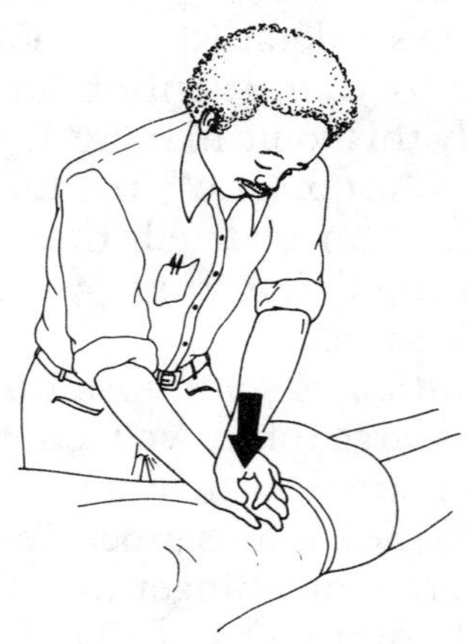

FIGURE 6–5 This is a simple direct thrust to the spine transmitted through the heel of the hand. These maneuvers must be done with care, as they can be irritating. (Reproduced with permission from White, A.A., and Panjabi, M.M.: *Clinical Biomechanics of the Spine,* J.B. Lippincott, 1990, second edition.)

Does It Work? Manipulation applies certain forces and movements to the spine. Within tolerable limits, these forces and motions are considered helpful. When tolerance limits are exceeded, spinal structures run the risk of damage. Our extensive, ever-growing knowledge of spine mechanics allows us to predict what changes spinal manipulations can effect. The theory that these forces relieve nerve pressure isn't compatible with our current information. Nothing suggests that manipulating a motion segment can move structures significantly into or out of the intervertebral foramen. This is the canal through which the nerve root passes as it leaves the spinal cord to go ultimately to the skin or muscle. (See "nerve root" Figure 2–6B, page 38.) The fairest summation is that at present there's no compelling theory to explain the mechanism whereby spinal-manipulative therapy relieves pain, if it does.

Is it helpful, then?

First, let's address the treatment of visceral disease, all diseases other than back pain. Starkly put, there's no clinical or scientific evidence to suggest that manipulation can help cure systemic diseases such as diabetes, ulcers, hypertension, and so on. Anyone who knowingly or unknowingly attempts to treat such diseases with manipulation renders a great disservice to his fellow humans.

On the other hand, myriad studies have examined the use of spinal manipulation on back pain patients, with and without leg pain or neurological problems. The messages from the more recent studies are as follows: There is a brief improvement and transient reduction of pain for patients who have back pain of short duration, say less than three months. If you have leg pain, numbness, or weakness, or long-standing back pain (more than three months), you're unlikely to get the transient pain reduction. The pain reduction may last for several hours or up to two days.

The Dangers of Spinal Manipulations. The greatest harm comes from inappropriately treating an infected or cancerous spine—or another disease, like diabetes—with spinal manipulation. Consequences are tragic when the disease could have been cured or controlled by a mainstream medical method.

Is manipulation itself risky? Sometimes. One publication reported four cases of patients who were paralyzed in the legs or developed other major neurological problems after a trip to the chiropractor. Whenever jostling the spine, disc, and nerves makes your condition worse, it doesn't matter who does the jostling. Other documented, though rare, dangers include manipulation-induced herniated discs and fatal brain hemorrhages, spinal cord injuries, and nonfatal bleeding caused by neck manipulation.

Conclusion. Recall that to be outstanding, a treatment must outperform the placebo effect of thirty-three percent success, plus nature's own healing rate of sixty to seventy percent. Spinal manipulation, then, comes out about even with other nonsurgical treatments, but its *subjective* results run a little higher. As a bottom line, consider spinal manipulation a justified alternative, provided you've been appropriately evaluated by a medical doctor and the manipulation isn't too vigorous. Prolonged, repeated, expensive manipulations that bring only transient improvement aren't the best use of your resources. The good news is that research now in progress in the United States and Sweden may soon give us more definitive answers about spinal-manipulative therapy.

The advice I give my patients is as follows: If you don't get distinct, lasting relief after several manipulations, don't continue them. If a patient has disc disease I advise him *not* to have spinal manipulation, because in my opinion there is a risk of potentially serious neurological complication.

Exercises

Exercise belongs to the pantheon of desirable states, alongside motherhood, peace, health, and love. Furthermore, it's a bona fide back-care therapy you shouldn't scorn. Even though exercises have been covered extensively in the preceding chapter, it seems worthwhile to return to the topic briefly here, from a slightly different perspective. Here we'll divide exercises into three categories: William's exercises, miscellaneous exercises, and truncal exercises.

William's Exercises. These exercises are mentioned briefly, mainly for historic interest. Their goal is to strengthen certain muscles and stretch certain ligaments in order to switch the spine's alignment from a swayback (lordotic) position to a straightened one. The assumption is that the straighter the spine, the healthier and more comfortable it is. Our theoretical knowledge lends some weight to this notion. A straighter position distributes the forces more evenly, reduces pressure on the sensitive facet joints, and discourages the backward bulging of the disc.

However, I have a real problem with the classic William's exercises. They're certainly not the best prescription for anyone with acute spine problems. The sit-up exercises, especially, are prone to irritate your intervertebral disc in the early stages of back disease, since the forces generated are equal to those caused by improperly lifting forty-four pounds. Would we ask someone with fresh, severe backache and sciatica to improperly tote around forty-four-pound weights?

Miscellaneous Exercises. Generally, these are exercises to strengthen the trunk muscles. They include back extension exercises, partial sit-ups, and range-of-motion exercises such as general bending, extension, sideways bending and maximum twisting motions, and general calisthenics. Improvement runs in the range of sixty to seventy percent. Complications are minimal, but some risks are incurred by back-arching and axial torque (twisting the shoulders from side to side with the hips fairly stationary). Toe-touching exercises can also irritate your back and cause leg pain, especially if you have sciatica.

When your back can tolerate it, good tone in the trunk muscles and those around the spine is a healthy goal. But these exercises should be reserved for your getting-better days, not for acute backache. Most important, avoid sit-ups with the legs straight if you have low back pain. Refer to Chapter V for a refresher.

Isometric Truncal Exercises. Remember how we compared developed abdominal muscles to an inflated football? The idea of isometric abdominal exercises is to compress your abdominal contents by tightening up your throat, holding your rectum tight, and pushing hard, as though straining at the stool. Do this at least ten or fifteen times, holding each contraction for about three seconds, three or four times a day. The result? Tightened abdominal and trunk muscles. Studies show that the pressure generated by compressing the fluid and air in the trunk adds considerable support to your spine, protecting it from forces imposed on it.

Any risks? If you have acute disc disease, these exercises can irritate the nerve roots. Avoid them, also, if you have either heart disease or a hernia; they can put too much pressure on your heart, interfering with its circulation, or enlarge a hernia. Otherwise, their great advantage is that you can perform them discreetly in the office, car, theater, or wherever, without equipment.

The McKenzie Program. In this exercise program, a patient, under the therapist's guidance, is put through various movements. These include flexion, extension, lateral bending, and rotation. Notations are made on which of these movements best "centralize" the patient's symptoms. During "centralizing," pain initially in the back, hip, leg, and foot gradually localizes to the back and hip. The patient is then advised to repeat the movement that has centralized the pain, and to do other exercises as well. Initial studies give this a favorable evaluation; however, more experience is needed to be certain of the therapeutic value of this program. The concept of "centralizing" pain is strictly theoretical and to my knowledge is without scientific basis. In its favor—it does no harm!

The Back School

The basic back-pain school was developed in Sweden by a physical therapist named Maryanne Zachrisson-Forssell, who assembled the best available knowledge into a packaged lecture-and-slide program. Since then the back school has been adopted and modified in many places. Most cities in North America have a back school of some type.

At Boston's Beth Israel Hospital we've supplemented the basic program with additional advice based on our own experience. The course comprises four one-hour sessions and relies on discussion and question-and-answer sessions between students and teachers, an orthopedist, and a physical therapist.

Beginning with a primer on back anatomy and the basic functions of the spine, drawn from recent research, we move on to more detailed biomechanics lessons and an enumeration of various back problems and their causes. What follows are a range of lessons, from isometric abdominal exercises to the translation of back-care tips into the common activities of daily life in home, office, factory, and playing field.

This is how one particular school works, but it's not unlike others around the world. The YMCA, for instance, runs a back-care class at various of its worldwide centers. Besides practical advice, the back school offers a kind of group therapy—the exchange of experiences, advice, and emotional support that may be a real solace to many a frustrated patient.

As a treatment mode, the back school has been proven superior to the placebo effect—and even to physical therapy. Volvo employees at a Swedish back school, observed in a controlled industrial study, returned to work sooner and reported sick less often than patients treated with physical therapy. Back schools have been effective in reducing medical expenses and industrial-disability claims. Moreover, function has been increased and recurrence decreased. But along with this upbeat information, there is the sobering fact that back school doesn't work for everyone. Those who happen to be drug-dependent or suffering from constant pain may not benefit. Also, one must understand what's being taught in the back school in order to reap the benefits.

Nonetheless, in case you haven't already detected, I'm a back-school advocate. Not only is it more cost-effective than most conservative therapies, it's complication-free. And it can head off more expensive treatment, like hospitalization and surgery, down the road. It's also a productive way to share information in an ambience of professional expertise and human understanding. In the ideal world there's a back-school program for the chronic as well as the acute pain sufferer, and there's a follow-up refresher "session" after several months for all students.

The following table is provided as a representative outline of a back school course.

I Anatomy
Function of spine
Cause of back pain
Who gets it
Treatment results

II Biomechanics of the spine
Effects of activities on disc pressure
Importance of controlling loads on low back

III Ergonomics (how to use your back safely)
Individual advice about work and recreational activities
Teaching back exercises

IV Review and summary
Instilling self-confidence
Encouraging: sports, activity, ingenuity, common sense, and having fun

Work Hardening, Functional Intervention Programs, and Pain Clinics

In the work-hardening programs, there is intensive physical training to improve strength and endurance. The patient/worker is also rehabilitated and reeducated to be able to perform tasks that are the same as and/or similar to his/her actual work. Specific advice as to how to best use the body in these tasks is provided.

The functional training is somewhat similar. The patient is reeducated and taught exercises, activities, and postures that will allow him/her to return to work. There is a rigorous selection process that eliminates all but the well-motivated and psychologically able. Group dynamics are involved to facilitate and sustain progress. We talk about "Low Back School"; some of these programs may be considered "Low Back Boot Camp": The strong survive and become successful combat personnel in the workplace. In a well-controlled clinical study, this type of program has been shown to be effective.

Pain clinics are designed primarily to teach the patient coping mechanisms for dealing with his/her pain. The cause of the pain, although it may be known, is not specifically treated.

CONSERVATIVE TREATMENT: PASSIVE AND INVASIVE

To complete our nonsurgical-treatment list we need to consider those approaches that "invade" the body in some way. Don't be put off by the word invasive; most of the following treatments are actually pretty mild. The needles used in acupuncture, for example, hurt no more than a pinprick and pose no danger. I should point out that invasive procedures used repeatedly and without proper indications may foster patient dependency and tend to prolong the pain. This is a kind of psychological dependency on the treatment and development of a "pain habit"—something we want to avoid at all cost, because it *will* cost.

Acupuncture

This procedure evolved out of thousands of years of Chinese history, culture, and tradition. Lately it has entered the West, charged with controversy and confusion stemming from our Western attempt to make it fit our own scientific models and biases. As two worlds mix and mingle, certain things are happening for the first time. Recently, experts from all over the world met in a congress to launch research studies to bridge some of our East–West gaps through collaborative research on the use of acupuncture.

Acupuncture is used in several contexts. One application is as an anesthetic. In China, in the fall of 1979, I witnessed a cesarean section performed entirely under acupuncture anesthesia, accompanied by a low-voltage electrical current delivered through the needles to the acupuncture points. This is called electro-acupuncture (EA). In my opinion, there wasn't a trace of hoax involved. It does work. Clinical studies have shown an increase in spinal fluid beta-endorphin levels (our own internal painkillers) after EA.

Acupuncture's other use is as a treatment for pain. Over thousands of years Chinese doctors have mapped out a complex system of "meridians," or lines of energy running up, down, and around the human body. We haven't found any analogues in our anatomy system. During acupuncture, thin needles are placed at specific points along the meridians in order to dull back pain, elbow pain, or whatever. Acupuncture is a common Chinese treatment for low back pain, with low-voltage electrical current often supplementing the needles. And of course, even here in the United States and in other Western countries, acupuncture is being used to ease back pain.

Does it work? While I haven't had acupuncture myself,

several of my patients have. As you'd expect, some felt they were helped and others found only transient or negligible relief. Complications are nil. The fine sterilized needles that are stuck in the skin carry no more risk of infection than a routine blood test.

The placebo recovery range is twenty-five to thirty-five percent; most studies show that acupuncture's success rate is not significantly better than this. The point is, then, that it probably does not have very much of a specific effect on the back pain condition to cure it or change it.

If you'd care to hear a traditional explanation of acupuncture's effects, refer back to Chapter IV's discussion of the gate control theory of pain. Presumably, the moving or electrically stimulated needles affect the central nervous system, blocking or dulling pain. It's also possible that acupuncture works through our system of internal opiates. In fact, some studies have shown acupuncture capable of stimulating endorphin production.

If you've decided after reading this that acupuncture is the thing for you, *a note of caution.* Discuss the treatment with the therapist and 1) make sure the needles are sterile, 2) make sure the needles are sterile, and 3) make sure the needles are sterile. There are several fatal diseases that can be transmitted through contaminated needles!

TENS (Transcutaneous Electrical Nerve Stimulation)

This can be viewed as a kind of Western medicine answer to the Eastern therapeutic modality known as acupuncture. Studies suggest that they both work by stimulating the body's endorphins or internal pain control substances. The theory and explanation are similar for both treatments. Small electrodes are placed on the skin and a low-voltage electrical current is emitted. It does appear to help control pain for some patients. There's no clinical risk. But it isn't effective for everyone. So, if it is not helping, stop it.

Trigger Point Injections

Sometimes patients point to a particular painful spot on their backs that, when touched, triggers pain even in distant sites in the back, hip, thighs, or legs. Some of these patients probably have the myofascial syndromes, fibromyalgia, or fibrositis. Some practitioners believe that injections of a local anesthetic, perhaps with cortisone or saline, relieves the pain. Supposedly the "trigger point injections" somehow break up the pain cycle.

There's little solid evidence for this notion. If it works for you and keeps your pain at bay, be happy. As long as the needles are sterile and you're not allergic to novocaine, there are no risks. If it doesn't work after one or two tries, however, you're probably wasting your time and money.

Deeper Injections of Cortisone and Novocaine

The assumption is that a long-acting local anesthetic agent will interrupt any pain cycle existing between the local pain and a secondary muscle spasm. Locally acting cortisone is also injected in the hopes of minimizing local inflammation.

Under the same theory, cortisone has actually been injected into the intervertebral disc in an effort to stop inflammation. And the same approach has been launched on the facet joints. Most rheumatologists and orthopedists advise against injecting cortisone into joints; this should also apply to the joints of the spine.

Unfortunately, I don't think any of these is a very good treatment for low back pain. Deep injections constitute an invasive and painful technique that is no more effective, according to the evidence, than milder therapies. In fact, cortisone may occasionally irritate structures with which it comes into contact, and we know that *repeated* cortisone injections into other joints can accelerate arthritis.

Epidural Steroids

It's not at all rare that one of our patients with low back pain due to disc disease, spinal stenosis, or some other cause will ask our opinion about epidural steroids. This is a procedure in which steroid in liquid form is placed in the spinal canal, using a needle or small catheter. The material does not go into the sheath or pouch where the nerves float in the spinal fluid; the cortisone is placed on and around the sheath (dura) that contains the nerves.

I rarely suggest this procedure, because most of the evidence indicates that it is not particularly helpful. Moreover, although complications are not frequent, they can and do occur. Some are not very serious, such as headaches, dizziness, or increased back and leg pain. Others are *very serious.* This group includes infectious and noninfectious inflammation of the nerves.

Chemonucleolysis

In the 1950s a prominent researcher, writer, and physician named Lewis Thomas was involved in an experiment in which meat tenderizer, injected into the bloodstream of rabbits, caused their ears to collapse. Why? Because the meat tenderizer contains *chymopapain,* an enzyme which dissolves mucopolysaccharides. These chemicals constitute a major component of the cartilage in the rabbits' ears and the nucleus pulpusus of the intervertebral disc. Recognizing that backache and sciatica may be caused by a herniated disc, Professor Carl Hirsch of Sweden suggested that chymopapain, injected into the disc, could dissolve some of it. Dr. Lyman Smith, of Chicago, popularized the idea in the United States, and chemonucleolysis was born.

Chemonucleolysis was very popular in the early and mid-seventies. As the patient lies under an X-ray machine, a needle placed into his intervertebral disc injects chymopapain into it.

The results? Patients with a distinct clinical picture of disc herniation, including back pain and sciatica, got the greatest benefit. Most studies computed chemonucleolysis's success rate at sixty to seventy percent—on a par with other treatments. But a few reported more glowing results. In one interesting experiment, chemonucleolysis was compared with surgery for lumbar disc disease—and came out on top. But I'm not convinced the surgical patients were properly selected.

The major, though rare, risk of chemonucleolysis is a severe, even fatal, hypersensitivity reaction. The material can also inflame the disc and cause scarring and inflammation around the lumbar dura and nerves if it comes in contact with them. Some studies show the substance is toxic to nerve tissues; others maintain that it is safe.

Chymopapain has been released for use in treating backache in the United States by the Food and Drug Administration. The concern is that it be used appropriately and not indiscriminately. How, you might ask, can you as the patient determine this? Here are two specific guidelines that should help: 1) Your condition should have all the indications that would make disc surgery the usual procedure (described in Chapter 6I); 2) You should have confidence in the advice of a well-qualified orthopaedic surgeon or neurosurgeon, and the agreement of another well-qualified spine surgeon (neurosurgical or orthopaedic) in the form of a *second opinion.*

When considering injection with chymopapain as an alternative to surgery, bear in mind that its success rate is about seventy to seventy-five percent, comparable to many other nonsurgical treatments. In addition, following injection, about fifty percent of those treated with chymopapain will have moderately severe to very severe back pain for three to twelve weeks.

Another potential difficulty is allergic reactions. If you are allergic to iodine or to any meat tenderizer, you should not be treated with chymopapain. You should not have a second injection of chymopapain, as the first injection will sensitize you to it and a second is likely to cause an allergic reaction. An allergic reaction that does develop can range from a simple rash with or without itching and edema, to anaphylactic shock, the most severe kind of allergic reaction. In fact, anaphylactic shock is a big-league problem. Many events occur in the body during this kind of reaction, the most deadly being a rapid drop in blood pressure that must be controlled if the patient is to survive. The chance of this kind of reaction is 1 in 100. Anaphylactic shock is ten times more common in women than in men.

In summary, then, this treatment does have a place in the management of herniated discs. Overall, it may be safer than surgery (Chapter 6I evaluates the risks of surgical procedures), and certainly it won't cause scarring, provided that it does not come into contact with the neural structures. However, it is not a risk-free therapy, and you should acknowledge that fact. Discuss with your doctor some of the problems presented here, discuss it with a friend, and if you decide to go ahead with it, maintain an optimistic, positive attitude. If it turns out not to help, you haven't burned your bridges behind you—you can still have the surgery; and if it does help, you will have allowed our hopes for this treatment to rise incrementally. Percutaneous discectomy may offer virtually all the benefits of chemonucleolysis, without its attendant complications. Let's review this procedure.

PERCUTANEOUS DISCECTOMY

Percutaneous discectomy is a technique with which it is possible to remove a portion of the nucleus and annulus of the intervertebral disc by placing a probe in the disc using X-ray control. Dr. Onik and associates in the United States invented a 2.5-mm.-diameter probe with a reciprocating suction cutter for dividing the disc material into small pieces and aspirating it from the disc space. (See Figure 6–6.)

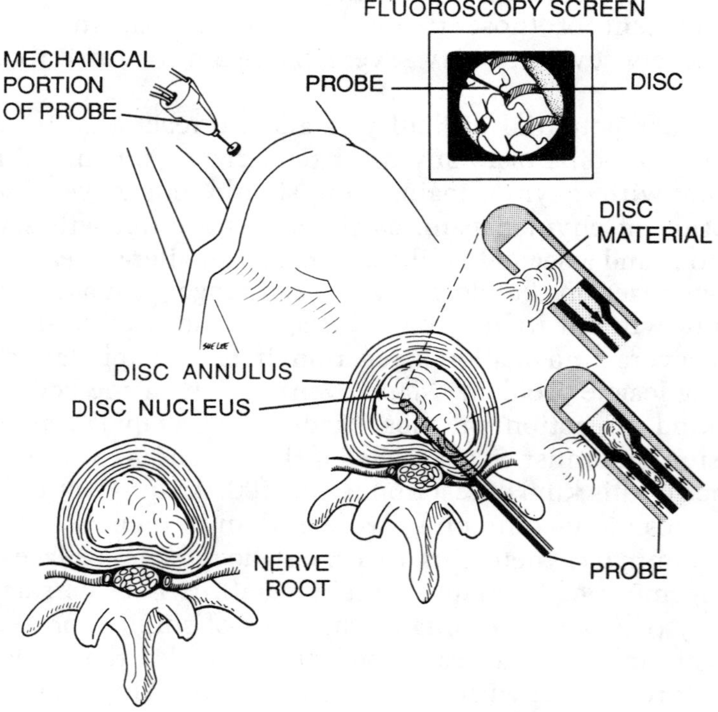

FIGURE 6–6 The patient lies on his/her side. A small probe, 2mm. in diameter, is inserted under fluoroscopic X-ray visualization and control through the skin muscle sheath, through the muscles into the central portion of the disc. With the use of an automated cutting/irrigating/suctioning device, some of the nucleus pulposus and annulus fibrosus is removed from the central and posterior lateral portion of the disc. The relationship of the protruded disc and the nerve root before and after percutaneous discectomy is shown. As a result, there is a reduction in both pressure and volume within the disc. This results in successful treatment in about seventy percent of patients.

Percutaneous discectomy was first performed in 1975 by Dr. Hijkata in Tokyo. He used long surgical instruments and worked through a cannula that he placed into the center of the disc. Several other surgeons in Europe and the United States have variations of this methodology. The Clinical Orthopaedics referenced in the Bibliography gives a good synopsis of the current status.

This procedure is done under local anesthesia and you may go home the same day or the next. You're probably thinking, "Sounds good—am I a candidate?" There are some specific factors to consider. You should have clinical evidence of disc disease, sciatica, physical exam findings to go with the sciatica, and imaging evidence—that is, your doctor should be able to see on a myelogram, CT scan, or MRI that there is a disc herniation. The abnormal disc should be at a level and on a side that fits with your physical examination. Then the imaging, preferably an MRI, should show that the herniation is likely to be still connected with the disc and not a "free fragment." A free fragment involves a situation in which the herniated portion of the disc is separated from the central portion of the disc. If this is the case the percutaneous discectomy will fail and is therefore contraindicated. You also should have given your back problem four to six weeks to heal under appropriate nonoperative care, something you're an expert on if you have read this far.

Now you may ask, "What is the chance of this thing working?" The evidence as of late 1989 is variable, but the success rate can reasonably be put in the range of sixty to eighty-five percent. You either already were or you now are (because you have read this far) a pretty savvy back patient, so you ask the next question. "What are the risks?" There is significantly less than a half of one percent chance of getting a disc space infection. There's a small chance (unquantified) that in theprocess of placement of the probe the inflamed nerve root could be irritated or damaged. If only irritated, this would be enough to cause some pain, numbness, or a tingling sensation for several hours or days after the procedure is finished. If damaged, one could have leg weakness. Also, there's the extremely low risk that an internal organ could be irritated or injured. Make sure you're not pregnant. If you possibly could be, discuss it with your doctor. Moreover, if you're sexually active, avoid exposure to conception from the time of your last menstrual period up to the time of the procedure. The reason for this is that the fetus is exposed to fluoroscopic radiation at the time of the placement of the probe into the disc. The routine procedure takes ample precautions to prevent these problems from occurring. Finally, as with any new procedure, there may be some complications that are not yet documented or recognized. For example, is there any long-range liability to removing a portion of the disc in this manner? On balance, however, used with appropriate indications, this quite safe technique merits a place among the armamentaria available to attack the ache in your back and/or leg.

Laser Discectomy

This too is relatively new. This methodology involves the use of vaporization to remove a portion of disc material. The technique is essentially the same as for the percutaneous suction discectomy described in the preceding section. The difference is that the disc is removed with laser energy rather than with suction nucleotome.

Patients appropriate for laser discectomy are the same as those for the percutaneous procedure. Essentially, the same precautions and risks of complications are involved, although we don't have as much information about the risks and benefits for this procedure. The risks associated with the probe and its placement would be the same; i.e., infection, nerve, and organ irritation. The benefit or clinical outcome *may* be different because of the amount of disc tissue removed. Clinical research is an ongoing endeavor that in time will be better able to answer these important questions concerning such risks and benefits.

SUMMARY: ALL NONSURGICAL TREATMENTS

For a listing of my opinion, based on the interpretation of the best current medical studies, as to how to select from the major available options of back care, see page 213, Chapter XII.

We've listed an awesome variety of treatments in this chapter, attempting to extract a sense of how their success rates, and risks, stack up. We found that most treatments fall into the sixty to seventy percent success realm. Chymopapain is *possibly* more effective.

Assessing what will help a particular patient, different physicians and therapists will choose different treatments, for complex reasons. One factor, of course, is their own familiarity with particular therapies.

How do *you* navigate the treatment maze?

The chart that follows summarizes the risks and benefits of the various treatments we've discussed. It will give you an idea of the likelihood of success to be had from several treatments, balanced against my opinion of their relative risks for the patient.

First, it makes sense to try two or three different conservative therapies. When one fails, it's possible another will succeed, as the sixty to seventy percent odds work in your favor. On the

RISK/BENEFIT CHART

		BENEFIT (*Rate of Success*)		
		OUTSTANDING (90 percent or better)	GOOD (70–80 percent)	AVERAGE (60–70 percent)
RISK	Serious	disc excision "conservative" selection McKenzie Program	chemonucleolysis	disc excision "liberal" selection
	Moderate		spinal manipulation percutaneous discectomy laser discectomy	rest analgesics percutaneous discectomy laser discectomy William's exercises drugs
	Minor		exercises patient education	heat and massage axial traction orthotics exercises McKenzie Program

other hand, don't search out and try every backache therapy on the planet, or you'll dissipate your time and resources. If, after giving two or three kinds of treatment your best shot, you're still stuck with intractable pain, you should consider one of two basic alternatives.

The first is surgery, discussed in the next chapter. But an operation is the answer only when you get a clear-cut diagnosis that calls for a specific surgical procedure. Your doctor can clarify your situation, and if you're still in doubt, try a second opinion.

The other approach is some kind of well-constructed program for managing chronic pain. I hate to see patients struggle along with an unsuccessful treatment after it has proven itself to be unsuccessful. There are no magic cures. Rely on a comprehensive, conservative back-pain management program, which includes a psychological and/or psychiatric assessment. I'm not saying the pain is all in your head. But when you've had severe pain for a *long time,* you may need emotional as well as medical or physical help to make yourself better.

COMMENT

Just a word about this risk/benefit chart. It's provided for you as a kind of basis for your thinking about what kind of treatment you wish to pursue. There is a tendency for the higher-benefit procedures to carry a higher risk. (The McKenzie Program is an exception.) To some degree you will only be offered treatment that is appropriate for your individual condition as regards risks and benefits. Obviously, you should not be offered surgery unless the time is right. Also, this chart is not based on a common diagnosis. Note also that "liberal" selection for surgery carries the same high risks but low benefits when compared with "conservative" selection. Conservative selection is where the patient has an imaging evidence of a distinct disc herniation, a physical exam which confirms this, and a trial of at least six weeks of nonsurgical treatment. Liberal selection is when one or more of these criteria are not present.

If things are not understandable to *you* about *your* back and just what to do, then I'll tell you. It's very simple. Get a *second opinion.* We will delve deeply into the important judgment calls about surgery in the next chapter.

Chapter VII

To Operate or Not to Operate?

The Risk/Benefit Equation

My task is a moral and legal one: to provide my patient with the opportunity to give informed consent. The gist of what we do for the patient here is to give an idea of what a) risks he/she is exposed to and b) what benefits are likely to be gained. The concept is expressed symbolically in Figure 7–1. This means looking some cold statistics squarely in the eye. We talk about the one or two patients out of forty-four thousand who do not wake up from their anesthesia; not bad odds, but nonetheless . . . We mention the possibility of pneumonia following anesthesia, and the remote chance that a blood clot in the leg will travel to the lungs as a dangerous pulmonary embolism. Then I must point out that one or two out of every hundred patients develops an infection at the surgical site.

I tell them that during surgery, the nerve root may be irritated, damaged, or lost, which, translated into the patient's terms, means numbness or weakness in a part of the leg after the operation. Some patients ask, "Could I be paralyzed by the operation?" This is asked when the patient fears the "helpless" situation where he/she cannot move arms or legs, or simply can't walk. It's fair to say that none of the operations discussed here could result in either of these tragedies. There is the risk of significant weakness, numbness, or tingling in one or both legs,

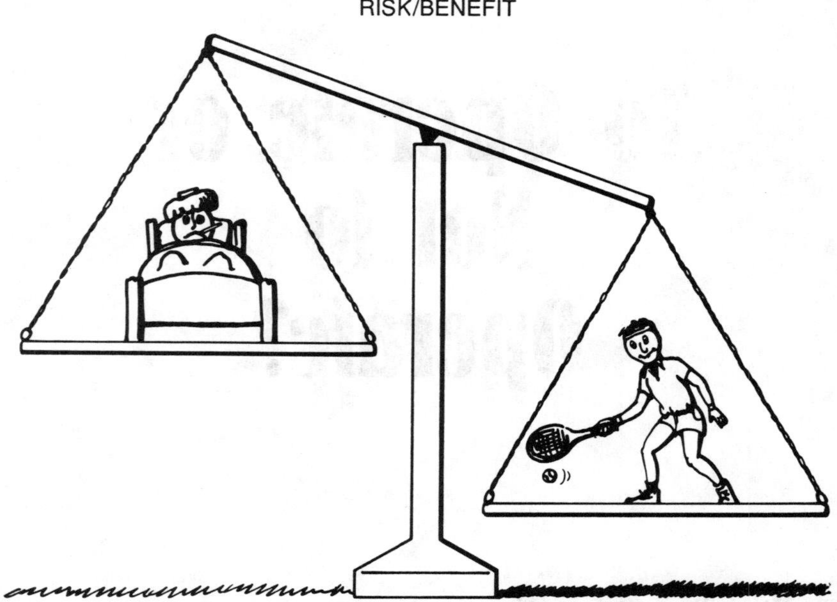

FIGURE 7–1 This cartoon attempts to be self-explanatory. Every operation is a risk but offers the possibility of benefit. The patient and surgeon must evaluate the situation and determine that the benefits "outweigh" the risks.

which is associated with some of the operations. I'll explain those as we come to them.

There's also a tiny risk of severe bleeding in the small vessels around the disc or in the major ones in front. Though the latter is a rare complication, it may require a lifesaving operation from the front to control bleeding.

Now, on the other side of the ledger, I reassure my patient. I review the probabilities of a good to excellent result. I point out that these major complications rarely occur. What I've given you is the most rigorous inventory of possible risks, and if I were talking to an extremely anxious patient, I'd try to transmit the essence without dwelling on rare, tragic possibilities.

Then I explain to my patient how his/her uniqueness bears on these gross statistics. That is, if you're a vigorous, assertive, positive, healthy person, you run a significantly lower risk than someone who is just the opposite. There may also be aspects of your particular diagnosis and condition that warrant more optimism. And I have no doubt that a positive, energetic attitude is one of the most favorable conditions for back surgery. Whatever his/her diagnosis and treatment, a patient without a sincere, realistic desire to get well isn't a good candidate.

All of this under our belts, I ask the patient whether he/she prefers surgery or continued attempts at nonsurgical treatment. In most cases, the patient has a clear-cut opinion. But sometimes the ball is returned to my court and the patient says, "You tell me what I should do, Doctor; I want to know what you think." At this point I'll share with him/her my best judgment, explaining why I think we should go ahead with surgery, or why we should wait.

I've decided to share the following surgical maxims with you for several reasons. First permit me to give some background. They happen to be orthopaedic surgical maxims that we use in our development program for young surgeons. In principle, the basic ideas are part of any high-quality training program. My reason for presenting them here is threefold: I believe that it will give you a sense of confidence, provide you with a better perspective, and perhaps suggest some questions that you may wish to ask.

Surgical Maxims

- Do the least amount of surgery that is necessary to solve the patient's problem(s).
- Each additional risk to the patient must be justified by substantial evidence of incremental benefit *for* the patient.

To Operate or Not?

In medical textbooks the terms of this dilemma are the *indications* and *contraindications* of surgery, and the question has been the focus of many a journal article, conference, and informal talk. Doctors, in fact, spend a good part of their careers figuring out how to select from among all the possible treatments the one that is best for a particular patient.

Indications for surgery? First, a specific, abnormal process in the spine should be identified and documented. And it should have been present long enough to assume that nature alone is not going to cure it. Finally, before anyone gets wheeled into the operating room, there should be reasonable evidence that surgery will correct, eliminate, or improve the problem.

When surgery isn't beneficial, or is likely to be harmful, it shouldn't be done. Of course, there isn't always a crisp, clean, yes-or-no judgment.

In this chapter we'll list the common low back operations, with the indications and contraindications of each. However, reading this chapter is no substitute for a thorough discussion with your surgeon if you're pondering a trip to the operating room. However, a review of its contents will equip you with the information you need to substantively engage in that conversation.

How to Choose a Surgeon

Things are getting serious. You need a spine specialist to evaluate and possibly treat you surgically. Here is a checklist to help you identify that person. The key questions are: Is this person qualified (i.e., adequately trained)? Does he/she care about me? Will this doctor explain what's wrong with me and answer my questions? That's essentially it. The checklist will help you to find a qualified, caring, explaining question-answerer.

Who should operate? Simple: someone well trained and experienced in low back surgery. Your surgeon should understand

CHECKLIST FOR FINDING A GOOD SPINE-CARE PHYSICIAN OR SURGEON

- Ask your internist or primary-care physician.
- Try a doctor referral service in your city.
- If one or more of the major hospitals in your city has a physician referral service, try that.
- Do you have a friend in the health care profession—doctor, nurse, administrator? Ask him/her.
- Make sure your doctor is board-certified. We've mentioned some publications to help you determine that.
- While there are good doctors outside university-affiliated hospitals, if in doubt go with teaching centers.

patients as people and be thoroughly knowledgeable about the diagnosis and management of lumbar spine pain. How do you know if a given surgeon is qualified? I'd recommend seeking one who is board-certified in either orthopaedic surgery or neurosurgery. (Your library has a *Directory of Medical Specialists* published by Marquis Who's Who. This book will tell you of your surgeon's board certification.) The hospital where a surgeon admits patients will generally provide board-certification information. Another useful reference is the *Town & Country*'s "Exclusive Directory of Outstanding Medical Specialists in the U.S." (Part I, October, 1989, and Part II, November, 1989), by Stephanie Bernardo Johns. Ask fellow back sufferers, listening for the kinds of traits we've mentioned. Don't hesitate to query your surgeon about how comfortable and experienced he/she is with your contemplated procedure if his/her training in a certain technique isn't evident. Nowadays this is perfectly acceptable patient-doctor etiquette. After all, it's *your* back. Finally, heed your gut feelings of confidence and rapport.

Now which should you choose, an orthopaedic surgeon or a neurosurgeon? If a spinal fusion is called for, I'd advise you to have an orthopaedic surgeon perform it. This is a procedure at which he/she is generally more experienced. But otherwise, either is fine. An Australian study compared a large group of low back pain and sciatica patients, half of whom were treated by orthopaedic surgeons and half by neurosurgeons, and found their success rates nearly identical.

If a surgeon seems to be rushing you into surgery, beware, unless you have the bladder problems we previously described. Also shun any self-proclaimed miracle worker. On the subject of doctors, let me tell you a little story. Apologies to any doctors who are reading this book, as they've heard it at least three times.

After bidding farewell to this good life, a woman finds herself outside the Pearly Gates, about to have her credentials checked by St. Peter. With her is a long line of prospective applicants, everyone on his/her best behavior. Then along strolls a tall, stately person in a white coat with a stethoscope around his neck. Without any timidity whatsoever, this self-possessed individual walks past everyone to the front of the line and enters heaven. "Who was that?" one person whispers to another. "That was God," the word filters back. "But why the white coat and stethoscope?" the people ask. The answer comes back, "Oh, He likes to play doctor sometimes."

Sometimes in our zeal to help, or laboring under an unrealistic belief in our own powers, we doctors can do *too* much surgery on backache patients. This is a consideration especially in the case of salvage back surgery, which we'll discuss later.

Disc Excision

Let's start with what is probably the most common operation for backache. The rationale for removing the intervertebral disc is that it's presumed to be the offending item and has become

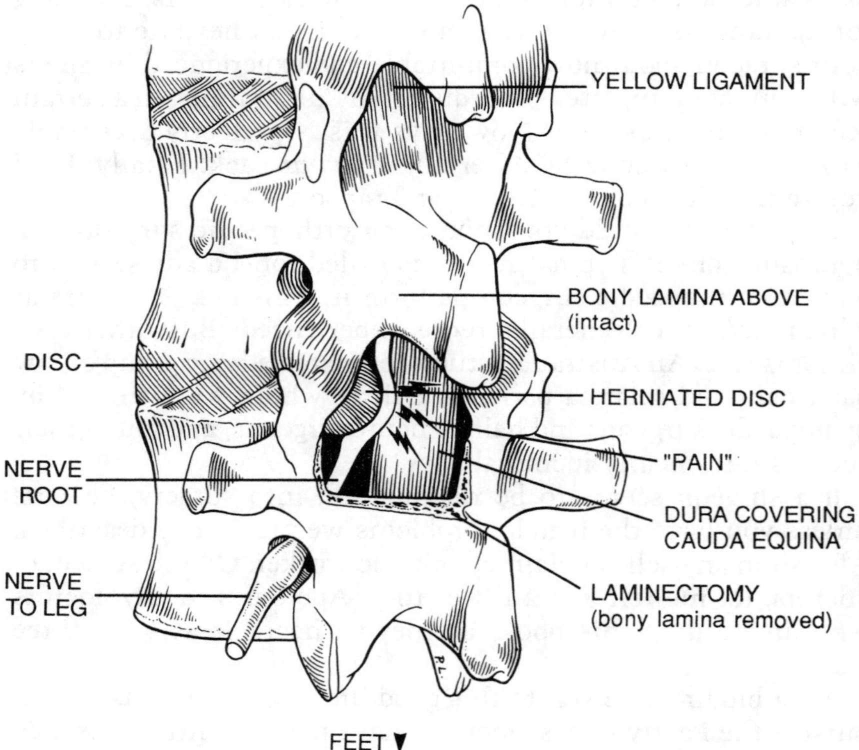

FIGURE 7–2 Here we see a "laminectomy." The operation called laminectomy is one in which part or all of the lamina (a portion of bone on the back of the vertebra) is removed. In addition, a part of the yellow ligament is removed, as shown here. The purpose is to get to the herniated disc. The herniated disc and additional portions of the disc are removed in order to relieve the irritation of the nerve root.

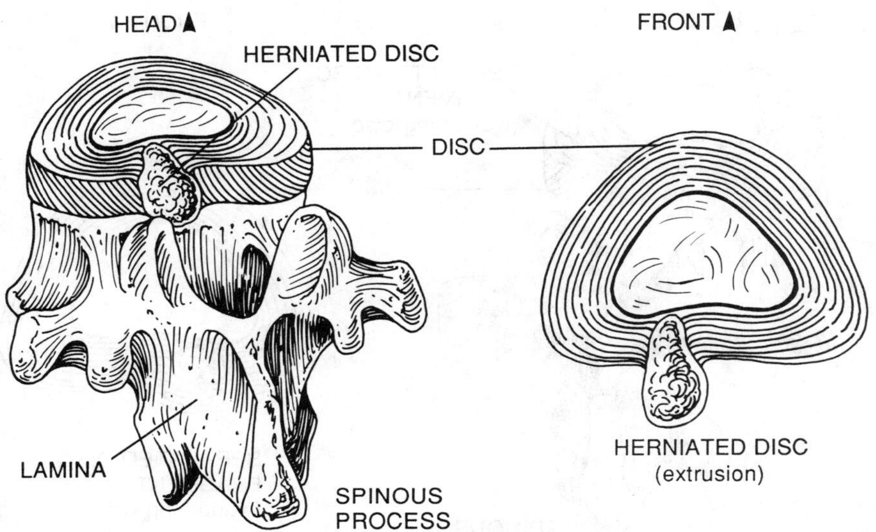

FIGURE 7–3 In this situation, there is a portion of the annulus that has isolated itself from the rest of the disc and all or part of it is displaced well out into the canal. This situation is the one that responds best to surgery. It may not respond to conservative therapy, including manipulation and even chemonucleolysis. (Reproduced with permission from White, A.A., and Panjabi, M.M.: *Clinical Biomechanics of the Spine,* J.B. Lippincott, 1990, second edition.)

abnormal. This is one of the first surgical principles, and it still holds.

What does the disc surgery consist of? Operating from the back, the surgeon dissects down the back of the vertebrae, making an entrance into the vertebral canal. He then moves the dura and the bundle of nerves called the cauda equina ("horse's tail") aside, exposing the disc itself. The important, somewhat sticky part of the procedure is to expose and protect the nerve elements and control the bleeding from the plexus of veins lying in this area. (Figure 7–2.)

Now the disc can be clearly identified. At this point one of three things happens. (1) If a portion of the disc has separated from the main part and moved from between the vertebrae out into the nerve canal, it's called a *free fragment.* (Figure 7–3.) It can simply be plucked out or dissected from the scar tissue and ligaments in the canal. (2) Or the disc may be incompletely displaced, with the fragment still partially within the space

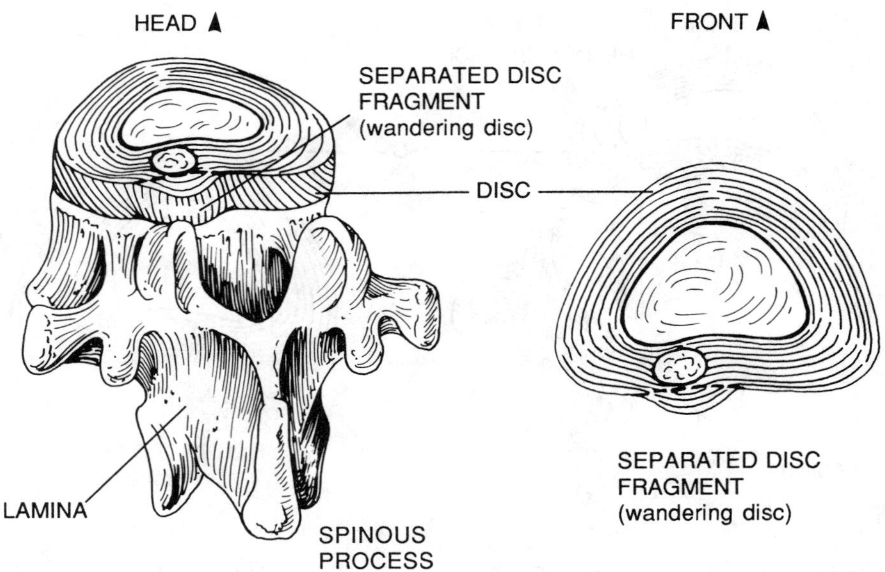

FIGURE 7–4 This one I like to call the "wandering disc." Some annulus fibers have isolated themselves, and wander about due to movement of the spine. In some positions they cause pain, in others they don't. Traction, manipulation, or chymopapain may help. The problem may suddenly come on following just a slight twist or bend, and it may go away almost as rapidly, following a fall, twist, or cough. Surgery is sometimes required, when severe pain and disability persists for three months or more. (Reproduced with permission from White, A.A., and Panjabi, M.M.: *Clinical Biomechanics of the Spine,* J.B. Lippincott, 1990, second edition.)

between the vertebrae. (Figure 7–4.) (3) The third possibility is that the disc isn't fragmented at all but simply bulging extensively. (Figure 7–5.) If either (2) or (3) is the case, the surgeon removes the bulging or displaced part and a part of the disc that lies in the interspace between the vertebrae.

What shape the disc is found in at the time of surgery has much to do with whether or not the operation relieves your leg pains (sciatica). The best prognosis—a ninety percent success rate—comes with complete disc herniation. When the disc fragment is not completely separated from the rest of the disc and the space between the vertebrae, the success rate drops to eighty percent. When only a bulging disc is found, success is in the range of sixty percent. Remember our discussion of the placebo effect? It may interest you to know that when the disc is neither herniated nor bulging nor abnormal at all, surgery still cures thirty percent of patients (an example of the placebo effect). The mind is a puzzling machine! Obviously, surgery should not be used for placebo effect.

Patients often ask, "Well, what happens when you remove the disc? Do you just leave nothing there? Nature must have put it there for some reason." That's a reasonable question, and the reply is that the patient, assuming disc surgery is appropriate for

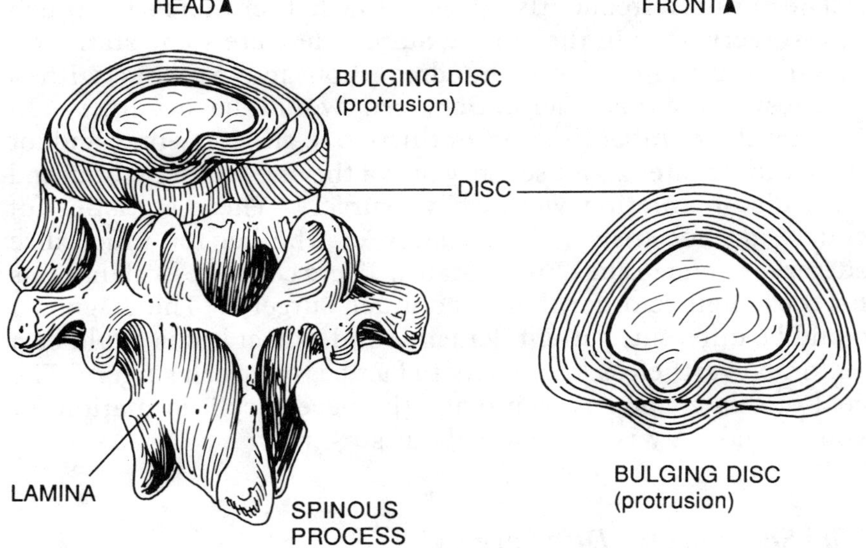

FIGURE 7–5 This we can call the bulging disc. Here the disc bulges enough to cause nerve root irritation and sciatica. These patients may be helped with traction, manipulation, and chymopapain. Surgery is sometimes needed if there is a positive myelogram and the back pain and sciatica do not subside in three to twelve weeks. The results are good with surgery, but not as good as when there is a significant fragment of disc out in the canal. Of all the situations that might respond to chymopapain injection, this type would probably respond best; however, this does not mean chymopapain injection would be the treatment of choice for every patient with this type of situation. (Reproduced with permission from White, A.A., and Panjabi, M.M.: *Clinical Biomechanics of the Spine,* J.B. Lippincott, 1990, second edition.)

him/her in the first place, is better off without the disc than with an abnormal one. You should know that most surgeons are aware that for good reasons the patient is best served by removing just the herniated part and a small portion of the remaining disc. And while the back is not restored to its original perfection, it's improved enough to be only very subtly different from a normal one. In most instances, of course, the patient has residual reminders that his/her back isn't quite its old self: When the weather is bad, a lift is not done carefully, or there's a long auto drive, there may be mild or moderate pain similar to what the patient felt before surgery.

The question frequently arises as to whether there's too much disc surgery done in the United States. Here are some statistics. In Great Britain, of one hundred thousand patients with a diagnosis of a disc herniation, ten would have surgery. In Finland the number is between thirty-one and forty-one, and for the United States about seventy out of the one hundred thousand with disc herniation would have surgery. These statistics, of course, *do not* answer the question of whether too much disc surgery is done in the United States. There could be explanations for these figures other than "too much surgery." The diagnoses could be different; patient demands and expectations could be a factor. Nevertheless, there may in fact be too much surgery. The goal of this chapter is to provide the necessary information for you to make a wise decision about surgery.

Who Should Have Disc Surgery?

For openers, consider a history of back pain that has lasted for at least six weeks. Now, much hinges on certain diagnostic tests, and this brings us to the matter of a thorough preoperative exam. If you're being evaluated for disc disease, several tests will clarify your condition.

First, your history and a few neurologic findings tell your doctor something about the state of your disc. One exam, called the straight leg raising test, is especially critical. Your doctor may recommend an electromyographic study (EMG) to help identify abnormal electrical activity in the muscles supplied by the sciatic nerve. This test sounds a bit tough, but is not usually bad at all, particularly if you can manage to relax. Very fine needles must be inserted into several muscles to pick up and record their electrical patterns.

Let me suggest a little "mental trick" that can make this test a breeze for you. Think of it as a little mosquito bite, followed by an "itch" or "tickle." I'm serious—the sensations are amazingly similar. You must faithfully convince yourself of that. People have trouble with these tests because they build up anxiety over the words "needle" and "electrical." The point is that the size of the needle and the magnitude of the electrical stimulus is such that it's like a mosquito and a tickle.

Abnormal activity suggests nerve root damage caused by an encroaching disc. There is something called a water-soluble myelogram, a technique that's more accurate than the older fat-soluble myelogram in providing visualization of a herniated disc. The difference between the two is the solubility of the contrast medium, or dye (see Chapter III for discussion of the myelogram). Happily, the water-soluble dye doesn't have to be removed after the test. This simplifies the procedure.

Now there are two additional studies that are useful in showing whether or not you have a disc herniation. These are called CT scans (Computerized Tomography) and MRI (Magnetic Resonance Imaging). The former exposes you to some radiation; the latter does not. The MRI is replacing the water-soluble myelogram and the CT scan as the best technique for imaging a disc herniation. You should know that MRI is not always available, and also there are times when your doctor will determine that one or both of the other two studies are best to evaluate your particular condition.

Expected Success Rate of Disc Surgery

Then your doctor can add up his/her evaluation of your history, the physical exam, and all the test results to gauge your odds of successful surgery. Bear in mind the correlation between disc herniation and pain relief. If you have a three-month history of back pain with sciatica and clear neurologic problems, an abnormal straight leg raising test, an abnormal EMG, and positive imaging studies (myelogram, CT scan, or MRI), your odds of being helped by disc surgery are around ninety to ninety-five percent. If the diagnosis of herniated disc is based on your history and neurologic exam alone, it may be only sixty percent accurate. Adding the abnormal straight leg raising test, we go up to seventy percent accuracy; with an abnormal EMG, to eighty percent.

Good news for the over-sixty group. You too can expect a favorable outcome with disc surgery when the proper indications are present. The data show that eighty-seven percent of patients over sixty will enjoy a good-to-excellent result.

Pros and Cons of Disc Surgery

Major complications of disc removal include damaged nerves in the lumbar area, damaged major blood vessels in front of the disc, and wound infections. Most of these complications are quite rare, although wound infections occur at a one to two percent rate.

Now it may occur to you to ask, "What will happen to me if I *don't* have the surgery?" A Swedish study addressed this question, dividing a group of patients with a clear diagnosis of herniated disc for six months into two groups. One group underwent disc removal and laminectomy (removal of the thin bone called the lamina that forms part of the spinal canal; see Figure 7–2), while the others were treated nonsurgically, with immobilization. How did they fare?

Well, those with definite disc prolapse, or herniation, who were operated on got quicker relief of their sciatica and returned to work sooner than the nonsurgical patients. But the experiment did show that nature can cure sciatica, too. Six months after treatment there was little difference between the two groups. But the patients' subjective self-evaluation differed. The surgical patients rated their condition as more improved and took less sick leave than those who'd been treated with immobilization, even though their tests of leg motor strength were identical.

Other studies from Norway show a superiority of surgical patients that lasts for two to five years. However, after ten years nonoperated patients do about as well as those who had surgery.

What does this all mean to you who are wrestling with the surgery-versus-nonsurgery decision? Once your symptoms are severe, and you have low back pain, sciatica, and a diagnosis of herniated disc, how long should you wait before considering an operation?

At this point, remember that ninety percent of patients recover in about eight to ten weeks with no treatment, because that's the natural course of the disease. The best information suggests that herniated disc patients who wait less than sixty days have a better surgical prognosis than those who wait longer. If you're going to have elective disc surgery the ideal time is at about forty to fifty days (six weeks) after the onset of leg pain. Timely and appropriate surgical intervention has the advantages of minimizing pain and psychological distress. Furthermore, patients who undergo disc removal after being laid up for a year are only half as likely to get pain relief as patients who have surgery earlier.

Even motor weaknesses, such as foot drop, can improve without surgery. So if the pain is improving or tolerated, the presence of weakness alone which is not progressing does not force our hand in surgery. This assumes we're still within the six- to twelve-week interval. If one watches a "foot drop" motor weakness too long—more than three, six, or nine months—it may not recover for one to two years after surgery, if at all.

It may be that the nerve roots are irreparably damaged during months of incapacity, for long-standing compression and inflammation can cause nerve root scarring. Over the years, I have detected scarring and other evidence of nerve damage in discs that have presumably been herniated for a year or more. There may be a curious psychological reason, too. We know that pain that has hung around for more than a year isn't usually completely banished when you correct the disease that caused it. It's as though the pain acquired a life of its own—and some psychological or emotional support may be necessary, in addition to removing the physical cause of the pain.

However, when it comes to you, the individual, don't interpret these statistics to mean that you must have the disc out by 11:59 P.M. on the fifty-ninth day of your illness. There are many intertwined considerations and few absolutes. If you can't spare too much time away from work, you should be seriously considering surgery around two or three months into your illness. But your particular surgical risks, your anxiety about or confidence in the scalpel, and the extent of your pain, disability, and life disruption must all be weighed.

There are two noteworthy exceptions to the two- to three-month principle. The first is the professional athlete who performs or participates in heavy-lifting, high-risk sports, and workers with strenuous lifting tasks. These individuals should lean more toward operative treatment. They cannot afford to wait to see if time will heal them spontaneously. During this time they will be out of work, out of competition, and eventually out of shape. We have developed a program for the well-trained athlete with acute low back pain (see Bibliography). Here we focus on the highly competitive athlete with low back pain and significant sciatica—more precisely with a herniated disc. We think that after six to eight weeks (in general) if these competitors are not rapidly improving they should have percutaneous discectomy, if appropriate, by MRI, or surgical discectomy. The problem (disc herniation) is removed and the athlete can begin his/her rehabilitation and return to competition. If there are any doubters as to the wisdom of this recommendation, consider the spectacular Joe Montana, who recovered from disc surgery and was rehabilitated to come back as a superstar quarterback of the National Football League.

The second exception is that of patients with severe sciatica who suddenly can't control their bladders. This suggests that they may have a large herniated disc fragment that has popped out. Sometimes there will be severe leg weakness or loss of the ability to control the bowels. In these instances, so much of the disc has been displaced that the nerves involved cannot function to provide the usual control of bladder, bowels, and legs. In this situation I view surgery as less *elective* and I would urge my patient to have surgery as soon as possible, provided the disc can be shown on a myelogram, CAT scan, or MRI.

There has been some gratifying feedback on our first endeavor to write a helpful low back book. The following vignette exemplifies a situation in which a reader converted herself into a heroine by applying this information about bladder control. Apparently our patient, who was reading the book, had a friend who had low back pain with sciatica, mild pain—but some slight weakness in the leg. She had been to see several doctors, and was being treated conservatively and appropriately. However, she began to develop some difficulty getting her urination started and had mentioned this to her doctor, who was not particularly alarmed. The reader of the book, being an intelligent and assertive person, suggested she contact her doctor again and reemphasize this particular symptom. This was done, and although the response was one of concern, it was not apparently one of recognition of the importance of this symptom. Our conscientious reader then insisted that her friend go and see another physician and again emphasize the problem. This was done, the physician ordered the appropriate imaging studies, and a large herniated disc was diagnosed and subsequently removed by a surgeon. The patient improved and her bladder function returned to normal. Again, my commendations to our patient, who acted with compassion, courage, and conviction on the basis of her knowledge.

Spinal Fusion

This is an operation in which bone from somewhere else in your body, or from a donor's body, is grafted into regions of living bone in the back. After a period, usually four to nine months, a natural process known as *creeping substitution* transpires. Though it may evoke scenes from *Invasion of the Body Snatchers,* all it means is that the bone graft is gradually replaced by living bone produced by the patient's own body. The result? A connection between two or more vertebrae, usually a strong, solid, stable union between the bones selected for fusion.

Your bone or someone else's may be used. Most evidence suggests that they are almost equally effective. Not infrequently, using your own will require a second incision and lead to possible complications of infection or a hematoma (a localized collection of blood in the tissues). Bank bone (someone else's) carries an infinitesimally small risk of transmitting a blood-borne disease such as hepatitis or AIDS.

There has been one documented case in which a patient contracted acquired immunodeficiency syndrome (AIDS) as a result of bone transplantation (bone graft) used in a spinal fusion. The bone was unwittingly donated by a patient with AIDS and the patient who received the bone developed the disease and symptoms within three weeks from the time of surgery. While there are some risks of using bank bone, if the allograph (bank bone) is obtained and managed according to

American Association of Tissue Banks'* standards for surgical bone banking, the risk is virtually eliminated. The most reasonable and balanced estimate is that of a risk of 1/250,000. Estimates by experts range from 1/75,000–1/500,000.

Processed human bone for spinal fusion implants is available for purchase from the American Red Cross Transplantation Services. This graft material is appropriately prepared and sterilized. Most important, the donors are very carefully screened for AIDS, syphilis, and other diseases that might be transmitted through bone grafts. This and other commercial sources are considered safe, but consult with your surgeon.

Safe bank bone has the previously stated advantages. We therefore recommend its use when available. Another safe alternative is commercially available: specially treated animal bone. This type of bone graft is thought to be almost as effective, if not as effective, as human bank bone.

The spinal fusion connection can be made either *anteriorly*—that is, from the front, between the vertebral bodies—or *posteriorly*—from the back, between the posterior elements of the two vertebrae. (Figure 7–6.) The bone used for the graft is often the ilium, the large pelvic bone, which you may be familiar with as the one that shows up in a slender bikini wearer. Or it may be the previously discussed *bone bank bone*—that is, bone taken from someone else and properly preserved until needed.

Why fuse bone, anyway? The idea is that fusing the bone reduces motion at an abnormal segment of the spine, and as a consequence the pain produced or irritated by excessive motion will fade. Normal motion of a diseased spinal segment, abnormal motion of a normal or near-normal segment, or an abnormal positioning between two segments can cause backache.

Who Should Have a Spinal Fusion?

First of all, should spine fusion be a routine fellow traveler on a disc-removal trip? The answer is *no.* In simple disc surgery, fusion is neither desirable nor necessary, unless there's some other abnormality. Where previous surgery has caused extensive

* American Association of Tissue Banks. Standards for surgical bone banking. Arlington, Virginia: American Association of Tissue Banks, 1987. (Revision to standards, effective January 15, 1988, section C1.330.)

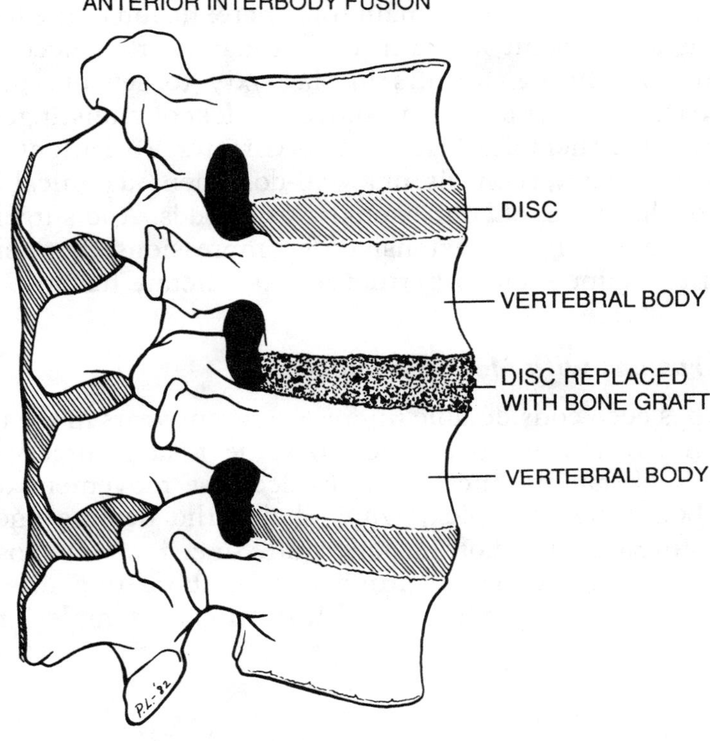

FIGURE 7–6 In an anterior interbody spinal fusion, the disc is removed and bone graft is substituted in the space. There are a number of variations on this basic theme. The variations have to do with the shape of the bone graft, how much if any of the vertebra is removed, and whether metal fixation or a spine replacement is used.

damage to the anatomic elements of the spine, or definite arthritis exists, spinal fusion may accompany disc surgery. Spinal stenosis may also call for fusion, but this will be discussed under a separate heading.

Otherwise, when is spine fusion a good idea? Sometimes considerable arthritis or damage from a fracture results in a definite instability of the spine, requiring a fusion. But these conditions aren't run-of-the-mill. A more straightforward case for spinal fusion is spondylolisthesis, or a slippage of the vertebrae. When spondylolisthesis causes severe back pain with or without leg pain, a spinal fusion may spell substantial relief, especially for younger patients.

But now we come to our main topic here: fusion of the lumbar spine as a treatment for pain. Unfortunately, the success rate isn't overwhelming. Results in the sixty to seventy percent range barely lift lumbar fusion above the host of undistinguished nonoperative therapies discussed in Chapter VI. Patients with spondylolisthesis, scoliosis, or a well-documented clinical instability of the spine, of course, enjoy rosier odds. And surgery for tumors, infections, or extensive decompressions that remove part of the spine's support structure may dictate fusion.

Spine Fusions with Metal Implants

There has been considerable interest in recent years in the use of internal fixation as an adjunct to spine fusion surgery. The rationale is that the metal devices decrease movement of the spine bone graft complex, which helps the healing and the successful maturation of the bone graft. Since it's quite possible that your surgeon may mention one of these implants or a similar type, I've provided some illustrations. Examples of four

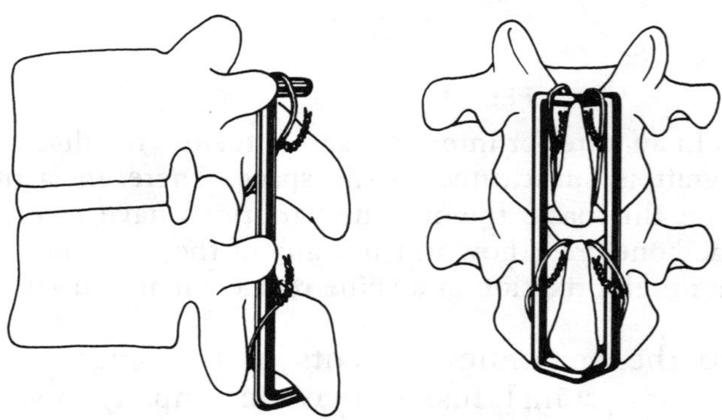

FIGURE 7–7 This is a technique for internal fixation of the lumbar spine. On the left is a side view of the heavy metal rectangle, which firmly holds vertebrae in place by connecting them through wires attached to the rectangular rod structure. The wires are passed around the lamina (back part of the vertebra) and the metal rectangle and twisted tightly. On the right is a view of the surgical construction from a posterior perspective. Bone graft is added to this construction. (Reproduced with permission from White, A.A., and Panjabi, M.M.: *Clinical Biomechanics of the Spine.* J.B. Lippincott, 1990, second edition.)

major types are presented in Figures 7–7 through 7–10. In the first one, Figure 7–7, the vertebra is attached to a rod by wire that must pass into the spinal canal. The second, Figure 7–8, called Harrington rods, is an instrumentation that was used

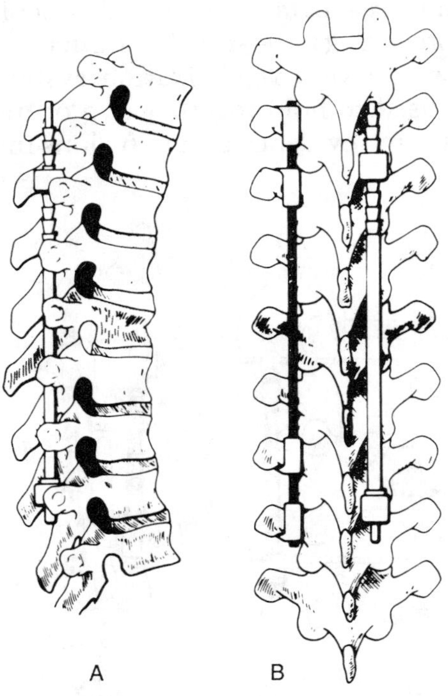

FIGURE 7–8 On the left we see a lateral view of the stainless steel rod with hooks applied to the back portion of the spine. These hooks go underneath the lamina of the vertebrae and are designed not to irritate the spinal cord. The rod is designed so that it can be cranked up (somewhat analagous to a jack on a car) to correct curvature of the spine, or to fix the spine by applying pressure through the tension created by the ligaments as they are stretched.

To the right-hand side of this picture we see a posterior view of the rod that we see on the left; we also see a Harrington compression rod on the left-hand side of the spine, and the distraction rod with the jacks on it on the right-hand side. The mechanics of these rods are somewhat complex, but it is only important that the patient understands that these are useful implants which provide some immobilizing capacity of the spine while a spine fusion heals and takes over the loads and forces from these instruments. These instruments are not needed in routine spine fusions, but there are situations in which they are helpful.

initially for scoliosis but is now used in lumbar spine fusions, especially for trauma. In the third, Figure 7–9, called internal fixitor, a screw is placed into the pedicle and the body of the vertebra and attached to a rod or plate. The fourth, Figure 7–10, the Cotrell-Doubisset apparatus, also used for scoliosis, combines concepts of the preceding two—that is, laminar hooks and pedicle screws—to provide a very rigid fixation system. These metal systems can be used to hold together two or more vertebrae if needed. There is some evidence that in fusions involving three or

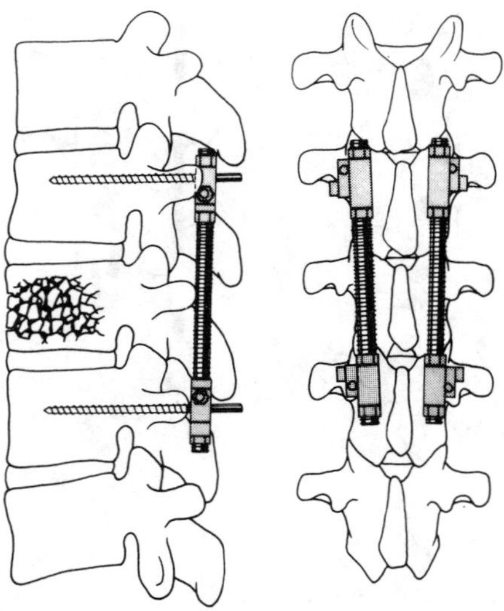

FIGURE 7–9 This is a specific device; however, it is a prototype of a transpedicular fixation device. The screw goes through the pedicle into the vertebral body and is attached to some kind of plate or rod, which connects to one or more additional vertebrae. This is shown on the left as a side view. The pedicle shown here from the side is well seen anatomically in Figure 2–6A, page 37. To the right the system is seen from behind the vertebrae. The pedicle screw is shown, but the heavy longitudinal screws (which are replaced by a plate in some systems) are seen here. These surgical constructs are augmented with bone and are thought to provide the most rigid immobilization. Note also the fracture (broken) of the vertebral body. This particular form of fixation is sometimes used to treat fractures of the vertebrae. (Reproduced with permission from White, A.A., and Panjabi, M.M.: *Clinical Biomechanics of the Spine,* J.B. Lippincott, 1990, second edition.)

more vertebrae, these internal fixation devices may help. However, the incremental benefit of using the hardware in addition to the bone graft has not been definitely determined.

Nevertheless, there are some circumstances, such as surgery

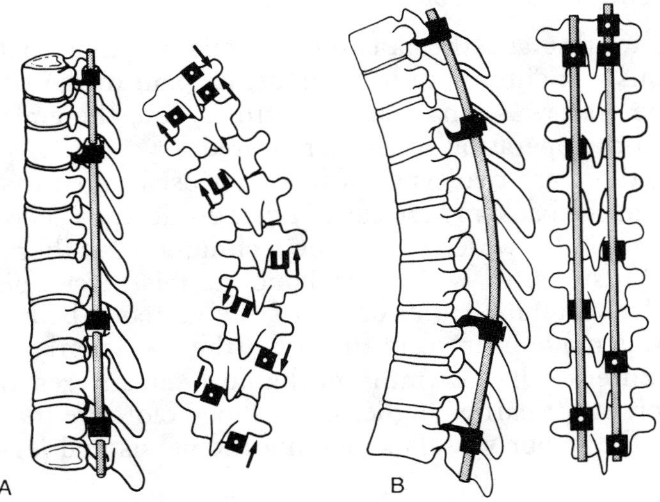

FIGURE 7–10 This is a Cotrel-Dubousset apparatus. This shows two views of the spine on the left (a lateral view and a posterior view), and then two views of the spine on the right (a lateral view and a posterior view). These rods are used primarily for correction of scoliosis, severe curvature of the spine; they are also used in some cases following trauma to the spine, and in some cases for other elective spine fusions.

First, on the left we show a lateral spine which is very straight. When the rods are applied on the right, the lateral view of the spine shows some curvature. This curvature is a more normal situation for the lateral view, so it is being corrected. Viewing again the posterior views of the spine, on the left we see a posterior view with the hooks placed in it, and on the right we see the posterior view after two rods have been applied and the correction has been made. The posterior view on the right shows correction of the scoliosis and correction of the lordosis—that is, too much extension of the spine. It is now flexed a bit, which is a normal position for the thoracic spine. Again, this is a bit complex, but it is important for the lay person to understand that these mechanical implants can sometimes be helpful in the correction and maintenance of correction of the spine. Ultimately, though, the longterm correction always depends on a satisfactory fusion of the spine.

for spine fractures, deformity, or tumors, in which the need for surgical instrumentation is different and the hardware is essential.

Complications of Fusion

Besides routine anesthesia complications, we must list wound infections and chronic mild to moderate pain in the site where the bone graft was removed. Sometimes, too, the graft doesn't take and the operation must be repeated.

Now, there are two types of fusion. Most lumbar fusions are done from the back and are called *posterior* fusions, as we noted. (See Figure 7–11, which shows the technique.) But there are also *anterior* fusions, in which the bone graft is placed either between the vertebral bodies or across the vertebral body, and the incision is made in front of the body (the abdomen).

The anterior has certain mechanical advantages over the posterior, but it carries higher risks. Blood clots are more apt to form in the major vessels supplying the pelvis and legs. Males

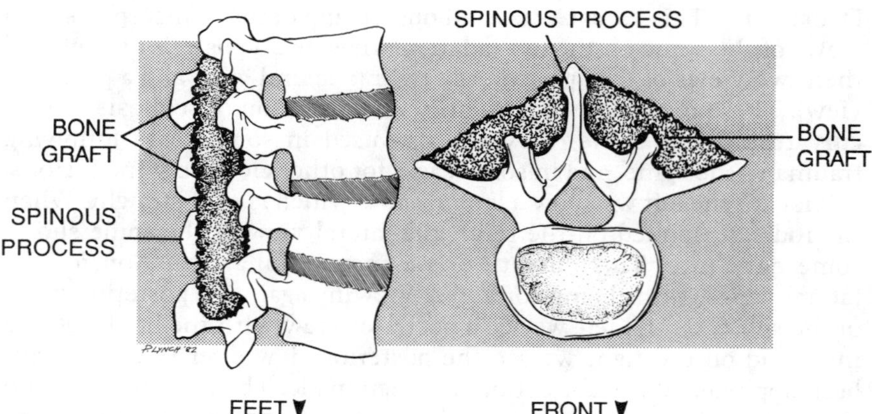

FIGURE 7–11 This shows two views of a posterior spinal fusion. Three disc spaces have been fused here. Usually only two disc spaces are included in a fusion. Our able illustrator is a more aggressive surgeon than the writer. The picture on the right shows an axial, or horizontal, plane view of the fusion—with the bone graft material posterior. This is the view one studies of the spine with a CAT scan. There are several variations of this surgical technique, but this is the basic idea.

run a very low risk, roughly 0.4 percent, of impotence or sterility if the nerves in the sacral plexus, which govern ejaculation, are damaged. Females are spared reproductive complications. Finally, gastrointestinal events may suffer transient interference several days after surgery. All these complications seem to hark back to the surgeon's frontal approach to the vertebral bodies. By the way, there is a technique for performing an interbody fusion from the back. This operation is known as the PLIF (Posterior Lumbar Interbody Fusion). However, the experience with this is not extensive enough to fully know its advantages and disadvantages. In my opinion, there are not enough advantages to this operation to justify the additional risks that it incurs. If you're a spinal fusion candidate, discuss all the options with your surgeon.

Before the following summary, you deserve to know about some of the complications that can ensue from the use of metal implants. There is the possibility of nerve damage or irritation associated with both of the devices previously discussed. The probability of infection is greater than with spine fusion without metal implants. Finally, for a variety of reasons it may be necessary to have an operation to remove the hardware. If internal fixation is recommended it may be quite appropriate. You should understand why and that the incremental risks are justified by sufficient benefits.

SURGERY FOR LOW BACK PAIN AND SCIATICA: SUMMARY

The discussion you've just waded through is extremely complex, so let's review the main points briefly.

Key Material or Indications for Most Common Low Back Operations

1. The surgery is elective, almost like cosmetic surgery. Its purpose is to improve the quality of life, not save your life. You don't *have* to do it. Your big question: Is the reasonable expectation of pain relief worth the risks?
2. If you're losing control of your bladder and have increasing leg weakness, we're no longer talking about elective surgery. You need urgent surgery.
3. If you think you want surgery, the longer you wait after two or three months of properly treated backache, the more you may dim your surgical prospects. We're speaking only of

selected, thoroughly diagnosed conditions that call for surgery.

4. If you're having disc surgery, know that it can help both your back and leg pain; however, you can expect most reduction to be in your leg pain.
5. You generally don't want to automatically have a fusion with disc surgery. If there is a good, clear reason to do so, your surgeon will explain it so that you can *understand* and *agree.*
6. In properly evaluated patients with disc disease, surgery is ninety to ninety-five percent successful.
7. When there is spondylolisthesis or some other cause of significant painful motion between vertebrae, spinal fusion should be considered, and on occasion there may be an *understandable, justifiable* indication for internal metal fixation.

SURGERY FOR SPINAL STENOSIS

Before we discuss surgery for spinal stenosis, I would like to emphasize a couple of points. First, this is a pretty important disease. It's important because it affects mainly our senior fellow humans, and there are happily quite a few of them and a lot more coming. The disease is fairly common among those sixty-five or older. The exact prevalence, to my knowledge, is undetermined. Now, the other point that is important before discussing surgery is that of nonsurgical treatment. For the sake of emphasis I've provided a conservative treatment checklist, see page 65.

As we've explained, spinal stenosis is a condition in which there is too little space in the spinal canal. Sometimes a person is simply born with an abnormally narrow spinal canal. Other times bony changes in the back of the vertebral bodies or in the posterior vertebral joints (the facet joints) may crowd the canal. A herniated disc or a bulging yellow ligament can contribute to stenosis, too. Finally, several diseases can compromise that space.

What does surgery accomplish? Any and all structures impinging on the nerves within the canal—and causing pain, weakness, or discomfort—can be removed surgically. The prognosis for patients having surgery for spinal stenosis is quite good: About eighty-five percent of patients have a good or an excellent result. Beforehand, radiographic studies, like a myelogram, CAT scan, or MRI, can generally unmask the identity of the encroaching structure. Then, the surgeon opens the spine from the back, usually removing the lamina and the spinous processes and sometimes a part (but rarely all) of the paired facet joints at one or more levels—i.e., L2–L3, L3–L4, etc.—of the spine. See Figure 8–1, page 224, for numbering of vertebrae. You can get a good sense of what is removed by a study of Figure 7–2. Here there is removal of lamina on just one side. For spinal stenosis, the spinous process would be removed as well as the lamina on the other side. This would then be done at as many levels as the imaging studies showed to be constricted, taking as much as needed of the facet joint to relieve encroachment. Sometimes part of the disc is excised, too. Depending on the patient's age, the extent to which important structures have been dismantled, and the surgeon's judgment, a fusion may be done to lock the spine in one position and prevent its displacing. The likelihood of displacement is proportional to the amount of bone and other anatomic structures that had to be removed to relieve the spinal stenosis.

Dear reader, if you're an elderly person with a documented case of lumbar spinal stenosis and you've tried conservative treatment without success, here's my suggestion to you. If your pain and difficulty in walking is such that you're losing your independence and are not able to socialize and otherwise enjoy life, consider the following: Unless you have some major illness that your physician thinks will make you an inordinate anesthesia risk, I suggest you explore the idea of surgery, which offers you about an eighty percent chance of improvement and perhaps as good or better a chance of keeping you from getting even worse. My point is that, barring major illness, your age alone is no reason not to give yourself a good chance to improve and/or preserve good quality of life. A reasonably healthy elderly person with lumbar spinal stenosis should not wait around to get worse and worse while assuming that he/she is too old to have surgery.

SURGERY FOR INFECTIONS

Infections of the spine can cause considerable back pain. Sometimes antibiotics alone can wipe them out, but surgery may be necessary. For example, there may be an abscess (a pocket of pus) or an area of chronic osteomyelitis (a region of infected bone, some of which is dead and some alive, with bacteria or fungus growing in it).

Surgery is performed to evacuate the abscess, remove the infected bone, and wash out many of the germs with sterile solutions containing antibiotics.

According to the circumstances, the surgeon may elect to perform some kind of fusion during this operation. Or he/she may clean out the infection first and carry out the fusion later. Each patient's problem is highly individual from the perspective of surgery and reconstruction. But the basic surgical principles are: to decompress the abscess; to remove enough bone to cure the infection while preserving as much of the spine elements as possible; then to use bone graft to fuse and reconstruct the spine.

SURGERY FOR TUMORS

To recapitulate Chapter II, when low back pain is caused by a bone tumor, its treatment depends on whether or not the tumor has originated there (a primary tumor) or has migrated from elsewhere (a metastatic tumor). When the tumor is primary, much will hinge on whether it's benign or malignant. Sometimes, metastatic tumors are better treated with radiation or chemotherapy, but surgery also sometimes offers benefits. This is particularly true when the tumor is very painful and aggravated by movement of the spine, or if the tumor is growing close to the nerves.

A tumor originating in the spine, with or without nerve involvement, is the most likely candidate for surgery. Here the principles governing infection apply again, except that the surgical challenge and risks are raised a notch or two. That's because the surgeon's mission is to eradicate *all* the tumor, plus an appropriate margin of normal spine. A great deal of spine may need to be removed, and a radical procedure employed.

Reconstruction

In this case, the spine may be rebuilt with bone graft, metal, and sometimes with a prosthetic replacement. The latter may be developed with *polymethyl methacrylate,* an implantation cement used in total joint replacement and spine surgery. This sort of extensive spine operation should be performed at centers with special expertise in spine surgery.

I'd like to reiterate here that malignant tumors that originate in the spine are extremely uncommon, so please don't start attributing every backache to cancer.

SURGERY FOR INJURIES

Most moderate spine fractures heal without very serious pain. Surgery for old fractures is probably unnecessary unless there's severe pain and the fracture can be reasonably identified as the culprit. Many surgeons first immobilize the patient in a body jacket as a trial. If the pain lessens, spine fusion can be expected to help. A posterior fusion is usually adequate, affording considerable relief.

What about recent injury? This is a complex and murky area and you should consult your surgeon about your individual needs and condition. Unless the vertebrae are extensively damaged, surgery isn't generally advisable. But if there *is* severe vertebral damage, especially in the lower spine, and associated neurologic problems (with fragments of bone in the spinal canal), the trend in recent years is to remove the bone from the spinal canal, immobilize the spine with metal implants (there are several types; see Figures 7–7, 7–8, 7–9, 7–10), and perform a spinal fusion. These rods are attached to the normal spine above and below the injury. They help to hold the spine in place while it heals.

NERVOUS SYSTEM SURGERY FOR LOW BACK PAIN

This surgery "interrupts" various parts of the nervous system in the hopes of alleviating low back and leg pain. We're really talking about a special class of salvage surgery, in my opinion, as these procedures have the same bleak odds.

The rationale? If you have pain in your back or legs, you can "turn off" the pain by cutting the nerve or the dorsal root ganglion, the site where the sensory part of the nerves from the back and limbs enter the spinal cord. The idea is that the sensation of pain can no longer be transmitted to the spinal cord and brain if the nerve has been severed.

Tractotomy

After the nerves enter the cord via the dorsal root ganglion, they travel up what is called the spinal thalamic tract to the brain. This tract, which can be quite well localized within the cord, can itself be cut in a procedure called a *tractotomy,* again with the goal of pain relief. These procedures are rarely done nowadays.

Rhizotomy

Cousin to the family of treatments that involve nerve interruptions is another back treatment called *rhizotomy.* By destroying the nerves around the intervertebral joints, the reasoning goes, you can deaden the pain that's presumably emanating from the joints. The nerves are eradicated either by direct surgical intervention or by a radio-frequency technique.

The tissues in the region around the facet joints where the nerves lie are electrically cauterized (seared). Temperatures of seventy to eighty degrees centigrade are achieved, which destroy the nerves and prevent transmission of pain.

Unhappily, rhizotomy hasn't been shown to be any better for backache than Mother Nature's own handiwork. In other words, my opinion is that it offers very little.

Why? Isn't it plausible that once the pathways to the brain are eliminated pain would no longer be felt? Yes, but it works out poorly in practice. Sometimes there's transient relief, followed by a recurrence of pain that is often more severe. The scarring and inflammation that surgery brings with it can leave the patient worse off than before. My impression is that these operations are performed rarely, and that's the way it ought to be—insofar as backache and sciatica are concerned, at least.

SALVAGE LOW BACK SURGERY

The term sounds like something the sanitation man picks up. But it refers to a patient who has had two or more operations for spine pain and is back for another. If you detect a subtle note of pessimism, you're absolutely correct. There's nothing more disheartening and sad than the all-too-common multiple-scar collector who suffers the dolorous cycle of spine pain, spine surgery, more spine surgery, more spine pain, more surgery, and so on, up to twenty or more operations.

The statistics are disheartening. After one operation, the chances of success from a second is thirty percent. The odds of the third dip to fifteen percent; of the fourth, to five. I might add that the fourth operation's success odds are equal to its prospects of making you worse. Some studies suggest that even the third operation has a reasonable chance of making you worse.

Having duly made my dreary forecasts, let me note that there are *extremely rare* circumstances that make salvage surgery a reasonable option. A specific cause of backache may be diagnosed and documented that a particular surgical procedure can alleviate. These are cases where spinal stenosis recurs, a disc herniates, or there's a well-diagnosed painful pseudoarthritis of the spine (when all or part of a fusion fails to take, leaving the spine painful and unstable). Perhaps I should add that a highly motivated patient who has had several back operations without fusion may benefit from a spinal fusion if the proper indications are present. Otherwise, additional surgery leads to a dismal outcome.

I recommend that any salvage spine surgery be carried out in a center that has spine-care specialists. It should never be done without a thorough psychiatric evaluation, as neurotic patients and "Poor Souls" have extremely depressing success rates from salvage operations. A second opinion is a must before having that third incision.

ON THE HORIZON ARTIFICIAL DISC

I don't know when I'll have the pleasure of doing this book for you again. Nevertheless, there's a chance that by the next edition prosthetic discs will be in use. At present they are considered experimental.

A prosthetic intervertebral disc is shown in Figure 7–12. It's a topic that has fascinated both patients and biomedical researchers for over twenty years. Patients ask, "Well, if the disc is the problem, isn't there something that can be put in there to replace it?" Surgeons and other researchers have experimented in the laboratory with a variety of materials and devices. As far as I am aware, the first published series of patients with artificial discs implanted comes from East Berlin. Professor Zippel there has implanted artificial discs of the type shown in Figure 7–12 in well over fifty patients. This is an intriguing new prospect. I suspect that we'll be well into the 1990s before any such device is used in North America. If you've read this and the preceding

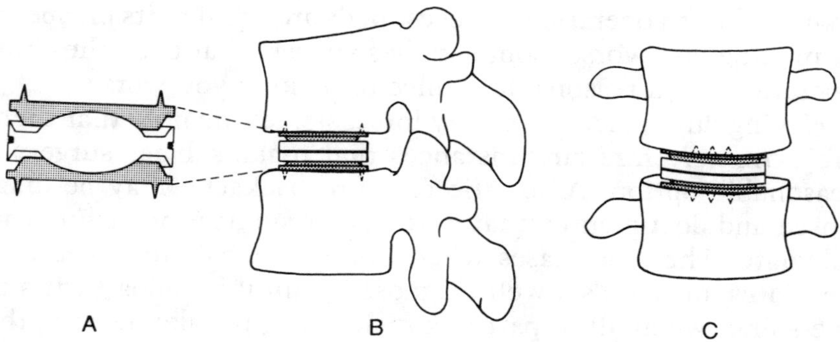

FIGURE 7–12 A) Shows a prosthetic intervertebral disc. This is probably the one used most in human patients. This device is made up of a plastic bicovex disc that articulates with a concave metal component on each side of the plastic disc. The metal components on either side of the plastic disc are imbedded into the vertebral bone above and below the disc space. B) Shows a view from the lateral perspective. C) Shows a view from a frontal perspective. (Reproduced with permission from White, A.A., and Panjabi, M.M.: *Clinical Biomechanics of the Spine,* J.B. Lippincott, 1990, second edition.)

chapter you can surely anticipate my closing suggestion on this: the advisability of having a new surgical procedure. Make certain that there is ample evidence that the added risks are fully justified by good evidence of significant benefits that will accrue to you. In other words, that your condition will be improved in a major fashion.

SOME SUGGESTIONS FOR POSTSURGICAL REHABILITATION

Comments from patients who read an earlier edition of *Your Aching Back* have been very helpful. This section was written in direct response to a request by a patient who observed, "One thing that you don't have any advice about is how to look after yourself following surgery." My theme for you after surgery is the same as it was before surgery: Do what you're supposed to do, be patient, and you will gradually get better.

Postoperative care really begins when you and your surgeon form a "bond," a "partnership," or a "team," and set as your goal your ability to get back to work on your pre-back-pain life and "have some fun." Remember that wonderful clause in the Declaration of Independence: ". . . that all men [people] are created equal and are endowed with the unalienable rights, that among these are life, liberty, and the pursuit of *happiness* [have fun]."

One additional component of preoperative and postoperative care is that the patient be knowledgeable about low back pain, anatomy, biomechanics, surgery, etc. This can be done by going to a "back school" or reading a good book on low back pain.

The basic rule is to follow your surgeon's advice. I will offer some general comments that may be of value. Please remember: If in doubt or if in conflict, follow *your* doctor's advice. No matter how we consider it, *your* surgeon knows *you* and *your* back infinitely better than I. In case you have no guidelines, I will provide some general points about postoperative rehabilitation.

We believe in the *liberal* use of pain medications to keep patients comfortable during the first few days after surgery. Especially during the first forty-eight hours, sometimes doctors and nurses may underutilize painkillers for fear of addicting patients. We don't worry about this. When someone is having postsurgical pain we provide what it takes to control the pain, and we know that this will not cause addiction. We even offer a system that allows patients to control the painkillers—yes, they medicate themselves as needed. We like to see the patients sitting up, standing, or walking a few yards, if possible, within the first forty-eight hours after surgery. There are some patients who for a variety of reasons should not or cannot be up that soon. Patients who have general anesthesia are strongly encouraged not to smoke. This is to cut down on developing problems with the lungs, such as pneumonia. We also encourage patients to try and drop the habit completely, as this can add several years to one's life. It's also important that the patient use an inspirometer (a bedside device. There is a mouthpiece, a tube, and a verticle volume indicator. The patient puts the mouthpiece in place and breathes in as rigorously as possible. The volume of air so inspired is measured on the indicator.) with the utmost of confidence for the first three or four days after surgery. We tell our patients that this is the most important thing they can do for themselves after surgery. This too helps to avoid postoperative lung problems.

We'll divide patients into three broad groups and discuss each. The three groups are a) routine discectomy or percutaneous discectomy; b) routine lumbar spine fusion without fixation and with fixation; and c) miscellaneous complex and reconstructive procedures.

Routine disc procedure patients are handled in the following manner: The percutaneous patients will go home either the day of the procedure or the next day. The patients with surgical discectomy usually leave the hospital on the fourth or fifth day after their operation. This group is advised as follows. Avoid prolonged sitting—that is, more than fifteen to twenty minutes. When sitting, the use of a *reclined* chair is preferable. Avoid bending, twisting, and lifting. Begin gentle walking inside or outside and gradually increase that as tolerated. After two weeks, stationary bicycling or gentle swimming as tolerated can begin. For the next four weeks patients are encouraged to continue any combination of gradually increasing amounts of walking, bicycling, or swimming. If more than minor pain in the back or the leg occurs and persists, the activity should be reduced to a better-tolerated level. Six weeks after surgery, management is more individualized, according to progress, occupation, motivation, sports, hobbies, etc.

The patients who have spine fusions with internal fixation may get out of bed the second or third postoperative day depending upon the fixation and the surgeon's opinion. The rest of the routine is similar to the discectomy patient's except that the progress is slower, extended for a much longer time (three to six months) and may include the wearing of a cast or brace.

If, however, there is no internal fixation, this is what we do. (Please understand: There are several different programs here that are acceptable, although quite different.) For patients with low back fusion operations in which no internal fixation is used, I think it is best to keep patients in bed for five to seven days; then a cast is applied. This cast goes from the nipples down to the hip, and includes one thigh (the patient usually decides, with our help), down to but not including the knee. This "extra length" or immobilization of one hip is required in order to control the spine. The goal is to hold the spine and fusion mass (bone graft) still for early healing. The cast is worn five to six weeks, which is the time required for mature fibrous tissue healing. The patient is back to see us after the next six to seven weeks, the cast is removed, and the exercise program is begun. This involves gradually increasing some combination of walking, biking, and swimming. It generally takes six months to a year for a lumbar spine fusion to heal.

Two questions that may be on your mind. The first: "What about removing the stitches?" The answer is as follows. Your surgeon uses absorbable sutures (we do), so they don't have to be removed, or the stitches are removed about two weeks after surgery. The second: "What about physical therapy rehabilitation and the like?" Again, lots of legitimate variation of opinions here. With a patient who is cooperative and understands what's going on, little in the way of special programs are needed. For a variety of other reasons some such program may be necessary. An obvious example is some useful form of a work-hardening program. (See page 170.)

RECAPITULATION OF MAJOR TREATMENT OPTIONS FOR ASSOCIATED BACK AND LEG PAIN

The following table summarizes the major therapeutic options for low back pain and leg pain. The various treatment modalities have been discussed individually in this and the two preceding chapters. To follow is a brief explanation of the table.

Column one: Recommended. There is good evidence that these treatments a) work, and b) are cost-effective, both in terms of risk/benefit to the patient and in terms of monetary and time expenditure versus therapeutic value. The listing presumes adequate diagnosis and indication for treatment (especially in the case of the surgical procedures). It also presumes that the treatments are appropriately executed.

Column two: Optional. These treatments may or may not be helpful, but the risks to the patients are minor and the time and money expended is not great. This deserves some additional comment. A patient should not have spinal manipulation if there is clinical evidence of even a small disc herniation. One should not repeat a given treatment extensively (not more than two or three times) if it is not obvious that the treatment is beneficial.

Column three: Not Recommended. The risks/benefits are not reasonable (chemonucleolysis) or the cost-effectiveness is not appropriate (chairs, beds, etc.).

SUMMARY TABLE

Recommended	*Optional*	*Not Recommended*
Bed rest forty-eight to seventy-two hours (study this book)	Heat or ice and massage	Vibrating chairs and beds
Aspirin, other anti-inflammatories	Special mattress	
Exercise	Corset, brace, cast	Chemonucleolysis
Appropriate seat: car, office, home	Seat accoutrements, standing desk	Implant artificial disc (more research needed)
Back school	Traction	
Work hardening		
Percutaneous discectomy	Spinal manipulation (some risks)	
Formal surgical discectomy	Acupuncture, TENS	
Lumbar spine fusion and/or decompression	Trigger point injection	
	Epidural steroids (some risks)	

Chapter VIII

Sex and the Aching Back

IF YOU have backache but no sexual problems, don't read this chapter at all. I'm serious about this; if you are not aware of any problems in this area then I don't want you to read this chapter and start thinking up problems for yourself. However, if you do have some problems, you have plenty of company, and a careful study of this chapter will give you some help.

I've done clinical work with spine problems for twenty-nine years, and only a handful of patients have ever asked about guidelines for sex during low back pain or sciatica episodes. How odd. Recently I've included the question, "Do your back or legs hurt when you have sexual intercourse?" in my patient questionnaires. A significant number of people answered yes. I now take more initiative in discussing sex with patients. Obviously, many low back patients who are experiencing difficulties with this rewarding form of human activity don't feel comfortable querying their doctors about it. And despite all the lovemaking manuals on display everywhere, little literature has been devoted to making love with a bad back. And so this chapter is born.

For starters, I'd like to share with you a patient's letter. Though I've abridged it somewhat, and changed certain names and identifying details, it speaks eloquently for many a low back pain sufferer.

> Dear Dr. White,
>
> I used to have an antidote for being under the weather: Get up, get moving, get busy, and everything will be all right. This worked for colds, pregnancy, nausea, sore throat, men-

strual cramps, the flu, etc., but not for low back pain. I'd trade a month of the flu for relief of my back problems.

As I lie here, I hear a crash and ensuing tears. I know one of the babies has fallen in the tub and I cannot move to soothe her, hold her, and wipe away the tears. Incidents such as these occur all day. Demands are placed on me continuously and I cannot respond. My mind responds, my body cannot. Arlene no longer comes to me when she falls. She knows I cannot pick her up. In her feverish state this week, she ran to Marian, our baby-sitter, for comfort. Marian brought her to my bed, but she didn't want to be with me. She knew I could not walk with her and hold her.

Susan smiles on me all day, comes to the bottom of the stairs and calls "Momma" if I'm up here. When I'm on the sofa she comes over and nuzzles me, filling my face with kisses. But Susan does not come to me when she is thirsty, hungry, or tired. Babies know who meets their needs and who doesn't.

Jane demands to see my incision to check my progress. It's visible evidence to a four-year-old that something tangible has been accomplished. She verbalizes, "*When* will you be better? *When* will you drive me to school?"

My husband expresses his aggravation with his short temper. This is a man who always relied on me, and now our roles are reversed. He's always trying to encourage me to get well, be happy, etc., but finds life pretty tough right now. Every now and then there is an outburst: "I'm tired this weekend, but how would you know what it's like to be tired? You're always in bed."

I guess it's all I can expect from a man who has lost an exciting sex life, has given up his social life (he won't go without me), has been under financial strain, has had his privacy taken away . . . and does not have the haven of a well-kept, well-organized home and family life after a long and arduous work week.

People—neighbors, family, "friends"—are tired of seeing me in a helpless, supine position. So am I. I tell everyone what a wonderful job they're doing so they will keep coming, tell my husband and children everything will be all right, and then, because I'm so helplessly frustrated and angry and distressed, I drown myself in music, books, and writing, and cry myself to sleep so that I can sanely face the next day with a smile.

I always face each day with a smile. I love the morning, to walk, go out, play with the children. I was so happy with my life, with myself and my accomplishments . . . but somehow I don't feel quite so good about myself now.

I cannot care for my family and my home. I cannot shake this damn disability and related pain no matter how many weeks (God, it's really been months now) go by. I've had to give up my job counseling new mothers, and my consultations for the Lexington schools. How can one be terribly happy when all outlets are taken away?

Sex is really a painful loss. We used to have an active, innovative, and exciting sex relationship. Amazing—after living with one man for ten years. What a great way to share feelings and release tensions.

The most aggravating part of sexual deprivation is knowing how long it took to reach the stage of being free and passionate [having spent] too many innocent years and the first ignorant years of marriage. . . . To be deprived of it now is really unfair.

I need and want sex, but I'm afraid of hurting myself. Prior to surgery, really active sex aggravated my condition terribly. Passive sex ("let-me-know-when-it's-over" sex) is very possible. So are alternative, less direct ways of being close, but really active sex (with lots of muscle involvement and orgasm) was terribly difficult prior to surgery, rendering me unable to walk for several days. Positioning is crucial (whatever is comfortable is fine), and the level of involvement is also a major problem—I'm too afraid of being hurt.

We have become awfully good friends. I have always cherished this thought: A helpmate surpasses a lover, and loving kindness surpasses love, even passion. . . .

I am usually reliable, emotionally stable, and basically positive, but not having control over my life pains me. My body won't do what I want it to. I'm at everyone's mercy for help and care. My independence has been taken away and my positive self-esteem lowered. . . .

Dr. White, this excerpt is rather personal and verbose, but I have decided to share it with you because I feel you are discreet and humane. I trust you, and perhaps it might provide some useful insights for your ongoing study of spinal disorders and their effects. . . .

Sincerely,
C.D.

This letter from a normal, intelligent, well-adjusted housewife depicts the devastating side effects of a chronic back problem. C.D. was spiritually, intellectually, and materially wealthy, in my opinion, yet only marginally able to cope with her shattered life. Finally, she did conquer her bad back, largely because of her own determination. Surgical removal of a lumbar disc helped. So did mastery of the principles for lovemaking with a bad back.

In conversation, C.D. confided that fear of hurting her back distracted her during lovemaking and interfered with her orgasmic response. This was a patient who had many things going for her, including sexual openness, a positive attitude, a happy marriage, and considerable resources, both material and intellectual. How do you think a neurotic, repressed, or unhappily mated person would fare?

Sex is only one of the activities that may be cramped by chronic back pain, but because it's right up there on the list of trouble spots, it deserves its own chapter. So here we'll take what we know about the pathology and biomechanics of back pain and translate it into guidelines for lovemaking. We'll start by setting out the general principles, then follow them up with specific recommendations for men and women with low back pain and/or sciatica.

Pain, Emotions, and Sexual Gratification

I would submit to the reader that a fully satisfactory sex life is no small achievement even *without* backache. One study of "normal," well-educated, happily married couples runs counter to the presumed happily-ever-after sequels to Cary Grant–Ingrid Bergman movies (and to our own dreams). Even though eighty percent of these people considered their marital and sexual relations happy, there were manifold problems. Forty percent of the men had problems with either erection or ejaculation, and sixty-three percent of the women expressed difficulty in "turning on" or climaxing. Among another group of family-practice patients, fifty-six percent had at least one lovemaking impasse. The real world rarely meets our romantic expectations.

The reason I'm presuming to add a couple of paragraphs to the thousands of pages already written about sex is to make the point that sex problems are by no means simple. I don't have to tell you that back disease isn't easy. As we grapple with the compound problem of sex and backache, we do indeed have a challenge.

Though I'd prefer to extol the beauty of sex and lovemaking, that is not the purpose of this chapter. In order to be helpful, I must focus on the problem. So let me offer a simple categorization of two types of sexual problems.

One category is exemplified by the person who tends to avoid sex—but doesn't *want* to avoid it. This is usually a virile, sensual person who loves sex but feels frustration both for him/herself and his/her partner. There is often an element of guilt to round out this mental anguish.

The other category includes the person who tends not to avoid sex, but doesn't enjoy it either. The lack of pleasure is based on some combination of mental and physical pain. While back pain could be a reason preventing enjoyable lovemaking, a person may also feel used or "locked in" by sex and therefore fail to get pleasure from it. One can readily appreciate the complexity of the mental and physical problems when we consider that the characteristic avoider occasionally participates in lovemaking and the traditional participant sometimes avoids it.

Emotional problems such as stress or depression and/or medications involved with pain management may result in male impotence or premature ejaculation. A female may be handicapped by frigidity or an inability to enjoy sex because of *fear* of pain as well as *actual* pain. Our patient C.D. springs to mind.

There's an oft-circulated story about a patient who asked his distinguished hand surgeon just before his operation, "Doc, will I be able to play my piano after you operate on my hand?" The answer from the confident surgeon: "Why, of course you will." The patient replied gleefully, "That's great, because so far I haven't been able to play the piano for the life of me!" The same principle holds here. This advice doesn't speak to any preexisting sexual problems, not even those that get channeled into the "backache." On the other hand, if you follow the suggestions for open, honest discussion about sex as it relates to your back, helpful communication about other sexual problems may surface and add to your overall satisfaction.

SEX AND THE BAD BACK

Here we'll analyze the sexual problems that stem directly from backache.

A sexually well-adjusted person with a short-term, non-chronic backache is obviously the most easily treated. You need only use proper body mechanics so as not to irritate your back during sex. When your back is acting up, follow this chapter's recommendations closely. If you fit into this category, I must warn you against falling into an enduring sexual-avoidance pattern as a backache side effect. Once set in motion, our habits have a way of sticking with us.

Most of us want to please and be pleased by our lovers. When sex is very painful or impossible because of a back condition, several kinds of emotional turmoil eventually affect both partners. Without clear communication, misunderstandings build. For example, the pain-free partner may become less physically affectionate out of consideration for the lover's backache, but the disabled mate may interpret this as rejection, punishment, or loss of love. The disabled person may then react with guilt, depression, or hostility—which, in turn, may provoke rejection or hostility on the part of the "considerate" nondisabled lover. A vicious cycle starts, which candid communication could have avoided from the beginning.

Or the sexually disabled person can sink into depression, anxiety, guilt, or hostility, irrespective of the mate's behavior. Here a more profound adjustment problem may be rearing its head, and specific medical or psychiatric therapy may be what is needed.

Sexual Maladjustment and Backache

Then there's the situation in which a preexisting sexual problem is worsened or revived by backache. Obviously, an already marginal relationship will be significantly penalized by a sore back. And it's also possible that the disabled person will consciously or unconsciously use the backache to escape from or manipulate the lover, as in the "Sorry, I have a backache tonight, dear" syndrome. This behavior pattern can lead you down the dismal path of guilt, anxiety, hostility, and depression.

Short-Term Versus Chronic Disability

Of course, it makes a world of difference whether your backache is short- or long-term. Short-term, in the medical universe, means six weeks to six months. Long-term, or chronic, means longer than six months. A short-term back patient can think in terms of carefully following this chapter's guidelines on a temporary basis, while a chronically disabled patient must consider revamping his or her sex life indefinitely.

The sexually active couple faced with a long-term sexual disability must cope with a potentially very serious problem. Over the course of my practice I've been made aware of two divorces caused by prolonged sexual disability—on the part of the man in one case, the woman in the other. The pain-free lover simply couldn't stand the deprivation for months on end. In both cases, emotional strain, distrust, and hostility culminated in a definite split. How can you avoid such a drastic state of affairs?

STAYING SEXY WITH A BACK PROBLEM

Let's now lay down a step-by-step plan for a more satisfying sex life for the backache sufferer and his/her lover.

PELVIC POWER . . . USE IT OR LOSE IT

Step 1: The pelvis and its dynamic muscles are an integral source of sexual satisfaction. The woman's pubococcygeus (P.C.) muscle, stretching from front to back, forms the "pelvic floor." It thereby helps support the rectum, uterus, and bladder, controlling urine flow and vaginal contraction. Isometric exercises can strengthen and create voluntary control of the P.C., intensifying the enjoyment for both partners.

Exercise:

First locate the muscle. Simply practice tightening the muscle you would use to stop the flow during urination. Now you've found it.

While sitting or standing, contract the P.C. twenty-five to fifty times twice a day (it shouldn't hurt your back). You can do it standing at the checkout counter or driving your car (no one will know). A variation is to contract for ten seconds, then release, continue breathing normally, and repeat several times. During intercourse the P.C. will contract around the penis percussively—thus the pleasure of pelvic power!

Step 2: Begin with the doctrine that if you ever "had it good," you can have it just as good again with a back problem. Moreover, if you've never quite experienced connubial bliss, this is a good time to institute some gratifying changes. So we start with a *positive* attitude: "I know it's a challenge, but after reading this I'm going to make it better."

Step 3: Talk to your lover. This is probably the most important advice of all. You can be "subtle." Place a bookmark on this page and leave the book on your pillow, the bathroom sink, or on your lover's plate at the dinner table. Or employ a more direct approach. Try to discuss the problem in a warm, clear, frank, relaxed, compassionate manner. But you must start communicating . . . now!

Step 4: You and your loved one must approach the problem with a sincere attitude of cooperation, a commitment to give and take. The goal should be the *most* pleasure (physical and emotional) and the *least* pain (physical and emotional) for all concerned. You might even reread the preceding sentence, engraving it in your mind. Other fringe benefits may flow from a save-the-back approach to human sexuality, and we'll detail them later.

Step 5: Expand your attitudes as well as your mind and heart. Noncoital sexual activities can be mutually gratifying experiences of love. Many sexual rewards may emerge from broader attitudes and more creativity and communication about lovemaking.

> *Step 6:* Commit yourself to understanding and following the specific practical suggestions about positions for lovemaking as well as the other recommendations provided in this chapter. The material presented here is based on the best contemporary clinical and scientific knowledge of the spine. I've searched the literature on general sex problems and those related to backache, culling the best data from body mechanics and from my own experience in advising patients.

Let's face it, there may be some rare situations in which you and your lover conscientiously follow all the advice here and there is no success. Then you should go to Step 7, which is to discuss the issue with a physician knowledgeable about backache and consider the advisability of a marriage or sex counselor. But *take heart:* It's only the very unusual "loving backache" that won't be helped by carefully following the advice on the next few pages.

HOW TO MAKE LOVE WITH A BACK PROBLEM

For starters, if what you're doing hurts, you can grin and bear it as long as there's more grinning than bearing. If not, you shouldn't be doing it. If what you're doing doesn't conform to the guidelines given here, but doesn't hurt, enjoy. Secondly, be innovative. Trying different sorts of lovemaking activities (just so they don't irritate your back!) can convert your disability into a romantic and sensual exploration.

Now you're ready for the basic mechanical principles for reducing the stress on your lower back during lovemaking.

1. Don't bend forward *with the knees straight,* even if you're lying down, as this position puts tremendous forces on the lumbar spine. (A review of Chapter II might be helpful.) It also stretches the sciatic nerve, possibly irritating it. Bending the spine slightly forward is okay, as long as you bend your knees.
2. Avoid swayback (lordosis) of the low back. In the next chapter, you'll read about how extreme back arching hurts dancers' and athletes' spines. Lovers run similar risks. Arch-

ing the back makes the disc bulge toward the back and places much stress on the posterior structures of the spine, such as the facet joints. (Figure 8–1.) A straight or slightly flexed (forward) spine is always preferable to an extended, or lordotic, one.

3. Stay away from positions—like lying flat on your stomach or back with your hips extended straight—that stretch, stress, or load the psoas muscles running from the front of the lumbar spine to just below the hip joint. To the extent that you flex

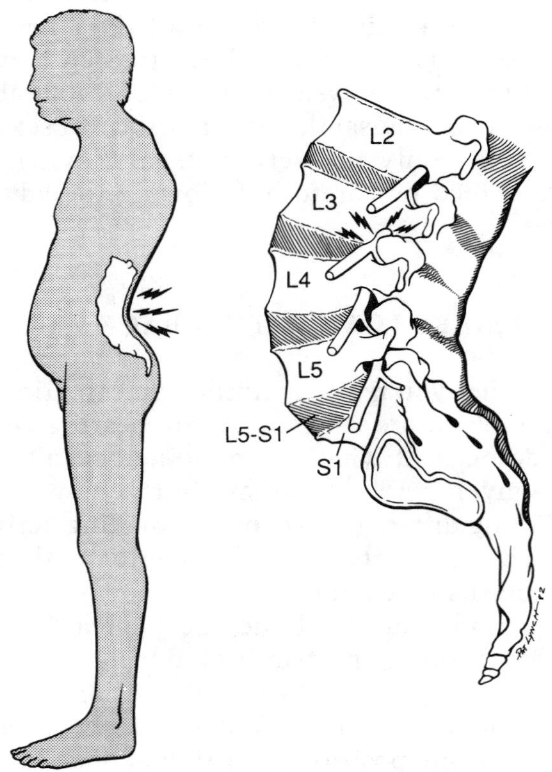

FIGURE 8–1 This important picture shows how a swayback or an extended lumbar spine does two things that are not likely to bring pleasure to the backache victim, even if he/she is making love. With this position the disc bulges posteriorly (upper sparks) between L3 and L4 and there are very large forces exerted on the facet joints (lower sparks) between L4 and L5, both of which can cause backache.

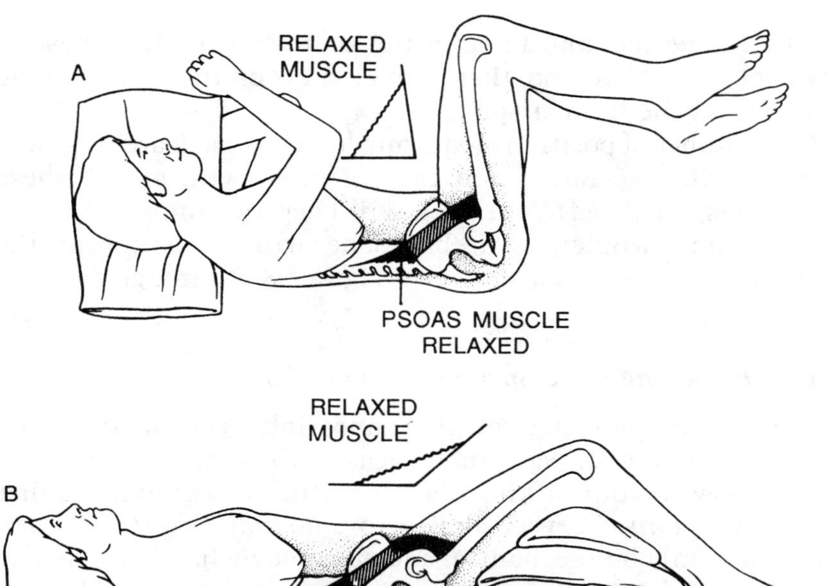

FIGURE 8–2 A) Lying on the side with hips and knees flexed relaxes the psoas muscle. B) Lying on the back with pillows or some other *support* for the legs, with the hips flexed, also relaxes the psoas muscle and the back. These principles are useful to think about for general back care and especially before lovemaking.

one or both hips, you relax those muscles and take the pressure off your lower back.

4. To the extent that you can flex (bend) your hips in a relaxed way you will protect your low back from irritation. (Figure 8–2.) This shows why the side-lying position and other hips-flexed positions are good.

Sexual Backache Care Specifically for Women

Start by assuming that the "missionary position" is probably painful to the lumbar spine if the woman chooses to be active. Why? Well, lying on your back and rotating the pelvis, either fore and aft or in a circular motion, extends the lumbar spine. To make matters worse, thrusting movements put demands on the abdominal and erector spinae muscles, which may be weakened and therefore uncomfortable in the acute or subacute phase of low back pain. Here, too, there is real stress on the psoas muscle and thus on the lumbar spine.

Any number of positions requiring lordosis (back arching) will also be irritating. But if you can get away with any of these maneuvers, go ahead. Your back will keep you informed.

In general, women with backache will do better in the positions of the women shown in Figures 8–3 through 8–6.

Sexual Backache Care Specifically For Men

Let me begin by asking you the impossible. You must temporarily suspend your ego, or at least mix your wisdom and creativity with your lurking macho attitudes. Bear in mind that you have a *temporary* disability to adjust to. Your bad back carries not only biomechanical and physiologic liabilities; it also has emotional side effects. Education and reassurance, plus the knowledge that your sexual problems are transient, should help.

All is not bleak. You may discover new patterns of sensuality. You may find that both you and your lover enjoy the novelty of your slightly more passive role. Remember, you're the same

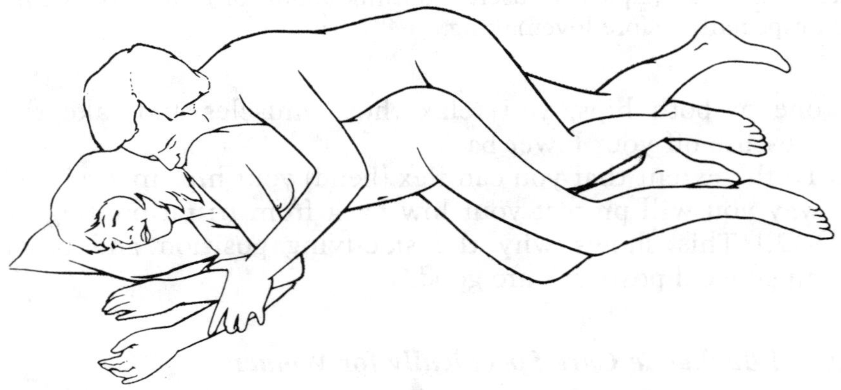

FIGURE 8–3 This is the basic first line of defense for the "loving backache" position. It's the best for the female or the male with back pain. Both partners have their hips and knees flexed. They are lying on their sides, so neither has to support his/her own body weight nor the weight of his/her loved one. The female should guard against getting into a swayback position here. This position is the one of choice if you want to make love in a fairly acute stage of backache.

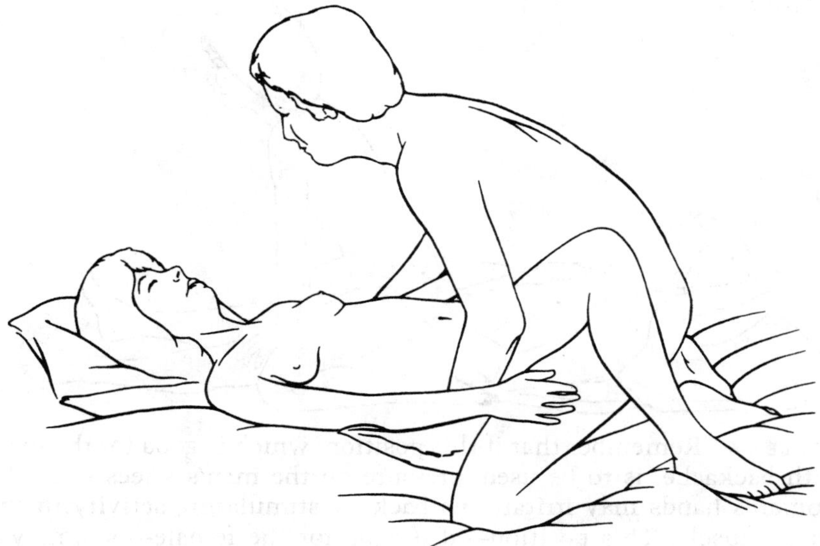

FIGURE 8–4 This position is good for the female with backache. It takes advantage of the principle described in Figure 8–2B. Care must be taken to support the woman's upper torso with pillows and her thighs with the male lover's thighs and arms.

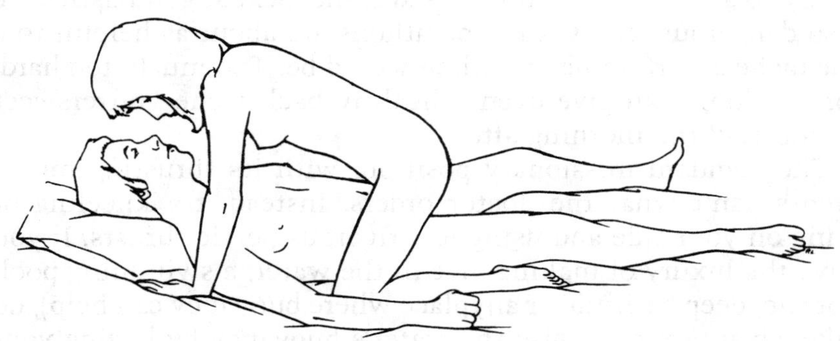

FIGURE 8–5 This position is good for the female with back pain. Like the male in Figure 8–3 her hips are flexed, she can avoid swayback, and she can support the weight of the upper torso on her hands.

This can also be a good position for the male shown here, should he have a backache. The upper torso should be slightly raised with a generous number of pillows so as to slightly flex the spine; and you must not be vigorous here, sir.

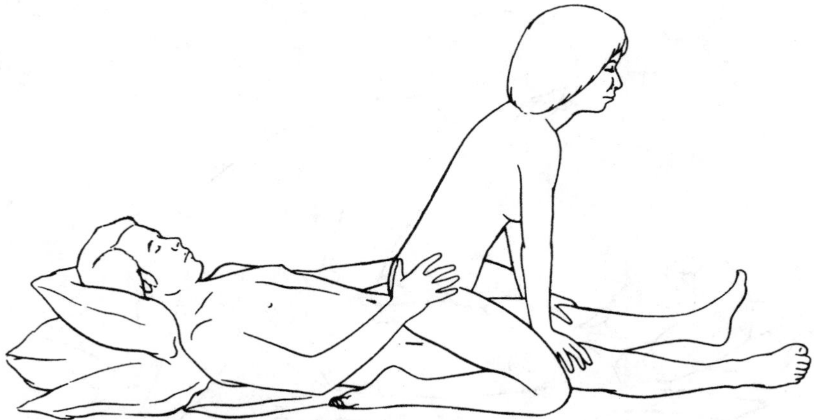

FIGURE 8–6 Remember that if this position, which is good for the male with backache, is to be used, pressure on the man's knees from the woman's hands may irritate his back by stimulating activity in the psoas muscle. This position—also good for the female—is simply a variation of Figure 8–5.

man you always were, but your back imposes some restrictions on your erotic athletics.

Be advised that the male's basic to-and-fro pelvic thrust is likely to aggravate a compromised spine. Sexual gymnastics are also dangerous, and sexual marathons are about as helpful to a backache as a running marathon would be. Too much, too hard, for too long, can give even a healthy back some "bittersweet memories" the morning after.

The standard missionary position, with its thrusting movements, isn't what the doctor orders. Instead, try kneeling or lying on your side and using less rigorous pelvic thrusts. If you have the luxury of making love in the water, a swimming pool, hot tub, deep bathtub, or anyplace where buoyancy can help), do take advantage of it. Use the water's buoyancy by having your feet flat on the bottom with hips and knees bent as in the sitting position. Your lover faces you and with the assistance of buoyancy sits on your thighs. Some additional positions suggested for the male are shown by the male in Figures 8–3 through 8–8.

There's another time-tested lover's formula that's as good for a bad back as for a robust one. I'm referring to what Lena Horne, in one of her songs, calls "Slow and Steady Wins the Race." It makes for graceful, athletic lovemaking that is good for your lover and for you. Your back will also appreciate it.

Sexual Positions That Respect the Back

A number of recommended positions for backache patients are illustrated in Figures 8–3 through 8–8. The drawings should speak for themselves, but the captions include some commentary that you should review carefully.

Use your ingenuity, as long as both partners are enjoying themselves without back pain. Admittedly, it's hard to be truly original in this ancient and profoundly expressive leisure activity, but who cares about authentic originality if a new variation pleases both of you? Remember, some of mankind's greatest discoveries have come about through trial and error.

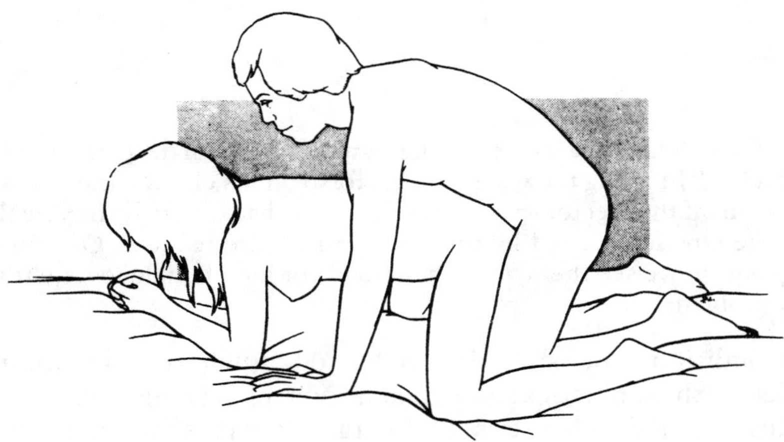

FIGURE 8–7 The position we find the male in here may be good for the male with back pain. The reason is that the hips are flexed and the male can and should support his upper torso using one or both hands resting on the bed or on pillows. Note that his back is slightly flexed, *not extended.*

A woman using this position may aggravate back pain if she is vigorously active, or if her lover puts too much weight on her. A variation that will help the woman with backache is to have both partners with their knees on the floor and the female's upper torso *fully supported* by a bed, couch, or chair.

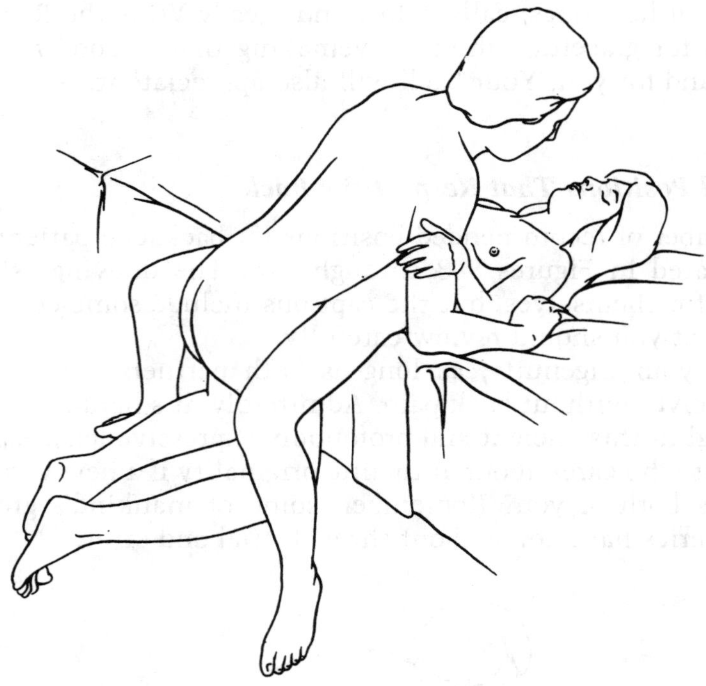

FIGURE 8–8 This is a position suggested for the male patient with backache. By resting the weight of the torso on his elbows, the stresses are taken off the erector spinae muscles in the back; also, by flexing the hips the stresses exerted by the psoas muscle are reduced. Of course, the position we see the woman in here is not for a female lover with a back problem.

In addition, you shouldn't have too much trouble finding books with sophisticated explanations of a range of sexual variations. This chapter's Bibliography lists some that may prove useful.

WHEN TO RESUME LOVEMAKING

Say you have to abstain from intercourse because of backache. When is it safe to go back into the bridal suite? First, some negative prescriptions. *Not* when you're still on complete bed rest and taking large amounts of pain medication. *Not* the very first day or night after you go off the preceding program. But one or two days after you've begun to feel better—when you can walk without much pain and require little or nothing in the way of painkillers—try a practice run. We refer to this as making love with the air, as you slowly try sexual maneuvers *without* your partner. If there's no pain, try it again with the air, a little more vigorously. Still no pain? Then try a dry run (still with the air) in one or two of the recommended positions. If you get a sore back, wait two days and resume the affair with the air. If you have no pain, break off the relationship with the air (with grace and kindness, as you may have to revive it). Now try gentle intercourse with your lover in one of the recommended positions. If it hurts too much, wait a day or two, touch base with the air again, and if there's no pain, try again with your partner.

Once you can make love without pain, or the pain is less than the pleasure and lasts no more than a few minutes afterwards, enjoy!

THE FINAL MESSAGE

Even if your backache has turned a once-exuberant sex life into infrequent, anxiety-ridden labor, don't give up. You may be able to put this chapter's guidelines to good use. A number of my patients—some of whom had virtually abandoned sex for months or years—already have, with success.

This isn't to say that life, with or without a sex life, is any picnic with backache, especially a chronic one. It's an uphill climb. But who knows? Your bad back may even translate into a rare opportunity for more sensitive, sensual, and communicative lovemaking.

Chapter IX

How to Avoid and Relieve Backache in Sports and Dance

WHY ARE athletes universally admired? After all, don't we reward our Olympic contenders, and even moderately successful Ivy League athletes, with high-paying corporate jobs? Don't professional athletes' salaries run ever more into the six figures—not including income from selling cologne, rental cars, razors, shaving cream, cereal, candy, televisions, and even alcohol? Savvy, powerful sixty-year-old men act like clumsy, excited kids in the presence of a twenty-year-old star athlete. And many people who can name all the Celtics, Bruins, Jets, or Pirates can't identify more than three Supreme Court justices, or three college presidents. How many heroes do we have, in contrast, among ministers, computer wizards, architects, or engineers?

Don't get me wrong. I too respect athletes. For better or worse, I probably spent as much time playing, practicing, and traveling as a member of my college football team as I did in the library.

But I would trace our adulation of athletes back to our more primitive hunting-and-gathering days. The strong man brought home bacon, literally, while the ninety-pound-weakling egghead-type couldn't protect family, village, or nation. Nowadays, of course, physical prowess doesn't count for all that much off the playing fields, and a physicist or mathematical genius can annihilate more of the enemy than all the finest warriors lumped together. Yet we still instinctively deify the athlete.

What does all this have to do with backache? Only that a glance at our societal reward system can give us insight into the athlete's consciousness and the way he or she copes with a physical problem.

First of all, athletes have hearty egos. It's not a good practice to prejudge human beings, but allow me a few generalizations here. Athletes are highly motivated, perhaps obsessively so. Because they use and train their bodies so vigorously, they're attuned to their most subtle twinge or twitch. Furthermore, they place very high, sometimes unrealistic, demands on their physical machine. So when it comes to back problems, athletes possess the *assets* of high motivation and a well-trained body, both of which would normally predispose one to "get well." However, there are the *liabilities* of heightened body sensitivity and the excessive physical demands that go with the trade.

Everything we've just said about athletes also applies to dancers, whose exquisitely trained bodies must meet equal or greater demands.

As a matter of fact, regarding endurance, strength, and flexibility, most serious dancers rank higher than most serious athletes. Dancers (professional and social types) rank very high in the forces they put into their lower spines.

Now where do athletes and dancers get into trouble, specifically?

Lifting

As we've said, those who do heavy labor are more prone to back trouble than insurance underwriters, and so are athletes, for the same reasons. The lumbar spine is the "workhorse" of the body. Remember that bending forward and lifting imposes heavy loads on the lumbar spine, especially if you do it the wrong way—that is, by bending at the waist without bending the legs. Male dancers, for instance, are at high risk. Pity the poor male dancer! When will choreographers "liberate" the ballerina, allowing her to catch a male dancer after a flying leap and walk around the stage carrying him?

Football players also incur lifting damage, and not just when blocking and tackling during the game. Did you ever think about the blocking dummies, the kind the coach stands behind during practice to see how hard you're really hitting? Gymnastics, rowing, and wrestling involve heavy lifting, too.

Twisting

One of this book's recurrent themes is that twisting motions are dangerous to your lumbar spine, and the deadly combo of twisting and lifting is even worse than just lifting. (Figure 9–1 explains why twisting can be a problem.) Baseball, bowling,

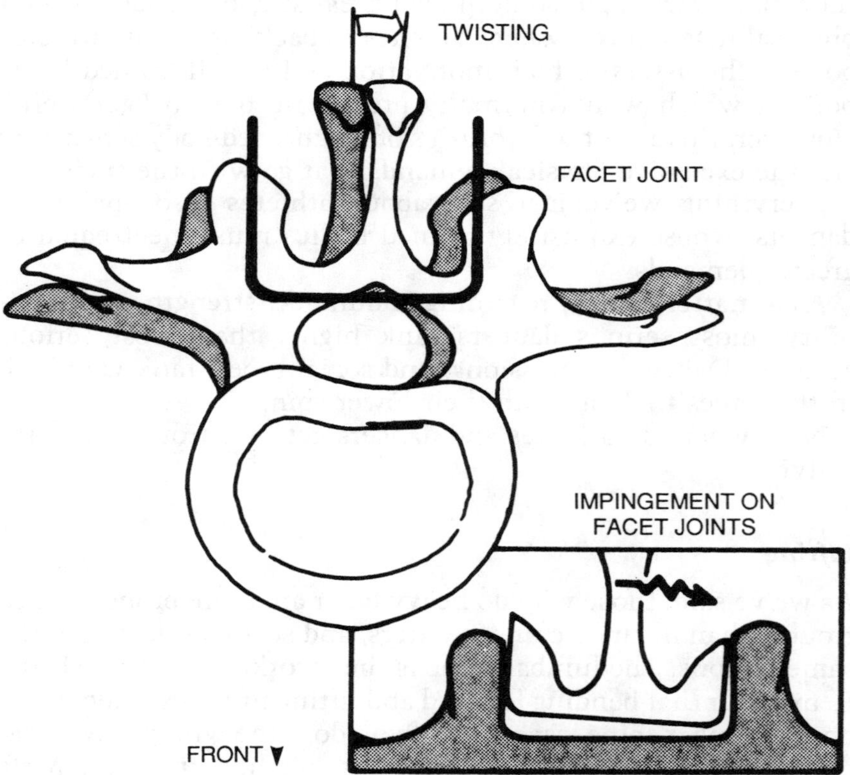

FIGURE 9–1 The facet joints in the low back are such that any twisting motion (axial rotation) may cause difficulty. After just a few degrees of axial rotation in the lumbar spine, there is impingement on the facet joints. This can result in irritation, injury, inflammation, and pain.

dancing, golf, gymnastics, hockey, lacrosse, sweep rowing, tennis, racquetball, squash, figure skating, and wrestling all involve some twisting. But of course much depends on the circumstances. You could twist your lumbar spine at a disco, dancing the twist to one of the oldies; or you could wrench your back by releasing a heavy bowling ball a little too late. Sometimes it's *how* you play, not what, that matters.

Besides having started in the African-American community and getting lots of play on television, what do the twist and break dancing have in common? Answer: They both can raise havoc with the back. I've discussed the twist and how it causes stress on the back by impinging on the facet joints (Figure 9–1). We should know that in break dancing, when one spins on the back, considerable bruising and painful irritation and even fracture of the spinous processes of the lumbar spine can occur. Happily, both dances are more or less "out of style." But it does alert us to pay attention to potential damaging activities to the low back and recognize that even popular social dances can take their toll on this powerful yet vulnerable region of the body.

Hyperextension

Another red flag for your back is the extensive lordosis ("swayback") of forceful hyperextension of the lumbar spine. If you're wondering what that means, picture how gymnasts, dancers, divers, and tennis players, when serving, arch their backs. Javelin throwing, pole vaulting, weight lifting (improperly done), swimming (butterfly or dolphin strokes), and wrestling (especially bridging) also involve a lot of back arching. So does pitching. You might be interested to know that contortionists who do lots of hyperextension suffer more spondylolysis—an anatomic gap in the back of a lumbar vertebra (see Figure 3–4)—than those who bend in the other direction.

Sports Injuries

There's no end to the variety of sports injuries. There are acute, specific injuries like fractures, and cumulative injuries, resulting from repeated damage. There are self-inflicted injuries and those inflicted by competitors. By the way, one of the least health preserving sports, boxing, more or less spares the back.

Acute injuries commonly crop up in connection with football, snowmobiling, tobogganing, and wrestling. Damage from repeated activity as well as acute injuries afflict bowlers, golfers, dancers, divers, football players, gymnasts, hockey players, rowers, weightlifters, and wrestlers. How do cumulative injuries happen? Well, usually lifting, twisting, or hyperextension is repeated until the bone breaks (it's called a fatigue fracture), a ligament or a disc fails, or you get wear-and-tear arthritis in a joint.

Now let me point out that sports can be *good* for you. Athletes usually have good muscle tone, or can develop it, and their bones and ligaments are stronger than those of more sedentary folk. Also, athletes' high motivation means they'll vigorously and conscientiously follow exercise programs and do everything possible to get well. But sometimes their zeal can be misdirected. We've all known jocks and jockettes who try to get back on the field (stage, court, rink, track, diving board) before their backs are ready—and reinjure themselves before adequate healing has taken place. This can lead to more serious problems.

RISKS OF DIFFERENT SPORTS

How does your favorite sport treat your back? What are its specific dangers? Is there anything you can do to protect your spine and keep on playing? Here I'll try to answer all your questions, sometimes with the support of epidemiological studies, sometimes from my clinical experience. To my knowledge, the backache risks of various sports have never been systematically compared in any one study.

Baseball

I'd rate it a medium-to-low-risk sport.

For starters, you have a straightforward twisting motion (axial rotation) as you swing that bat, and your contracting muscles exert large forces to accelerate the twist. (Figure 9–2.) At the moment of impact, the forces required to swing the bat must be high, because they're operating well away from the pivot point (your spine). Then the twist must stop at some point, whether or not you've made contact with the ball. And this sudden stop

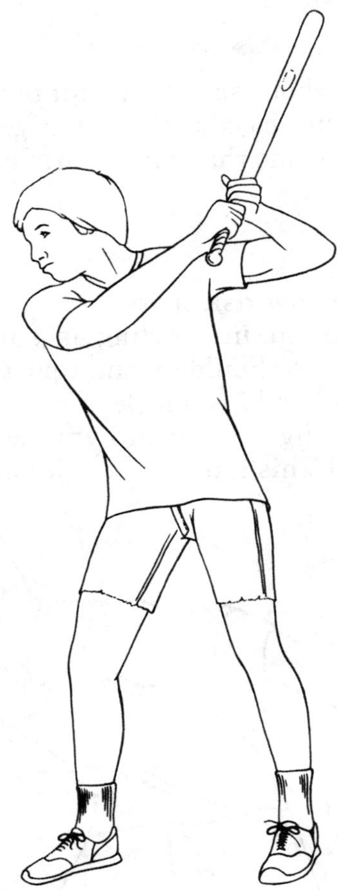

FIGURE 9–2 In going from this position to a full swing of the bat, the spine goes through considerable axial rotation (twist), which can be irritating or damaging to the disc or the facet joints.

applies pressure to both the disc and the spine's facet joints. The ensuing wear and tear can result in disc disease or arthritis of the spine. Or sometimes a particular motion, usually a swing and miss, can provoke back pain. Pitchers, who arch their backs extensively, run an additional risk. What can you do for your back if you're a baseball aficionado? First, concentrate on developing a smooth, even swing. Come out of it by decelerating gradually and twisting your hips and knees to absorb some of the twist. Don't use a bat that's too heavy for you. If you pitch, smooth out your technique, avoiding extreme arching.

Basketball

How can you write about sports and not mention the big round ball? Well, simply put, basketball players get backache, but the sport seems not to be one that particularly puts the back at risk.

Bowling

Another medium-to-low-risk sport.

The twisting motion in bowling is similar to batting in baseball. The bowler's shoulders and upper torso twist in one direction while his/her hips and legs twist the opposite way. He/she is also bent slightly forward with a heavy ball at arm's length. (Figure 9–3.) This motion provides an efficient mechan-

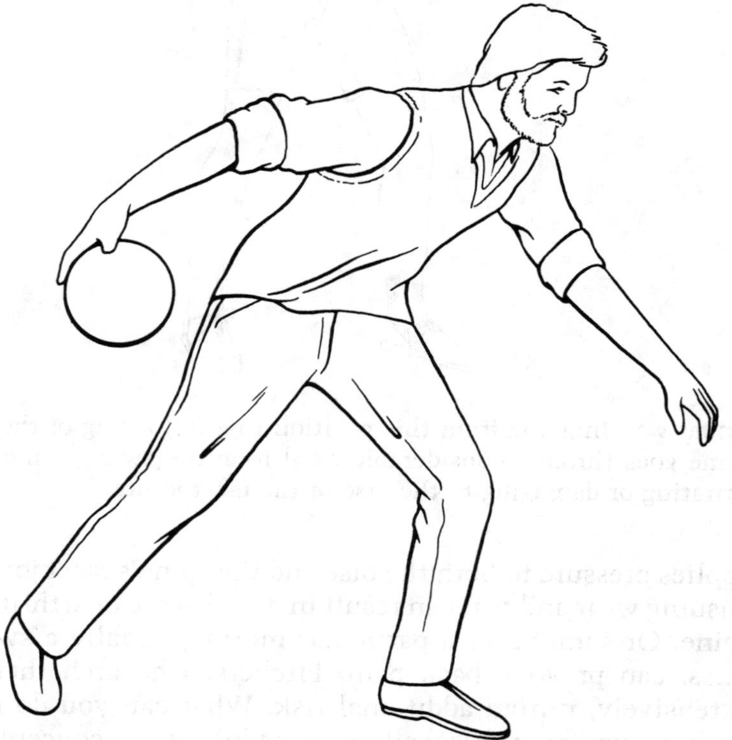

FIGURE 9–3 From this flexed starting position to the twisted release position there are considerable forces exerted on the spine. The forces are compression and shear, both of which can be damaging or irritating to the spine.

ical advantage—exerting very high loads on the spine and stressing the disc and facet joints.

You can protect your back by developing a good technique. Try for a smoothly accelerated delivery and avoid releasing the ball late, which transmits heavy stress to the spine and results in injury or excessive wear. Don't use too heavy a ball or one that doesn't fit your fingers. The latter can cause a jerky delivery, a delayed release, and a sore back.

Cycling

This sport is generally not devastating to the back-pain-prone athlete. In fact, it's a good option for the jogger. It provides the leg exercise, the cardiopulmonary stimulation, and the change of scenery of jogging, but without the repeated impact-loading. It also has the advantage of being a bedroom sport, if you use an Exercycle.

Dance

Medium-risk, depending on the kind of dancing.

I won't attempt to separately classify classical ballet, modern dance, jazz ballet, slow dancing, and folk dancing, but of course some are more dangerous to your spine than others.

The women's movement notwithstanding, the male dancer's back bears the brunt of the action. It has been noted that there are more low back problems among ballet dancers than among modern or jazz ballet dancers. The dancer can't very well lift the ballerina according to the best biomechanical principles. How often would you go to the ballet if the male dancer lifted his partner by firmly planting his feet on the floor, squatting slowly in front of her, keeping his back straight and his buttocks placed on his heels, wrapping his arms around her knees, and grunting? While you're deciding, let me say that few choreographers have planned it that way.

The ballerinas still go flying through the air, to be caught at chest level by the male, or they're lifted high overhead while both dancers arch their backs gracefully. I'm assuming that the lovely creatures being lifted rarely weigh more than one hundred twenty pounds and are jumping like hell to help their partners. Still, even fifty pounds, improperly lifted, can mean the imposition of forces four or five times heavier on the lumbar spine. This clearly puts the back at risk.

The dancer's risks relate to back arching and various pelvic motions that impart twisting and flexion to the lumbar spine. Naturally, these pelvic movements account for much of dance's sensual and aesthetic appeal, and I wouldn't want to tamper with them. But dancers pay a price in wear on the disc and other structures, and in injuries from the muscle forces required to start, stop, or modulate movements to fast, complex rhythms. You'd have to do a lot of bowling, golfing, or baseball playing to swing your hips as forcefully and frequently as a performing dancer.

How can you save your back if you dance? Good conditioning, pacing yourself in rehearsals, and cutting down on routines that obviously hurt your back can help. If a particular routine is causing a lot of backache in the troupe, perhaps the dancemaster or dancemistress could be persuaded to drop or change it. This advice won't win me a place on the board of trustees at Juilliard, but it's good preventative medicine. I'm assuming a well-trained dancer has already developed optimum muscle control, strength, and suppleness. There's nothing more I can suggest to help your body do what it *wasn't designed to do.* We appreciate and enjoy your contribution—just be careful.

A precautionary note—beware new social-fad dances. Think about them, apply the principles, and decide for yourself whether or not the dance may aggravate your back. Remember the "twist" and "break dancing?" Well, neither was a friend of the low back.

Diving

Medium-risk.

The main danger in diving comes from arching the lumbar spine as the diver snaps in and out of the dive's various maneuvers. (Figure 9–4.) Hitting the water wrong—jacknifing the lower torso into a hyperextended position as the upper torso is being decelerated by the water—can also hurt your back. Acute injury or progressive wear of the spine's posterior elements can result. Repeated wear can cause spondylolisthesis. (See Figure 3–4.)

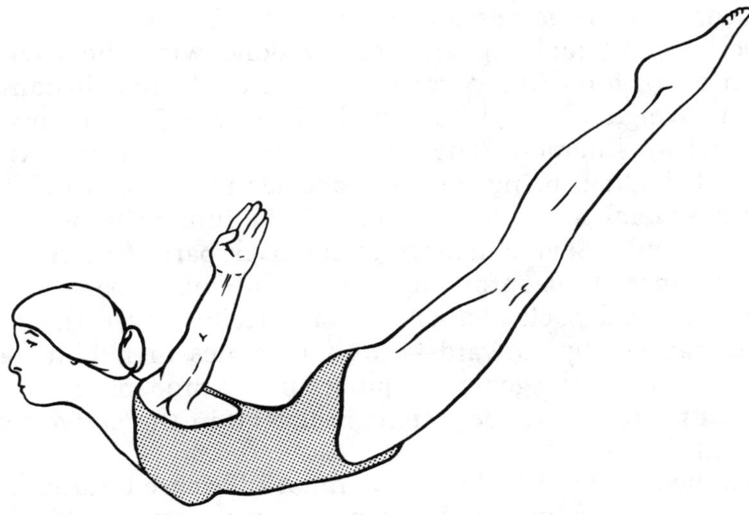

FIGURE 9–4 The forceful hyperextension as the diver goes through various maneuvers can irritate the low back.

Good conditioning and careful attention to technique are your best allies.

Forgive me, but I can't resist this opportunity to practice a bit of preventative medicine for the neck, as opposed to the back. One of the most comon causes of broken necks and paralysis of the arms and legs is diving—diving in unknown waters. Folks, it's preventable if you follow this simple rule: *Never*—I repeat, *Never!*—dive into unfamiliar waters, and don't let your friends do it either, no matter how many or how few cocktails they may have had. If we would all follow this safety rule, so much sadness could be avoided. End of sermon.

Football (American)

A high-risk sport. Besides the United States and Canada, only one other country on earth has adopted football, and that is the nation known for hara-kiri and kamikaze pilots. I enjoy and respect football, but I believe you ought to know its dangers.

Football players engage in frequent heavy lifting in less than ideal ergonomic circumstances. Linemen are especially burdened, both in games and in practice. You may notice that blocking and tackling are usually done with the back in a position of forty-five degrees or more of flexion (bending forward). Weights being lifted are the 200- to 300-pound bodies of competing linemen. The lift is usually performed with an extended spine, using the back and leg muscles, which places forces several times body weight on the lumbar spine.

The result? Severe damage to the back part of the vertebrae, for instance. Is it surprising that spondylolisthesis—in which the destroyed back elements of a vertebra cause the lumbar vertebrae to slip forward—runs four times higher in football players than in the general population? It's probably the number one cause of severe, persistent backache in the active teenage football lineman.

To the list of football woes we must add acute injuries, for the impact to the spine in this contact sport may result in spine fracture. When there's severe back pain immediately after an impact injury, fracture is the prime suspect. Quarterbacks, running backs, and pass receivers are vulnerable to a semipassive twisting injury. It occurs when the upper part of the torso is being twisted in one or more directions by tacklers while the lower torso is being held fast or twisted in the opposite direction by other tacklers. The resulting twist injures the spine.

And we're just talking about back injuries, which account for only one in twenty football injuries. The neck and the knee are even more vulnerable on the gridiron. Knee injuries account for about twenty-five percent of all the injuries in this sport.

What precautions can you take? Get in the best shape possible, not neglecting a good weight-lifting program. Then develop blocking and tackling techniques that respect your back a little. This is easier said than done, I know. But while lifting helps with blocking, it's not absolutely essential. It's not altogether necessary to lift while tackling, either, though it is one of the lineman's few plays for the grandstand.

If you have a persistent severe lower backache for fourteen days with no improvement, have it checked for spondylosis or spondylolisthesis, either of which should be treated before it gets worse. Spondylosis is the result of two defects (cracks) in the back part of the vertebra; spondylolisthesis results when a cracked vertebra slips forward and out of place. (Figure 3–4.) When you have a sore back, remember that you may be awkward, weak, and prone to a more severe injury if you insist on playing. Sometimes your doctor may let you resume playing in an appropriately prescribed brace.

Golf

Medium-to-low-risk. Those who've been around golf much at all know that back pain goes with the turf. (Figure 9–5.)

The twisting motion accompanying the drive is the dangerous part of golf, as it can damage the intervertebral discs and the facet (intervertebral) joints.

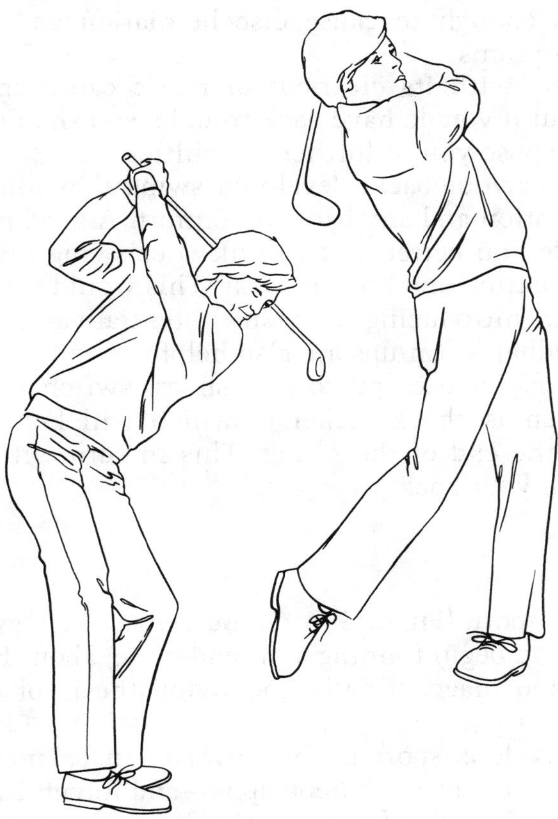

FIGURE 9–5 This shows quite clearly how a full golf swing can result in a considerable axial rotation (twist) to the lower back. This can irritate not only the facet joint but also the disc. Smooth out the swing and rotate the hips to reduce the stress on the back.

I had occasion to meet an avid golfer who for twenty years after a disc removal and spinal fusion had done very well, playing golf regularly. Then one day he completed a long driving swing with a number two club and fell to the ground with excruciating back and leg pain. At the hospital, a myelogram revealed a large disc extruding just above the fused area of his spine. He had immediate surgical removal of the disc. After his recovery, he was advised to stay away from the green.

What had probably happened was that his very efficient twisting swing was accentuated by the stable fusion beneath his normal disc. Over the years, the efficient, progressive wear and tear on the disc adjacent to the fusion had damaged it. The final swing was enough to cause disc herniation and the golfer's drastic symptoms.

This case, with its clear-cut dramatic cause and effect, is unusual, but if you do have back trouble, you should know that golf may expose you to further difficulties.

To pamper your back, develop a swing that minimizes the twisting motion and any back discomfort. A good pro could no doubt guide you better, but I think your swing might involve more hip rotation and knee motion. This would stress the back less without introducing too many potential variations in your swing. Gradual warm-ups are also helpful.

Finally, if you use spiked golf shoes, switch to *nonspiked* shoes or tennis shoes, either of which will help reduce the impact at the end of the swing. This in turn will reduce the irritation to your back.

Gymnastics

A high-risk sport. (Figure 9–6.) In Bulgaria, where gymnasts are identified and begin training at a tender age, about fifty percent suffer back damage, usually spondylolisthesis of the lumbar spine.

This marvelous sport is the ultimate in balance, strength, coordination, courage, choreography—and forceful hyperextension of the spine. The forces involved in arching the back—on the mat, the uneven parallel bars, and horse or vault—are of a very high magnitude. Indeed, one of the criteria of perfect form is a beautifully arched, extremely extended lumbar spine. The ability to snap into this position with almost imperceptible

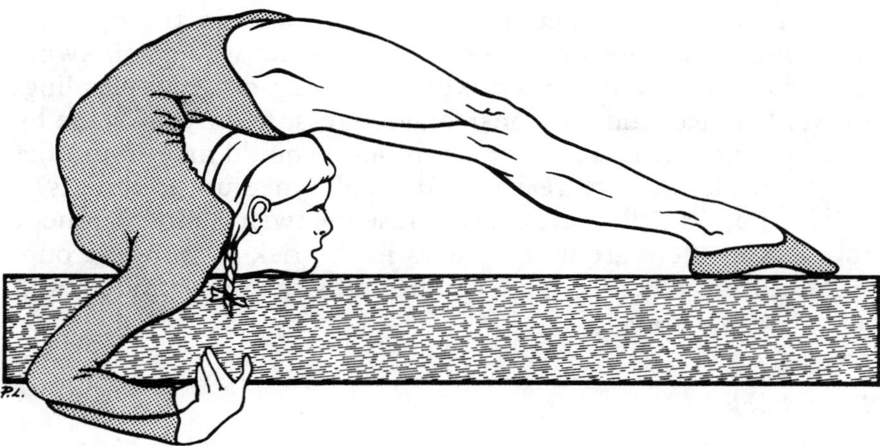

FIGURE 9–6 If golf is the prototype for the twisting problem, gymnastics is the prototype for the *hyperextension* problem. This position causes large forces on the facet joints, the posterior part of the vertebra, and the disc.

speed and agility impresses the judges—and hurts the back, particularly the immature, developing spine of the youthful gymnast.

Fracture of the *pars interarticularis,* the posterior part of the vertebra where one finds the cracks of spondylolysis, can result in severe back pain. The gymnast's risk of spondylolysis, the defect in the spine's posterior elements, is four times higher than average. These athletes also have more disc disease and facet joint arthritis. Until the rules are changed to deemphasize the importance of hyperextending the spine, there is little the competitive gymnast can do other than to be careful and minimize the hyperextension—at least in practice. If you have prolonged, severe, and unimproved backache, seek appropriate medical care.

Hockey

Low-risk.

The sidearm shot, which requires twisting with a very large torque combined with leaning forward, is hockey's main "backbreaker." The arms and shoulders are twisted in one direction as the hips and legs either hold steady or twist in the opposite direction. This shot hurts the back the same way a golf swing may, except that in hockey you also hang out in a bending-forward stance, and put considerable pressure on your spine by contracting the erector spinae muscles. I should mention to the careful reader that the reason I rated golf "medium-to-low-risk" and hockey only "low-risk" is because the twist is more frequent in golf and there are more golfers in the risk-prone age group.

Precautions include good conditioning, good technique, and adequate warm-up.

Horseback Riding

The risk is inversely related to the cumulative skills of horse and rider.

Through alphabetical positioning this sport almost appears next to jogging. The trouble with both sports is vertical impact-loading—or, in the vernacular, the bumpy up-and-down motions in the saddle that jolt your spine. If you have real back problems, you should drop riding, at least until you've been pain-free for six months. In this sport you're *sitting,* a position that imposes large loads on your back to begin with. Also be careful about your back in the work positions and activities involved in grooming your horse.

Javelin Throwing

Medium-risk.

This is another sport that is believed to lead to developing back pain and spondylolisthesis. The twisting and hyperextension of the upper body is the probable cause. The solution is good technique and good conditioning.

Jogging

Medium-to-low-risk.

Working with these athletes, one rarely encounters indifference. Joggers, in particular, often evince an enthusiasm bordering on the fanatical—which is great, in my opinion, since there's already too much subtlety in life.

However, vertical impact-loading, or the bump-bump-bump as the road's vibrations are transmitted to your spine, can damage the discs and other structures. Fortunately, there's quite a lot you can do about it. The magnitude of the bump-bump-bump depends on your weight, your conditioning, your fatigue or lack of it, the smoothness of your stride, and the ability of your leg and other muscles as well as the hip and sacroiliac joints to dampen the impact. Your shoes and the surfaces you run on also count.

Happily, few people who jog remain obese for long, but weight may handicap the beginning jogger. Start slowly, gradually adding to your distance as you shed pounds. Actually, starting with marathon distances isn't advisable for anyone, obese or svelte. The tissues of the spine—its bones and ligaments—strengthen with practice and adapt to the rigors of this most ancient of man's sporting activities.

If you feel tired and notice that your weary muscles are allowing your legs to flop around a bit, or if you're stumbling, you're clearly in the fatigue range and susceptible to injury. This brings us to the matter of technique. The runner with smooth, excellent form is at lower risk than the clumsy runner. Read a good book on jogging, concentrate on your form, and observe well-trained runners.

Avoid running at night on anything but smooth, familiar surfaces. Irregularity in the terrain can hurt your ankles, knees, hands, and face if you should stumble—and unanticipated surface irregularities can transmit sudden shocks to your spine. Also, you should remember that unexplained knee pain without knee swelling or aggravation by knee motion can be caused by a herniated disc. Grass, wood, cinder tracks, sand, and soft ground are more forgiving surfaces than concrete and asphalt. Hard surfaces can damage your muscles and tendons, and produce fatigue (stress) fractures in your bones.

Hundreds of pages have been written about running shoes. In brief, a good running shoe should (1) comply to the foot's contour; (2) be made of material in the heel and sole that will absorb energy; and (3) allow the foot to breathe. It doesn't necessarily follow that the most expensive shoe is the best.

Some people think jogging is good for the back because the forces applied to the disc contribute to the physiology of chemical exchanges and improve their nutrition. Moreover, good athletic conditioning is said to increase endorphin production (see Chapter IV), and these morphinelike substances may be the physiological basis of "runner's high." These theories are reasonable but not overriding. If you enjoy jogging and it doesn't hurt your back, continue. If you're jogging and having back trouble, try eliminating the risk factors we mentioned.

I sometimes ask joggers with back problems why they didn't consult a doctor earlier. Often they respond, "Well, I didn't go to a doctor because I knew a doctor would tell me to stop jogging, and no jogger wants to be told to stop." I can understand this sentiment. Some joggers don't want to give up their passion, and we doctors should try to help them continue jogging while reducing the stresses on their backs. If you're a jogger with a backache, know that your back condition is unlikely to cripple you or threaten your life. But you do need to examine your pleasure-pain ratio. If you subtract your back pain from the pleasure of jogging, is there some net pleasure left over? If so, good luck, be careful, and if you must jog at night, use reflectors.

Before leaving this subject, I'd like to offer a bit of information to female joggers. If you're training to the point that you've developed amenorrhea—that is, your periods have stopped—you may be losing some bone mass. Female runners and athletes have sustained up to fourteen percent decreases in bone density in association with the hormonal changes.

Lacrosse

Low-risk.

Lacrosse was invented by the North American Indians, whose casualties, in games of eight hundred to a thousand players, included broken legs and even deaths. Nowadays, lacrosse is mostly limited to private secondary schools and colleges in Canada and the Northeast, and, happily, deaths rarely or never occur. I've never understood why lacrosse hasn't caught on more widely. It is fascinating to observe a situation in which it is socially acceptable for one player to take a stick and hit the other player on the head, before they run down the field together. How strangely marvelous!

In any case, the twisting motion lacrosse requires for the "side shot" resembles the side shot in hockey and poses identical risks to your back. As the shoulders and arms twist vigorously in one direction to execute the shot, the hips and pelvis are stable or turned in the other direction as a stabilizing counterforce. If you stay in excellent physical condition and develop a technique that minimizes the side shot's twist, you'll protect your back.

Pole Vaulting

This beautiful sport involves a maneuver that is potentially irritating to the back. During the ascent of the vaulter to the bar there are several phases: the run, the jump, the pull with the arms, and the lifting of the legs up as they are virtually snapped, kicked, and thrown over the bar. This lifting over of the legs requires tremendous action of our old friend the psoas muscle, which attaches to the femur (thigh bone) just below the hip joint. And you know what that does. It's analogous to sit-ups with legs straight and feet held down. The psoas contractions needed to throw the legs up put very large forces on the low back, the other points where they attach. Thus the back may be irritated.

Good conditioning and smooth execution of technique should reduce the risk and allow a pole vaulter with back pain to spring back, neither pun intended.

Rowing

High-risk.

There are two types of rowing—*sculling,* where a single rower uses two oars and pulls his back in the direction he's rowing, and *sweep rowing,* or team rowing. In sweep rowing, half the rowers extend oars on one side of the boat, half on the other. The sweep rower must pull the oar with both hands, from way off to one side of his body onto his chest. This process constitutes a twisting motion as well as a forceful extension of the body. Consequently, there is a forceful twist and extension of the spine, two maneuvers that are unfriendly to the ailing back.

Both types of rowing pose risks to your back. But because of its characteristic twisting motion, sweep rowing is probably more dangerous than straight sculling, which involves only spine extension. This little logical gem I learned from a rowing coach. With sweep rowing, have the athletes alternate sides of the boat as much as is feasible, as this will decrease considerably the concentration and accumulation of forces on the involved anatomic structures (mainly the facet joints and discs). I don't think that this involves significant training problems as regards the development of muscle strength and endurance for competition.

What can you do about the risks? Stay in condition, concentrate on technique, and hope your coach employs careful fatigue management and training. Some training exercises that involve simulated rowing are stressful to the back, and should be kept to a minimum. When a rower's back aches, it's often hard to distinguish spine problems from the soreness of any athlete's overworked muscles. But when there's associated leg pain, the possibility of nerve root irritation or significant damage to the spinal elements looms large. A doctor should be consulted.

Let me share a case history with you. A patient of mine, a vigorous, nineteen-year-old Olympic-class rower on the Harvard team, started having back pain while rowing. Soon it began to crop up between rowing sessions as well, and he developed pain in his right leg. On the recommendation of an orthopaedic surgeon, the young man rested and stopped rowing, and first his leg pain, then his back pain, subsided. When he went back to rowing after several weeks, he turned to sculling because summer vacation had arrived and his teammates were away. It caused no problems. In the fall, however, when he resumed sweep rowing, his severe back and leg pain flared up once more. Intrigued, the student did an informal survey of his rowing friends, quite a number of whom also complained of back and leg pain. Not only did he note that those who did sweep rowing had more pain than those who sculled, but the teammates who pulled oars on the right side of the boat had pain in the left leg, while those who pulled on the left had right leg pain. This anecdote perfectly fits the mathematical model and the experimental studies of the spine as it relates to body activities and disc problems.

I learned from a female rowing coach that it's good to develop *both* sides of a sweep rower. How ingenious. This provides balanced muscle development and distributes the stress on various parts of the disc and the facet joints more evenly.

Sailing

Yes, there is risk here too. When crewing on a larger craft there is simply the hard work of lifting that goes with the job. However, there is a more subtle problem that the small-craft sailor should be aware of. When you must hook your feet under a stable structure on the boat, extending your torso well over the side of the boat for balance, you certainly risk irritating an underlying back problem. The reason is the same reason you should avoid sit-ups with knees straight and the feet hooked under the bed. In both circumstances considerable stress is exerted on the iliopsoas muscle (Figure 5–14) and therefore on the lumbar spine to which it attaches. This may truly cause your back to ache.

If you need this maneuver as a competitive sailor or in an emergency, you probably have to pay the price. Otherwise you can improvise, or simply not allow yourself to get in that situation, letting a crew member with a good back do it.

Scuba Diving

There is a very rare situation with scuba divers in which they have low back pain following too rapid decompression. Unfortunately, this pain can be the beginning of a severe neurological problem in which there is spinal cord and nerve damage due to gases in the neural structures. This must be treated promptly by hyperbaric oxygen therapy.

Skating

Three skating activities are potential back aggravators. The basic skating position with the spine slightly bent forward is the first. The other two liabilities are related more to figure skating; the various spins are one problem, and landing after a jump is the other.

What can we do about it? The recreational skater can take it easy and skate as upright as possible if he/she has a back that's acting up. The figure skater must be ever so careful with the twists and ever so graceful in the jump landings. And if backache does hit, I suggest knocking it off for a few weeks until the back settles down.

Skiing

Low-risk overall.

The main bogey here is the mogul that appears out of nowhere, or the jump in which you don't land just right. Other stresses are the parallel skier's repeated twisting (Figure 9–7) and the chronic back strain endured by downhill and cross-country skiers as they hold their torsos in a slightly flexed position. I suggest that if you're a skier with a back problem, avoid twisting your shoulders in the opposite direction in which you're twisting your hips. Keep them as parallel as possible to avoid torque on your low back.

Another suggestion: If you ski and want to spare your back, develop your quadriceps muscles (so named for their "four heads"), the ones running from your hips to your knees in front.

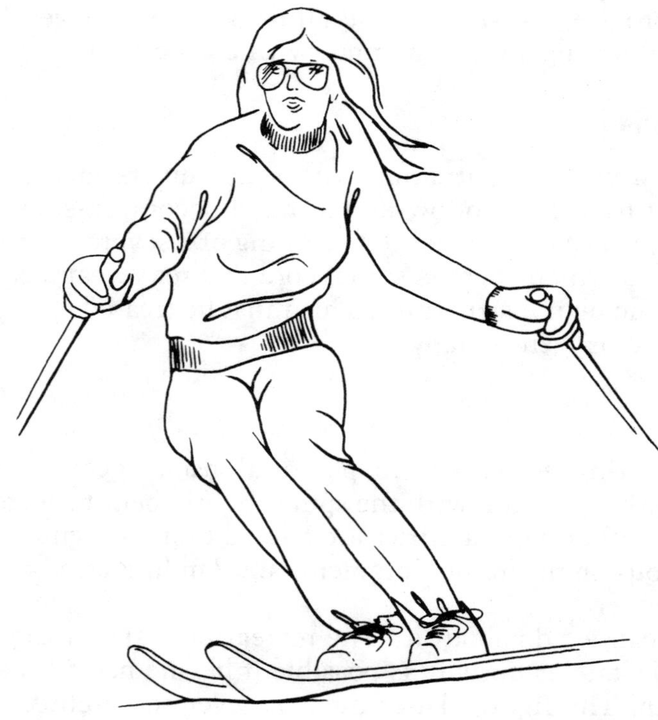

FIGURE 9–7 Here again, axial rotation or twisting of the spine is a contributing factor in the skier who develops low back pain.

They're critical shock absorbers, balancers, and controllers of the skiing body. When strengthened, they can take up much of the energy that might otherwise jolt the spine.

Here are some quadriceps-strengthening exercises. Begin exercise *number one* by standing with your back against the wall, making sure that the floor isn't slippery and that you're wearing rubber-soled shoes. Now carefully slide down the wall, moving your feet out gradually from the wall as you go—all the way down to the point where your hips are ninety degrees flexed, your knees are bent ninety degrees, and your feet are flat on the floor. You end up in the position of a person sitting erectly in a chair, except that there's no chair and your derriere rests on air. You're supported by your feet and by your back resting against the wall. So what's the force that keeps you from sliding down the wall? The sustained contraction of your quadriceps! You'll feel it immediately. At first you'll be able to sit there for a few seconds only, but try to gradually increase your endurance to between one and two minutes.

If the wall-sitting exercise makes your knees hurt, don't do it. Do exercise *number two* instead. Take a ten- or fifteen-pound weight and attach it to your foot or ankle. You can improvise the weight in several ways; a sack filled with large, weighted pebbles, a pillow slip holding full food cans, or a sandbag will do. Two bags or pillow slips containing weights can be tied together and draped over your ankle, one on each side. Or you can go to a sports store and buy a shoe attachment that allows you to apply measured weights in various quantities.

Now sit on a high counter or table, or a low bedside. If you're sitting on a counter or table, rest your weighted ankle on a stool; if you're sitting on a low bed, rest it on the floor. Start the exercise with your knee bent about thirty or forty degrees (not ninety degrees), then slowly extend the knee of the weighted leg fully. Gradually work up to doing this twenty-five to fifty times for each knee, once a day. After two or three weeks your quadriceps will be strengthened for better, injury-free skiing. If both exercises cause severe knee pain, reduce the weights or the number of repetitions. If there's still pain, desist.

You can add extra protection to your back by doing the back exercises in Chapter V.

"When can I go back to the slopes?" is the question I most often hear from dedicated skiers. A quick, accurate, unfacetious answer is, when you can make love without back pain, and when you've done some basic back and quadriceps exercises. Then *gradually* work into skiing—sticking to the intermediate slopes for a few days if you're an advanced skier, to the beginner slopes if you're an intermediate. Though your ego may be begging for more, don't deceive yourself about how tired you really are.

There is no agreement as to the status of cross-country skiing as a back-pain-risk sport. My suggestion is that if you want to do it, try it and see how your back tolerates it. If you have a backache and you're looking for a sport, then I'd say this shouldn't be high on your list.

Snowmobiling

Medium-to-high-risk.

This delightful recreation contributes to both sides of the pleasure-pain equilibrium during the winter months. The threat to your back is that of injury, pure and simple. Because snowmobiling is done at high speeds, spine fractures can result.

Commonsense precautions are advised. Don't snowmobile "under the influence" or speed in crowded or hard-to-maneuver places. Manufacturers could help greatly by designing seats that absorb a maximum of impact, sparing the spine. Repeated jostlings and high vibrations that don't cause immediate fracture can sometimes cause cumulative damage.

Squash

Similar to tennis as a sport and in the movements that may irritate the back. The twisting motion involved in the backhand can be the cause of an injury that results in backache. Conditioning and the technique of using the arms more than the trunk in the backhand will help.

Sumo Wrestling

I started to leave this one out, because it's pretty much limited to Japan. Then, thinking about global markets, patriotism, and the popularity of sumo wrestling in Japan . . . I decided to include it, in order to help the trade balance. But seriously, the *real* reason for including it is that this is such a marvelously fascinating sport, historically well entrenched in the finest of Japanese culture, and a brief discussion allows us to reemphasize certain points for any backache-prone athlete. Contrary to what you may have thought, these athletes are not fat, out-of-shape, over-the-hill wrestlers of the type that you may see in the ring on your late-night TV entertainment. They are exquisitely trained, powerful, lightning-quick competitors who work out early every morning almost 365 days a year. The afternoon is spent eating and sleeping to develop that very large and powerful stomach. Why? Because the idea of the sport is to keep from being thrown out of a rather small circle while lifting your 250- to 350-pound opponent and throwing *him* out of the ring. The large abdomen also serves as a fulcrum and lever to accomplish the task. Balance, style, reflexes, and strategy are the highly tuned skills employed.

Since you're now a scholar of the backache, you know that possessing a large abdomen and lifting heavy objects out in front of your body is not good for your back. Among sumo wrestlers, there is a high incidence of spondylolysis and spondylolisthesis.

Swimming

Very low-risk. Swimming is excellent exercise for backache sufferers, because you get a workout of virtually all your muscles, and cardiorespiratory conditioning as well. All this, and it doesn't put undue gravitational loads on your spine.

Sometimes, however, a patient complains that swimming irritates his/her back condition. If you have a fairly severe back problem, the breaststroke and crawl could aggravate it, perhaps because you hyperextend your back when you execute those strokes. If so, I recommend the sidestroke. There are, however, some very sensitive backs that would be uncomfortable in any swimming activity.

What about vigorous, competitive swimming? The breaststroke, particularly the dolphin breaststroke (butterfly), involves tremendous flexion and hyperextension of the spine, and should be considered a risk for those with back problems. Otherwise, swimming offers good therapy and very few opportunities to hurt your back.

Tennis

Low-risk.

Tennis gained considerable popularity in the seventies as North Americans became more fitness-conscious. Not only is tennis stimulating and exciting, but it's a great equalizer. An eleven-year-old girl can have a good game with her sixty-year-old grandfather. A fifty-year-old female college professor can teach a twenty-year-old male student a few lessons. Husbands and wives, fathers and daughters, friends and lovers can all get out on the court with reasonable chances to win or be competitive.

Two parts of tennis can cause backache, however. These are the serve and the backhand. Some serving styles load the lower back as you extend your back and uncoil arm and racket to hit the ball. (Figure 9–8.) This exerts great pressure on the spine. The follow-through is down and around to the opposite side of your body, which means a slight twist. If you have back trouble and you're using an Australian-style or American-twist serve, try changing your serve so as to eliminate the hyperextension. If back pain occurs only occasionally with your serve, do some exercises to strengthen your back and abdominal muscles and stabilize your spine.

As for the backhand, this involves standing with your legs and lower trunk held stable while your shoulders are turned. As you swing, your shoulders, waist, and arm are uncoiled with great force, and then there's the impact of hitting the ball. This coiling and uncoiling exerts twisting forces on the back.

What should you do about your backhand, which is many players' most vulnerable point anyway? Ask a pro to teach you the best technique and hope it will let you carry out the stroke in a more relaxed way, minimizing the torsional forces. If that doesn't work, you may have to evaluate the game's pleasure-pain ratio. Or perhaps you could go back to running around your backhand.

In general, conditioning and good technique help your back. Because tennis is a "social" game, most people start playing without an adequate warm-up. Try doing these warm-up exercises. *Number one:* Stand and spread your legs to about the same width as your shoulders, then gently twist from side to side (Figure 2–8D). Begin *number two* by sitting on the ground with

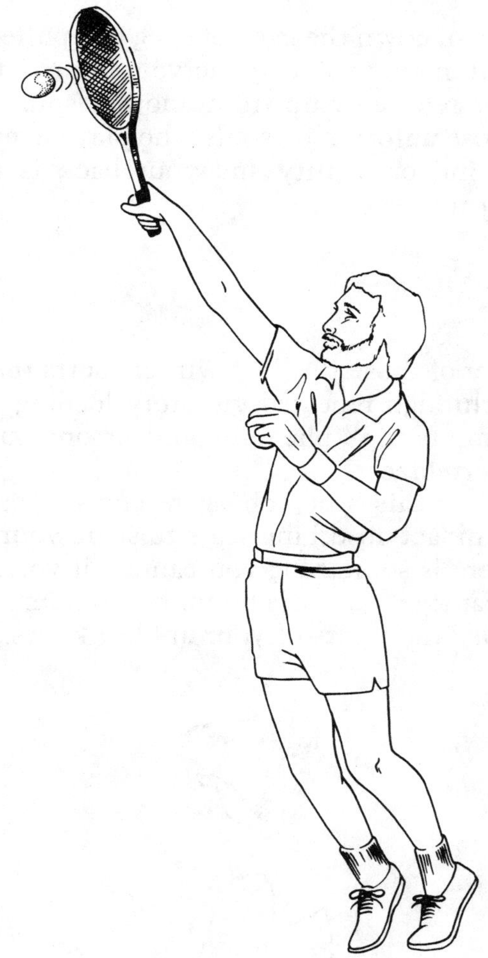

FIGURE 9–8 It's the hyperextension arch in serving that can do it to the tennis player. Occasionally, the twist associated with the backhand will cause the tennis player to have back trouble.

your legs stretched out straight. Now come as close as you can to touching your toes. This stretches your hamstring muscles and helps keep the spine in a better position. (If you already have a back problem, though, don't do this exercise. It may irritate your spine.) For *number three:* Do at least ten push-ups.

If your backache is associated with leg pain, seek medical attention. Weekend athletes, especially if middle-aged or older, often attribute pain down the back of a leg to a pulled hamstring muscle, when it may be due to nerve-root irritation from a damaged disc or referred pain from another spine problem. If you're one of those unfortunate souls who plays winter tennis in a rather chilly indoor facility and your back is hurting, try playing in a warm sweater.

Tobogganing

Low-risk.

This is another of those thrilling winter sports that does back damage either through repeated vibratory loading of the spine (the "bump-bump-bump" phenomenon) or one sudden injury that fractures vertebrae.

Unfortunately, at this time, toboggans and sleighs don't come equipped with impact-absorbing seats to spare your spine some jostling. But there is something you can do. If you sit properly, you can significantly reduce the bump-bump-bump transmitted to your back. Use the joints of your ankles, knees, and hips to

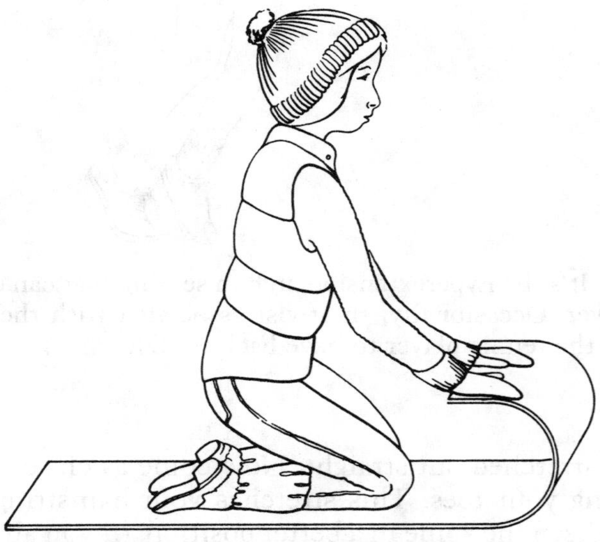

FIGURE 9–9 By utilizing this position, actually sitting on the heels, you take advantage of the shock-absorbing capacities of your knees and ankles. This reduces the intensity of sudden impact that would otherwise be transmitted to the spine.

dampen the loads that ultimately reach the lumbar spine. I advise sitting as shown in Figure 9–9. As a second precaution, use common sense and don't sled or toboggan "under the influence."

Weight Lifting

High-risk.

Weight lifting exerts immense stress on the lumbar spine. Evidence of spine damage—spondylolysis—runs as high as forty percent among young Japanese weight lifters. But don't be discouraged. Most weight lifters are well-conditioned athletes who have carefully studied lifting techniques.

The first back-saving suggestion is to master your technique and train appropriately. Avoid jerky movements and lifting weights from the floor. Other no-no's are movements in which the spine must go from a flexed to an erect or hyperextended position. If you lie supine or semireclined and use your shoulder, arm, and chest muscles for lifting (bench pressing), you'll spare your back much stress. And there's an excellent theoretical and experiential basis for the use of belts in both practice and competition. By increasing intra-abdominal and thoracic pressure, belts contribute to stiffening and unweighting the spine, which diminishes the strains on it.

It has been observed that highly competitive, poorly supervised, teenage–weight lifting can result in a type of fracture of the vertebral body in the region of the growth plate. If this information is relevant to you or anyone you know, use it!

Wrestling

This is one of those sports with a factor X—for unknown. That means that though you can protect your back with careful conditioning, your opponents constitute factor X. Their moves remain a source of potential injury.

In wrestling there lurk several potential stressors to the lumbar spine. For one thing, wrestlers spend a great deal of time trying to lift each other. And each also plots to make lifting as awkward and inconvenient as possible for the opponent.

Stamina is a major factor in survival, and in protection from injury. A wrestler needs superb overall conditioning, together with excellent strength and endurance in all his/her muscles. Diligent sparring and shadow practice is critical, and in sparring the use of difficult lifting moves can be controlled.

Whenever you have severe pain that lasts for several days, hold off on any training activity that aggravates the pain. This great sport has a certain baseline injury potential that is difficult to minimize.

SOME PARTING SHOTS

Of course, we haven't covered *all* sports. If your favorite has not been included, let me suggest that if it doesn't hurt your back, fine. If it does, then you should get in the best possible shape. Try to figure out what particular activity in the sport irritates you. Discuss it with a fellow sportsman, coach, or pro, with the idea of altering your activity so as to maintain your competitive edge while alleviating the pain.

Since some of you readers are likely to be serious athletes, let me share this with you. Say you're doing your sport, and you have a backache. But you want to go to the limit to gain maximum abdominal strength. Here's how to do it: Use the medicine ball. You know what I mean, the big heavy ball (it comes in two sizes) that boxers whip into each other's abdomens to strengthen the abdominal muscles so that they can take a body punch. When you can take the medicine ball twenty-five to one hundred times in the stomach, two to three times a week, you'll have an abdomen that will support any grieving back handsomely.

You may have noticed that each subheading of this chapter contains admonitions about fitness and good conditioning. Good muscle tone and endurance are of the utmost value to your health in any sport. For some sports we've suggested that you follow the basic back-pain exercises. Properly done sit-ups should be a part of most training programs, and good abdominal tone and posture mechanics make for a healthy back.

An excellent, well-coached technique in your chosen sport improves your performance and minimizes the risk of injury. Good coaching, conscientious practice, and in some cases, videotapes or careful reading of the right book can help sharpen your skills. Sometimes you may be able to modify your technique to spare your back. If your tennis serve, for example, causes backaches, you could work with a pro to develop one that's kinder to your spine.

Coaches can help in another way. When aware of a particular sport's risk potential, a coach can cut down on its most dangerous elements. A football team's full-blast practice scrimmage might not include a lot of kickoff plays, for instance. In this chapter we've pinpointed some of each sport's backache-inducing activities. If these can be kept to a minimum, so much the better.

Of course, one must be circumspect about suggesting rule changes; I certainly wouldn't want anyone tampering with "my sport." But as my goal is your back's well-being, I've taken the liberty of sounding a few warnings. If this book were written by a cardiologist or an ophthalmologist, you'd be reading a different set of tips.

One more point. People often say, "Use a little common sense." My recommendation is that you use a *whole lot* of common sense, especially when engaging in recreational sports like skiing, tobogganing, snowmobiling, and diving, where you may be tempted to perform after a few drinks. Common sense is also helpful to the weekend athlete who may become overexhausted, or the football player who's trying to excite the grandstand with an overhead lifting tackle.

We've mentioned the pleasure-pain ratio. Simply put, if the pleasure derived from a sport exceeds the pain incurred, then "batter-up," "serve 'em up," or whatever. Backache in the absence of leg pain usually has as its sole liability the misery it brings; it's not likely to result in any terrible disease or further injury. If there is associated leg pain, however, it's possible that it's early disc disease and that if properly rested, it will have a better outcome than if it is repeatedly irritated by some athletic activity.

After following all the recommendations in this chapter, you're probably safe in regulating your sports activities on the basis of the pleasure-pain equilibrium. Good luck!

Chapter X

Answers to Some Backache Questions Patients Frequently Ask

FOR A moment pretend you're a student at our Low Back School. Now you have the chance to ask any question and to be enlightened on any point that still puzzles you. Unfortunately, books aren't an interactive medium, so you'll have to hope your questions coincide with some of those we've collected here. But since back patients tend to have similar problems, chances are you'll get yours answered. For your convenience, we've grouped the questions by topic.

DIAGNOSIS

Q. *When and how should I ask for a second opinion?*

A. Whenever you feel like it. Consider it seriously if (1) your doctor seems to rush you into surgery or gives you a heavy sales pitch; (2) you've already had one operation on your back; (3) your surgeon *promises* you an excellent result from surgery; (4) the proposed surgery and its basic techniques, risks, and benefits haven't been explained lucidly in nonmedical language; (5) there is compensation or litigation involved in your case and you don't believe you're being treated fairly; or (6) you're being treated by someone you believe is racist, sexist, or otherwise discriminatory.

Where racial, religious, ethnic, or other such factors are concerned, you may be more comfortable and confident if you seek out a physician of your "own kind" through friends, contacts, and so on. Or ask any doctor or your county medical society for a referral. Don't neglect to check for the appropriate specialty board certification.

On the lighter side . . . there's the story of the patient who sat down in the psychiatrist's office, and within three or four seconds the psychiatrist glared at him and said, "You're crazy." The irate patient retorted, "I want a second opinion!" There was a brief contemplative pause before the psychiatrist accommodatingly rejoined, "Okay, you're ugly too."

Q. *What should the workup consist of? Should my doctor take X rays? Must I have a myelogram?*

A. A thorough medical history and physical exam are usually enough to categorize (though maybe not diagnose) your back pain. Routine X rays aren't essential (especially if you've had pain for less than seven weeks), but by the time you've been referred to a specialist, he'll probably ask for recent X rays or take a new set. Some doctors routinely perform a series of lab tests, including a complete blood count, a uric acid test to rule out gout, a sedimentation rate (blood test) to check for an inflammatory process, and a serum test to rule out lupus erythematosus and ankylosing spondylitis. Other physicians feel confident in diagnosing low back pain on the basis of your history and physical exam, putting the X ray off for a while. As a matter of fact, an extensive review in 1988 of all the best clinical information on back pain led to the recommendation that no X rays or laboratory studies are needed during the first seven weeks of a back problem *unless* something specific in the patient's *history* or *physical* exam so indicates.

Myelograms, CAT scans, or MRIs are rarely done unless surgery is proposed (the myelogram has been virtually replaced by the MRI). Their purpose is to confirm the diagnosis, usually of a herniated disc, and to precisely locate the abnormality. Be leery of any doctor who offers these procedures and surgery early in the nonoperative treatment process. Most people recover spontaneously after two or three months.

Q. *I feel terrible. What did my doctor mean when he said my spine was degenerating?*

A. He or she probably didn't say the spine was degenerating, but rather that your spine showed *degenerative changes* or *degenerative arthritis.* What this means is simply wear and tear wrought by age.

As you get older, your spine's structures undergo inevitable wear changes that aren't nearly so dreadful as the word *degenerative* seems to imply (see Chapter III). These changes happen to everyone at different rates, just like gray hair and wrinkles. Some people get back pain in the process; others don't. And even though they're described as "progressive," degenerative changes don't necessarily result in worsening symptoms. Also, don't be alarmed if you see your X rays and there is evidence of degenerative changes. This doesn't mean that you can't get better. Actually, many people see extensive degenerative changes on their X rays, yet experience little or no back pain.

Q. *What causes low back pain in children?*

A. When a child who has not had a specific injury has persistent low back pain for one or two weeks, get him/her to a doctor. Though teenagers occasionally get low back pain and disc disease, it's uncommon, and usually occurs as an aftereffect of a distinct injury, such as a sprain or twist. Disc disease can sometimes go undiagnosed in children for a long time, because it's rarely suspected. Most of the other, more serious diseases we worry about in adults also afflict children. Though cancer is less frequent in children, it does occur. But again, rest assured that low back pain rarely means anything dire. Don't be alarmed. Merely have your child checked by a doctor if he/she gets no better in a week or two.

Otherwise, most of what we say about back pain in adults applies to children. It is less common in children and the psychosocial considerations are rarely factors in childhood low back pain.

Q. *Could very large breasts be the cause of my back pain? Would a breast reduction help?*

A. Mechanical and postural changes caused by excessively large breasts can provoke several clinical aches and pains. These include neck strain, headache, aching shoulders, pain and tingling in the fingers, and deep bra-strap furrows, as well as low back pain.

The added weight and the shift of the center of gravity forward can put additional strain on the muscles of the low back and more force on the upper and lower spine. Moreover, a self-conscious woman may try to minimize her prominent breasts sometimes by rolling her shoulders inward and rounding her thoracic (rib area) spine. This adds to the mechanical problem and further stresses the back muscles, joints, and nerves. Very large breasts are a mechanical liability, requiring great muscle force and stress on the lumbar spine to maintain erect posture. So it's no wonder that a large-breasted woman may fall into the posture described above, which shifts the center of gravity backward toward a more natural position. Initially voluntary, this posture can turn into a fixed deformity. Its disadvantages include lordosis (swayback) of the lumbar and cervical (neck) spine and a rounding of the thoracic spine—and compromised muscle control and balance.

Would breast-reduction surgery relieve your back pain? There's no real proof, but it seems reasonable. If you're considering this operation mainly to help your back pain, you can get a better prediction from a doctor who specializes in low back problems, in consultation with a plastic surgeon.

Q. *Tell me about myelograms.*

A. From time to time we run across a patient who simply says, "Do anything you wish to me, Doctor, but please don't give me a myelogram." Usually such a patient has had severe pain during a previous myelogram or excruciating headache or backache afterwards, but more likely he/she has been exposed only vicariously to the exaggerated "horrible reputation" of this procedure.

Myelograms are routinely carried out on most patients without any complication or difficulty. Since the procedure does pose certain risks, however, a myelogram probably shouldn't be done unless you and your doctor have decided to proceed with surgery if it shows an abnormality. It takes about an hour to do, and the cost, including the radiologist's interpretation, is $572.

One of two types of dye is injected into the *subarachnoid* space around the spinal cord and the nerves of the lower spine. The injected dye is called a *contrast medium* and shows up on X rays as a dense white image. When it surrounds the spinal cord and nerves, anything that is pressing on them looks like an indentation in the column of dye. The indentation you see on the X ray may be a disc, a tumor, an infection, or another disease process. Your doctor must interpret it.

What are myelography's risks? You may be allergic to the dye, especially if you've been found to be allergic to iodine, shellfish, or a previously administered contrast medium. Hypotension, or a drop in blood pressure, may occur during the test. The water-soluble dye can inflame brain tissue if it's allowed to run too high in the neck-area canal. Sometimes the lower back gets inflamed. The most serious complication we worry about with the water-contrast dye is *anaphylactic shock*, an acute, generalized allergic reaction that on extremely rare occasions can be fatal.

Q. *What is a venogram?*

A. This is an X-ray test in which a contrast dye is injected into the lumbar spine region through the spinous processes of the vertebrae or through a large vein in the thigh. Then it's picked up by the veins in and around the spinal canal. An abnormal distribution pattern in these veins can sometimes reveal whether or not a disc is herniated. This test is one that may be suggested when the myelogram is normal but your doctor thinks you may have a disc or something pressing against your nerves. Though considerable radiation exposure occurs, the only real risk of this two-hour procedure is an allergic reaction to the dye. The procedure can be painful.

Q. *What is a discogram?*

A. In this diagnostic procedure, a needle is inserted through the lower back, flank, or midback into the intervertebral disc. A dye is then injected, and its distribution may reveal a degenerated disc. The *amount* absorbed by the disc can also hint that it's degenerated, as degenerated discs tend to accept more fluid. Finally, the particular location and kind of pain you report during the test itself can help your doctor determine whether the disc space is causing your backache. Cortisone and novocaine may also be injected to reduce pain and inflammation. When the pain is eliminated in this way, it indicates that the disc receiving the injection is the one causing the problem.

While all this seems logical, a number of flaws detract from the test's accuracy. For one, most people don't remember, localize, and describe back and leg pain very precisely. Not all grossly degenerated discs are painful, either. And the injection may cause placebo pain relief.

Discograms are rather controversial. There is vigorous disagreement about this procedure among spine specialists. There are arguments about when they should be done, how they should be done, if they should be done, who should do them, where they should be done, and how they should be interpreted.

Okay—what is my advice, then, on discography? Maintain a significant level of skepticism, and if your doctor feels that it's really needed, he/she should explain the reason(s) satisfactorily.

Q. *What is a bone scan?*

A. This X-ray technique has the advantage of little radiation exposure, but it takes four hours to complete. Because it requires you to lie facedown on the table for as long as an hour, it can make a back patient quite uncomfortable. We like to make back patients lie immobile on their stomachs as seldom as possible.

The bone scan can diagnose recent fractures, as well as tumors and infections. It's half as expensive as a myelogram, and is thought to expose you to less radiation. This test gives information about the possibility of tumor, fracture, infection, or arthritis in the bone and joints of the spine, whereas the myelogram tells you if there's something abnormal, such as a herniated disc, in or near the spinal canal. The radiation exposure for this study is about 1/10th of what is involved in routine low back X rays.

Q. *What is a CAT scan? Can it diagnose a herniated disc?*

A. Computerized Axial Tomography—a CAT or CT scan—is an exciting new development in diagnostic radiology. Through sophisticated imaging it can "photograph" the spine clearly in several cross sections. The diagnostic value of being able to look right down the spinal canal is wonderful! (Pages 64 and 66, depicting examples of spinal stenosis, shows one of the views a CAT scan can give us.)

Depending on the technological capabilities of the scanner used, a CAT scan can rather reliably reveal a herniated disc. It's of great value in diagnosing spinal stenosis. The CAT scan is supplanting the myelogram as a diagnostic tool in many circumstances. In some centers, where the appropriate machines are available and the experience of the doctors in using CAT in place of myelograms is ample, they do the CAT scan before resorting to the myelogram. When you have a myelogram or discogram, you're usually given narcotics and other medications, which can cause other side effects in addition to those the dye may provoke. The CAT scan, in contrast, requires no drugs or dye, and hence causes no side effects. Some doctors, however, will suggest using the contrast dye along with the CAT scanner for enhancement and better visualization.

At present it takes about twenty minutes for the CAT machine to X ray the lumbar spine regions where a disc is likely to occur. During that time the patient must lie flat on an X-ray table—no small chore for the normal person, let alone a back-pain patient. Its cost is about the same as that of a myelogram, its radiation exposure slightly less. However, the radiation involved with a CAT scan is approximately two or three times as much as is emitted by regular

X rays of the low back. In general, it's fair to say that a regular CAT scan, even with lying on the table, is less painful than a myelogram. Of course, it's difficult to predict precisely in the case of any given individual which of these procedures would be more painful. This study, including the radiologist's interpretation, costs about $696. If combined with a myelogram, the cost is about $1,018.

Q. *What are EMG studies?*

A. EMG stands for electromyelography, a test that takes about an hour and a half and involves no radiation but can be moderately uncomfortable.

The doctor, usually a neurologist, attaches little pads to the skin over your muscles or, sometimes, inserts very fine needles into the muscles. Once the pads or needles are in place, we can study the pattern of electrical recordings caused by nerve conduction. Changes in the electrical patterns and the speed of nerve conduction can help uncover various kinds of nerve pathology. Irritation of the nerve roots in your lower spine will show up as abnormal electrical responses. So the EMG can help us recognize when a disc is encroaching on the spinal canal's nerves.

Q. *Tell me about this MRI.*

A. MRI means Magnetic Resonance Imaging. This is a noninvasive system of imaging that is capable of depicting the spine in many planes—that is, from different views: front, side, as well as looking down the spinal canal to see if the disc is herniated or if something else is irritating the nerves. Various anatomic structure, such as normal and herniated discs, spinal nerves, the dura, the intervertebral joints, and tumors can be imaged. Not only can the technology provide excellent images, but it also has some capacity to characterize certain biological activity of some tissues. This technology (which assays magnetic fields within the body and radio waves) is only in its infancy and is already replacing myelography to a considerable extent. MRI, with some variations and use of biomechanical agents, is likely to provide some major advances over current knowledge of low back pain. At present this is an appropriate test to utilize if you and your doctor think that surgery is a consideration for disc herniation or for spinal stenosis. This test, including radiologist's interpretation, costs $825.

The test is not painful. You merely lie still on your back in a hollow tube for thirty to sixty minutes. There's also a noticeable popping sound of the machine at work. If you're claustrophobic, let your doctor know, or just relax and keep your eyes closed. Think pleasant thoughts, or, better—fantasize.

Q. *How useful is DSSEP (Dermatomal Somato Sensory Evoked Potentials) in the diagnosis of slipped discs?*

A. This test is in its very early stages of development and has not yet been proven to be a sure and accurate method for diagnosis of disc herniation. The myelogram, CAT scan, and MRI are the most reliable tests. The DSSEP is an electrical test in which the skin of the foot is stimulated and the response of brain waves are recorded. An abnormal recording suggests that something, presumably a herniated disc, is interfering with the signal being transmitted from the foot to the brain.

SELF-CARE

Q. *Doctor, couldn't this just be a bad "muscle pull"? It hurts in the muscle and I'm getting lots of muscle spasm.*

A. If so, you're fortunate, as a muscle rupture should heal in one to two weeks. Frankly, the muscle spasm you're having is not well understood. It will gradually subside. Rest, relaxation, heat or cold, and massage are all likely to help. On rare occasions, muscle relaxants are prescribed.

Q. *Do you recommend special beds or mattresses?*

A. The text of Chapters V and VI covers this question in some detail. If you're sleeping fine on a soft mattress and it doesn't hurt your back, enjoy it. If you want to test the idea of a harder mattress, try sleeping on the floor on a stack of blankets for a few nights. A recent study showed that a firm mattress is probably better for your back.

Q. *Someone told me that bucket seats were not good for people with backaches. What do you say about that?*

A. Certainly a number of people with or without backache find bucket seats uncomfortable. This is due to the fact that the classic bucket seats have nothing in the way of lumbar support. On the basis of the principle that lumbar support is a desirable support, the idea of a bucket seat with no lumbar support comes up short. If you have a back problem and are considering a new car, you *ought not* to buy one with a bucket seat unless it has a distinctly comfortable lumbar support. However, if you have been riding or driving in a bucket seat for an extended period of time and it does not interfere with your back or cause you backache, then the thing speaks for itself; but you are the exception. Truck-stop stores often have high-quality lumbar supports that are readily transferable to a variety of motor vehicles.

Q. *Does wearing high-heeled shoes hurt my back?*

A. Wearing high heels tends to shift the back into a slightly swaybacked position. Traditionally we have thought that high heels aggravate backaches, and maybe they do. A recent study has shown that high heels up to 4.5 cm., or 1¾ inch, do not increase or cause a swayback position. The best answer is to test yourself, "objectively." That is, if wearing high heels definitely *does not* increase your backache, then "go for it." If it does, then I usually recommend wearing the high heels for shorter periods, which may give you a tolerable pain range.

Q. *How do I know if I'm going to have a second attack?*

A. Your doctor can best answer this, but in general there is a tendency for recurrence. Statistics show that about sixty percent of patients with acute, incapacitating low back pain are likely to have another attack within two years.

Q. *Every time I glance at a magazine or newspaper I see an article about some new breakthrough or cure for back pain. I'm confused. How do I know what to believe? What sort of treatment should I spend my money on?*

A. Consider all claims of great medical advances in advertisements with the greatest skepticism. News reports of medical events merit interest and follow-up inquiries, but don't believe everything you read or hear right away. Ask your doctor about these different "cures." Don't blame him/her if he/she is prudent and doesn't immediately try out the latest vogue. The new devices and treatments you hear about are usually in the experimental stage, at best, or at worst aren't even solid enough to reach the experimental stage. It generally takes years for a new cure to prove itself to be better than the placebo effect and the self-limiting characteristic of the problem.

When treatments are cheap, noninvasive, and riskless, it makes sense to try some of them. But do so under your doctor's supervision.

Q. *What is your opinion about stretching exercises?*

A. Well, first of all, virtually any exercise is good for you if it doesn't hurt your back. But stretching exercises sometimes do hurt your back, and for those patients who experience pain they should be discontinued. These are usually patients with new, intense backache associated with severe sciatica.

The theory of the stretching exercise is that it loosens up the ligaments in the back part of the spine, as well as tight hamstrings, making it easier to carry the spine in a straighter position, as opposed to a "swayback" or lordotic position. This is a reasonable hypothesis and is adequate to justify the inclusion of stretching exercises in an exercise program—provided they are not irritating.

Q. *I've got sciatica, and when it's necessary to bend over to put on or tie my shoes, my leg hurts. Can I do anything about that?*

A. Yes. There's a simple, practical solution: Wear shoes that don't have to be tied, and use a long shoehorn.

NONSURGICAL TREATMENT

Q. *What is Rolfing and do you recommend it?*

A. Ida Rolf, an organic chemist, began practicing "connective tissue therapy" in the 1940s. It's a very vigorous, even painful, sort of muscular manipulation. The technique is supposed to reorder the myofascial (muscles and the connecting fascia) system, realigning it with gravity and thus achieving better balance. Like any other treatment, Rolfing has succeeded most with people who believe in it religiously. In my opinion, Rolfing's premise is unsound. It's an unscientific, nonmedical treatment unlikely to have any value beyond the laying-on-of-hands and placebo effects. I don't recommend it.

Q. *How would you compare the relative efficacy of transcutaneous electrical nerve stimulation (TENS) with that of acupuncture in relieving low back pain?*

A. Most likely the mechanism for the two forms of treatment is similar. That is, it works through some combination of counterstimulation closing "the gate" for the reception of pain signals and stimulation of endorphins (the body's own morphinelike pain-control substance).

A study (E. S. Fox and R. Melzack, *Pain,* 2:114, 1976) comparing the two methods of treatment shows a significant amount of pain reduction (about thirty-three percent) with both techniques. This reduction of pain was achieved in a majority of the patients (seventy-five percent) treated with acupuncture and slightly fewer (sixty-six percent) of the patients treated by electrical stimulation, and those treated with acupuncture apparently enjoyed more prolonged pain relief. The average was forty hours with acupuncture and twenty-three hours with electrical stimulation. But these "differences" are not significant when analyzed statistically.

This particular study did not evaluate the usefulness of acupuncture supplemented by a small electrical current running through the acupuncture needle. That technique may or may not be superior.

Q. *Should I wear a lift in my shoe?*

A. Of course, if it helps—assuming one of your legs is longer than the other. While it's controversial as to whether or not a leg-length discrepancy is causing your backache, it may nevertheless make you comfortable to correct it. Test the situation by having a cobbler do a crude adjustment on an old pair of shoes. Leg-length differences as a cause of back pain is by no means as common as some practitioners would suggest.

Q. *What do you think of DMSO for back pain?*

A. DMSO is an acronym for dimethyl sulfoxide, a substance that has been used in animal treatment for many years. More recently, it's been used to treat various human musculoskeletal disorders, especially arthritis. Athletes have used it for muscle tendon and joint pain. Its believers claim it can decrease inflammation, ease pain, and speed the healing of musculoskeletal conditions. But so far there's no proof.

When you put it on your skin, DMSO is absorbed and transmitted throughout the body. This makes for some problems. Its ease of absorption raises the possibility of toxicity. You can have a severe allergic reaction to it. Possible side effects include visual disturbances, headache, nausea, diarrhea, and dermatitis (pain, irritation, or itching of the skin). It has caused cancer in some animals.

In my opinion, DMSO's possible, unsubstantiated benefits for pain and arthritis don't outweigh its risks. In short, it probably shouldn't be used for backache, as there are safer methods for gaining relief.

Q. *What about gravity boots?*

A. This is a technique that involves turning the patient upside down—that is, in the vertical position with the head *down* and the feet *up* (in boots). This has been very popular, a virtual fad among back pain sufferers. Unfortunately, the benefit is unproven; moreover, there are risks of its causing sudden increases in blood pressure, as well as heart rate. The nerves in the region of your ankles can be irritated or damaged by the boots. There is also a significant risk of its causing bleeding in the back of the eye, the medical term being retinal hemorrhage.

SURGERY

Q. *How do I know when I should have surgery?*

A. For the sake of this discussion, I'm assuming you have severe low back pain with or without sciatica, and that you're considering surgery for pain relief, rather than to make a diagnosis, biopsy a tumor, or treat a tumor or infection. The recommended surgery, in your case, is probably a laminectomy with disc removal and/or fusion. Or the surgery under consideration may be a fusion needed to treat spondylolisthesis (a slipped vertebra).

First make sure you're under the care of a spine specialist and that you've given conservative treatment a fair try. This means two to three days' bed rest and analgesic medication and a reasonable period of some combination of physical therapy, traction, rest, and medication. A "reasonable period" means six to eight weeks for disc surgery and generally three to six months before a spinal fusion, at least. Then your doctor must have diagnosed a genuine abnormality, and you should have a positive myelogram, CAT scan, or MRI before surgery if it's for disc disease, or X-ray evidence of spondylolisthesis if it's for that problem.

Anesthesia, surgery, and hospitalization carry certain inevitable risks. To justify them, your pain should be severe, incapacitating, and compromising to your quality of life. (See Chapter VII for a more detailed account.) Every patient is different, and there are situations in which you may elect to have surgery before two or three months are up.

Ultimately the decision rests on you. If you're confused, get a second opinion.

Q. *What about my second, third, or fourth back operation?*

A. I suggest you get a second opinion for a second operation, a third opinion for a third operation, and a fourth opinion for a fourth operation. If you get unanimity you may be on the right track. If you don't get unanimity you may need a tie-breaker opinion. This is a little bit facetious, but the point is, if you're having multiple back operations you should, if you do it at all, do it with extensive consultation. The second, third, or fourth spine operation is rarely—I repeat, rarely—indicated, or successful, in relieving the pain and returning the patient to work.

Make sure your doctors have made one or more specific diagnoses. X rays, and possibly EMG (electromyelography) studies, should probably be done. Your doctors should be able to clearly explain what is wrong and convince you it's surgically correctable.

You must accept the fact that a second operation may not help you or may even make you worse (though the odds are still slightly in your favor). Your chances of getting better with a third operation are about fifty-fifty, and they're lower with a fourth. Don't *ever* allow yourself to have multiple operations for compensation or legal reasons.

I don't mean to sound too discouraging. In some rare circumstances, a person can benefit from a second or third operation (see Chapter VII). I even know a prominent orthopaedic surgeon who benefited from a fourth. However, the message is, be very hesitant about that second, third, or fourth operation.

Q. *Will I be completely cured by surgery?*

A. Surgical cures for back pain are generally presented in terms of success, or in terms of good and excellent results. The percentages we have discussed throughout the text are the probability of a good or an excellent result. I generally tell patients this translates into their satisfaction and their opinion that it was worth it all to go through the experience.

I also like to remind them that they won't have a new back, or a perfect spine, and they may not be quite as good as they were before they ever had a problem.

Q. *How much of the disc do you take out?*

A. Most surgeons do not remove the entire disc, nor do they even attempt it. Our practice, which we believe is justified by our collective experience and the medical literature, is to remove the offending part of the disc and a margin beyond that. This usually means taking all of the extruded part of the disc and perhaps twenty percent of the remainder. This is a good compromise in terms of maintaining some mechanical integrity of the functional spinal unit, avoiding any complications that could occur should one rigorously attempt to remove the entire disc, and removing enough to minimize the likelihood of subsequent herniation of material within the disc. We also make a point to carefully remove all *loose* material inside the disc space.

Q. *Will my back collapse if you take out my disc?*

A. Sometimes with an attempt at a total discectomy, there is some collapse of the interspace. Also, disc degeneration and partial removal of the disc can sometimes result in some narrowing of the disc space. This in and of itself is not a problem.

Sometimes this question is evoked by the patient's worry that the unseparated vertebral bodies will be scraping together after the disc is removed. This is not something that one need be concerned about. Even if there is some collapse, there is not necessarily a problem with the bones scraping together.

Sometimes, however, in association with mechanical changes, disc degeneration, and/or disc removal, there are changes in the facet joints (the posterior intervertebral joints of the functional spinal unit). When this occurs it may be arthritis, and there may be pain and difficulty.

On rare occasions, a spinal fusion is required some years after partial removal of a degenerated disc. This problem can also develop without associated surgical disc removal.

Q. *Can I give my own blood for surgery?*

A. Yes. Most major hospitals do have programs in which you can donate your own blood for transfusion. If for any reason this does not work, is not available, there are administrative problems, the timing is inappropriate, etc., consider this: Although it is more of a risk than auto-transfusion, we believe it is in your best interest to sign a release allowing your doctors to give you a transfusion from a donor if they deem it in your best interest as regards risk and benefits. Nevertheless, it is preferable and desirable to avoid the exposure to diseases that can be transmitted through transfusion, even with the careful screening methods that are now available.

Q. *How big will my incision be?*

A. "Just right!"

I am glad you asked that question, because I think it is an important one, and this answer should be helpful to you.

I will begin by suggesting that cosmetics are very important to many individuals. No one *wants* to have any scars on their body. Many think the smaller the better. Let me attempt to put this in some perspective.

The size of the incision is not a reliable measure of the seriousness, danger, extent, efficacy, or desirability of any particular operation. Please read that sentence again, as it is important. I believe patients, as a result of some medical marketing, perhaps, put too much emphasis on the length of an incision.

It's quite possible to perform a huge, lousy, and ineffective operation through a rather small incision. Conversely, it is possible to do a neat, safe, and quite effective operation through a very large incision. Clearly the least amount of incision that is compatible with a safe and effective operation is desirable. However, one should never compromise in any way an operation in order to have a tiny incision.

Now, let's return to the issue of cosmetics. A vertical, well-centered, midline incision in the lumbar spine is not at all cosmetically offensive. The other important issues in cosmesis of an incision are the type of suture that is used and the techniques that are used for closure. Generally, where cosmesis is of major importance the surgeon attempts to avoid crosshatching scars from sutures. Ask your surgeon about a "subcuticular closure" if cosmesis is important to you.

Midline lumbar spine incisions, both short (5 cm., or 2 inches) and long (10 cm., or 4 inches), are readily acceptable and compatible with everything from string bikinis on up.

Q. *What about this microsurgery procedure? The one where they claim it is possible to take out your disc through a 1-inch incision?*

A. It is true that this procedure involves less surgery than the usual laminectomy for disc excision. The question is whether the benefits of that smaller amount of surgery outweigh the limitations of the procedure. They rarely do.

If you have a very specific kind of disc problem—that is, one where there is a clear-cut displaced fragment of disc that is lying in just the right place so that the nerves can be moved out of the way and the disc can be easily removed—

then the positives of this procedure may outweigh the negatives.

If, on the other hand, in the usual situation where the offending pathology does not turn out to be there, but is slightly up, down, or to one side or the other, only part or none of the offending disc can be removed through this limited access. In this case the negatives will outweigh the positives.

Because there are so many factors that can compromise the efficacy of this method, I believe that traditional formal exposure is to be preferred.

Q. *If I have spinal fusion, will it interfere with my lovemaking?*

A. The answer is yes and no. A mobile lumbar spine definitely contributes to the pelvic motions in sex, just as in dancing. You'll be only minimally compromised if your fusion involves just one motion-segment—that is, two vertebrae fused together. Perhaps if two levels—two segments of functional spinal units—are fused, you'll experience some limitation. But we're speaking of a trade-off. The issue is not the pelvic motion of a fused back versus that of a normal back; the comparison is between a disabled, painful back and a fused back. So there's likely to be a *net benefit* if one is trading some loss of motion for loss of severe pain. Discuss this issue with your surgeon before your operation.

POSTSURGERY CARE

Q. *In terms of my physical activity, will I be able to do as much—or even more—than prior to surgery?*

A. The answer here is that we always attempt to rehabilitate our patients back to whatever level of activity they aspire to. We think it's prudent before answering his/her question to ask the patient if he/she was a decathlon champion *before* having the back problem. We do think a careful rehabilitation program after good surgery can get people to very high levels of achievement—witness Joe Montana, National Football League quarterback and Super Bowl champion, following lumbar spine disc surgery. Sometimes, though, the gradual rehabilitation process does not get patients up to the level they had hoped for. Nevertheless, the patient whose outcome is successful can do a great deal more than before the surgery, and is often able to find a level of activity that is appropriate.

Q. *When can I take a shower after my back operation?*

A. Unless there is some complication with your incision, you may shower on the tenth postoperative day, provided you are able to walk in the shower, balance, stand, etc.

SOCIAL AND PSYCHOLOGICAL ISSUES

Q. *How do I know when to go back to work after an acute attack?*

A. This is a complex question, and you'll find a more detailed answer in Chapter V. The bottom line is to rely on your doctor's advice. Remember, too, that while you need to protect yourself and your earning power, you don't want to turn into a chronic "compensationitis" sufferer. It's certainly best for you as regards overall quality of life to *prevent* chronic disability and long-term pain. Let your disease process, and nothing else, dictate your work activities. Recent programs being developed in Sweden advocate the concept that getting back to work can be therapeutic for the back pain patient.

Q. *What should I do if my doctor tells me my pain is all in my head?*

A. Psychiatrists tell us we shouldn't tell you your pain is all in your head even if we think so, since this tends to make patients angry, resentful, and uncooperative. When someone is told his pain is imaginary, he may go about consciously or unconsciously trying to prove it's real. This makes the pain more deeply ingrained and harder to dislodge. Then, of course, we may be wrong. In any case, we shouldn't operate on you when we think your pain is psychological.

There's a difference between having your pain strictly in your head and having your backache affected by what is going on in your head. What is occurring in your life, on the job, and in your family can certainly aggravate a backache.

If your doctor says your pain is psychological, don't feel ashamed. Realize that emotional problems, especially in our stressful society, are every bit as painful and as noble as a broken leg. There are numerous medical channels for getting emotional support. You may wish to schedule a consultation with a psychiatrist, and with another orthopedist as well. Try to avoid getting angry and to remain cooperative, as ninety-nine times out of a hundred your doctors are truly interested in helping you.

Q. *How do I know if the pain is in my head?*

A. Some pain is imaginary, and some pain is stimulated or made worse by tension, sleep deprivation, and morning lethargy. If it appears when you're frightened, guilty, angry, stressed, or tense, your pain may be to some extent psychological. Such pains are often subconscious, and it's difficult to recognize their pattern. Does your pain, for example, gain you more attention from your family, or let you avoid certain things like household chores, work responsibilities, sexual commitments, and so on?

Several psychological tests are designed to detect the psychological roots of a pain syndrome. The MMPI (Minnesota Multiphasic Personality Inventory) is perhaps the most common psychological screening test. A wealth of experience and data back up its accuracy. It provides a personality profile that may reveal evidence of depression, hysteria, or hypochondriasis, which is the tendency to focus on or exaggerate physical complaints. There are also many other psychological tests, such as the "mini-mult" (a short version of the MMPI), the Middlesex Hospital questionnaire, and the Cornell Medical Index. Much can be deciphered from the way you describe your pain, your choice of words, and the overall content.

Of course, any pain has some psychological components, and some of them are helpful. *Beneficial* psychological factors may include a particular philosophical outlook, religion, mysticism, autohypnosis, and the conscious utilization of the new science of endorphins (again, natural painkillers produced by your central nervous system).

Undesirable psychological factors are depression, guilt, hostility, and anxiety. These are negative in themselves; moreover, they tend to aggravate and prolong back pain.

A final option is psychology or psychiatry. A skilled psychiatrist can offer an opinion about the role of psychological factors in your pain.

Q. *Is there too much surgery done for backache?*

A. That's a tough question. Let's examine some figures. In Canada and the United States, 760 people out of a million have disc surgery annually, compared with 125 out of a million in Sweden and 110 out of a million in Great Britain. In South Africa, 360 out of a million whites (although only 0.5 out of a million blacks), have back surgery each year. These numbers raise some interesting medical, social, economic, and political speculations.

It appears that in countries with socialized medicine there are perhaps *too few* back operations performed, and *too many* in countries where there's a fee involved. Then, too, cultural demands and expectations of bodily comfort may be higher in North America than in Sweden or Britain, and U.S. and Canadian patients may demand more aggressive treatment. Medical care is more readily available in some countries than in others. There are waiting lists for elective surgery in countries with socialized medicine, such as Britain and Sweden—and South African blacks, it would appear, are virtually excluded from elective back surgery.

Since back surgery is elective and intended to improve quality of life, it's a subjective matter, making it difficult to say how much pain is enough to warrant surgery. But if you follow this book's suggestions, you needn't worry about having unnecessary surgery.

Q. *If I have a fresh, severe low back problem with or without sciatic pain (leg pain), will an orgasmic experience irritate the situation in any way or will it cause any harm or be painful?*

A. No. It will not irritate the situation. It will not cause any harm and it will not be painful. The physical activity involved in the process of achieving an orgasm may cause pain and irritate your back. But the orgasm itself is without liability. See Chapter VIII for ways to avoid irritating your back while making love.

DOCTORS AND THERAPISTS

Q. *Can non-M.D. practitioners, such as osteopaths, chiropractors, acupuncturists, herbalists, or faith healers, help my back problem?*

A. Some of this is covered elsewhere in the text, but let me review some of the principles.

Now, we know the placebo effect can crop up in connection with any treatment. And the natural course of acute back disease is such that ninety percent of patients will be better within two months. So, say you go to an herbalist, faith healer, or some other practitioner and get well during that period. You may believe the healer performed the miracle. Maybe he/she did, but obviously you had a ninety percent chance of getting well "on your own," provided you waited eight weeks.

But let's not neglect psychology. Whatever his/her background, training, and tools, any practitioner can potentially use his/her personality to make you feel better. This is especially true when your major problem is pain. Anyone who exudes warmth, concern, confidence, and a positive attitude will inspire faith in the afflicted person, and this alone can ease pain.

Naturally, I can't write without bias, given my training and experience in scientifically based Western medicine. I think a good, well-trained M.D. can offer you treatment founded on solid science and adequate diagnostic and treatment procedures. This protects you from being inappropriately treated for the wrong disease while your real disease gets worse, possibly even endangering your life.

The liability of a nonmedical healer is the possibility he/she will do more harm than good by misdiagnosis. The "quack" isn't just a figment of the AMA's imagination. There are real-life con artists in the health profession, as in any other, and the stereotypical used-car dealer doesn't just turn up around defective Chevys and Cadillacs. You can waste time and money (as well as your health) on ineffective treatments.

Some osteopaths are qualified M.D.'s as in California and several other states where they practice medicine. Chiropractors come good and bad, careful and careless. Some are ethical, some aren't. However, there's no scientific basis whatsoever for the theory that all diseases emanate from subluxations of the vertebrae (see the next question).

Now for specifics.

Spinal Manipulation, practiced by chiropractors, is a legitimate form of symptomatic treatment for certain appropriately diagnosed spine conditions. When done carefully, it can temporarily relieve pain, though its benefit hasn't been proven to outdo the combined benefits of the placebo effect and natural healing. Of course, the same is true of most conservative back treatments.

For some patients, chiropractic treatment is inappropriate, even dangerous. Don't stick with it for long periods if you're not getting any prolonged, objective pain relief.

Acupuncture can treat idiopathic low back pain (pain not linked to a specific disease process) without risk. Again, though, it makes no sense to continue acupuncture for long if it's not helping. A well-controlled clinical study in 1983 showed the results to be the same as with a placebo. At that time there were seven high-quality studies in the medical literature. *Two* of the studies showed acupuncture to be superior to the placebo; in the remaining *five* there was no difference.

Herbal Therapy raises the same points. A qualified physician should check your back first. If your herbalist is careful, your risks are very minor. But whenever you're introducing substances into your body, you can run into complications.

Faith Healing, again, shouldn't replace medical diagnosis. As long as you're not spending exorbitant sums, spiritual help is probably good for you.

Q. *What is subluxation? What is chiropractic adjustment?*

A. Subluxation can be defined as partial dislocation, a situation in which X rays allegedly show an abnormal positioning between two adjacent vertebrae. The displacement must reach a certain point before it's called a subluxation. It may or may not cause pain. The subluxation that the chiropractor refers to cannot be seen by independent observers. This has been one of their major problems.

In chiropractic manipulation, the vertebrae are supposedly manipulated back into their normal position. The chiropractic hypothesis is that as a vertebra slips out again, you have pain and it must be put back once more. This process can go on *ad infinitum,* and manipulations are sometimes sold in prepaid packages of a certain number.

What bothers me is this: If a vertebra is simply pushed back into place, why assume it will stay there? And why would continually pushing it back *ever* make it stick? It's awfully tempting to suppose that the treatment's "success" is related to the placebo effect and/or the natural course of the ailment. Though the pain probably was never related to "subluxation" in the first place, manipulation gets the credit for relieving it.

You may have heard the story of the man who comes in hunched over with terrible pain and muscle spasm, then has a spinal manipulation and walks away from the table standing erect and feeling wonderful. No doubt such phenomena occur, but just about any sort of practitioner using his/her favorite "treatment" can relate similar tales. Obviously, we're looking at a complex psychophysiological problem that responds dramatically to what we dub the "treatment situation." This is the mystery and misery of low back pain.

Q. *What kind of doctor should take care of my back? When do I need a consultant or a specialist?*

A. It's a good idea to start with a general practitioner, family-medicine doctor, or internist who has known you and your family for a few years. But it's not the only way to go. Group practices and health care organizations are a viable alternative.

If you have back pain associated with leg pain, go to your family doctor, internist, health care clinic, or a spine care specialty facility. They will take a medical history, examine you, and manage your ensuing workup and treatment. Most back pain is the idiopathic type, and analgesia, rest, and various forms of physical therapy are considered the best prescription.

If you haven't improved after three to six weeks of the above regimen, you may want to see a specialist. I'd recommend a board-certified orthopaedic surgeon or neurosurgeon. The choice between the two is largely dictated by convenience and your own gut feelings about a particular doctor.

It's fair to say that orthopaedic surgeons are generally more knowledgeable about the conservative care of spine problems. Their training includes more attention to the mechanical, structural, architectural, and intervertebral joint factors related to the spine. However, a particular doctor's knowledge, experience, and manner are more important than his/her specialty.

MISCELLANEOUS

Q. *Will disco, social, and ballroom dancing give me a backache?*

A. Let's start with disco, the most vigorous—and the sort most often done by untrained, occasional dancers. Twisting and jerking motions, and arching of the back, often irritate low back pain. The high heels women wear for ballroom dancing may also hurt one's back.

If you don't have back pain while dancing, go ahead and enjoy. Nature is helpful. If you hurt a little, slow down or stop. When you feel better, gradually work back into it, staying in good condition and pacing yourself. Sometimes, though, your back won't warn you. Also, we know that a few drinks not only loosens up social inhibitions, but in addition may reduce the protective mechanisms of the muscles that support the spine. There's also a "morning after" type of backache you can learn to avoid by pacing yourself during the "midnight hours."

Q. *Can my problem recur?*

A. This patient is usually asking about a herniated disc, and the answer, of course, is that it can recur. It can happen at a new level or it can happen again at the same level. The latter is very unlikely, but nevertheless possible. Generally, when that occurs it is managed the same as if it were a fresh disc herniation.

It is probably also reasonable to assume that all other things being equal, a patient who has had one disc herniation is a little more likely than the average person who has not had a disc herniation to have a new or recurrent disc problem.

Q. *How much does everything we've said about backache apply to neck ache?*

A. A great deal. It's much the same, except that there are fewer visceral diseases that cause neck pain, and its overall prevalence is lower. Since we know less about the biomechanics and ergonomics of neck pain, we have less advice to offer about its management.

Neck-disc surgery is similar to back-disc surgery, though it's generally done from the front and more often calls for a fusion.

We don't see as many totally disabled neck-pain patients. For some reason, in this society, the work environment especially fosters back pain, though half of all people with work-related backache have neck pain, too. Your posture while reading, writing, or working at a desk can mean a pain in the neck, as can tension and anxiety. Neck pain gained considerable attention and notoriety in the medicolegal field with the phenomenon of whiplash, which fortunately has been reduced by an increase in the use of car headrests.

Treatment of neck ache, like treatment of backache, should first exhaust the reasonable steps of conservative therapy. It calls for surgery only in specific correctable situations.

Q. *What does it feel like to be in a body cast?*

A. Body casts vary. Some immobilize and encumber the patient more than others. Some cover just the middle part of the body, from the pelvis to the rib cage. Others extend from the nipple line down one leg to the knees. Usually, a large hole is cut out to allow your abdomen to expand.

Most patients have no problem with a cast. But some adults have trouble adjusting to its constraints. They may have anxiety, frustration, or simply be very annoyed that they must wear it.

If this is the case with you, discuss it with your doctor beforehand and during the cast period. Even those who don't like casts generally manage to adapt with some support from doctors, nurses, friends, and relatives. If you're in a body cast and start vomiting repeatedly, get in touch with your doctor immediately. It may be a sign of intestinal problems caused by the cast. (See Chapter VI.)

Q. *What is Stoshak-Mortimer Syndrome? Perhaps you know of it as "jean-seam coccygodynia."*

A. This is a rather unusual medical condition in which someone, most likely an adolescent female, presents with low back pain. On careful questioning the pain is localized mainly or in part at the coccyx or tail bone (see Figure 2–1, page 30). The patient is likely to be wearing tight-fitting jeans with a hard reinforced midline seam, and sitting in a fairly hard seat at school. The solution is not to take a vacation from school, but from the hard-seam jeans. The pain will disappear in two to three weeks.

Q. *Is the back-pain problem hereditary?*

A. Again, this question usually comes from a patient with a herniated disc. There has been some recent evidence that perhaps within some families there is a higher than expected prevalence of problems of disc herniation. This has not yet been precisely documented and proven, but should be considered a possibility at this point.

Q. *The doctor told me I had not one, but two or three degenerated discs. Does this mean my whole spine will degenerate?*

A. The appropriate medical term for changes within a disc is "degeneration." Unfortunately, this carries rather threatening connotations and is bad-sounding to many of us. I like to point out to patients that as bad as the word sounds, disc degeneration is a natural process that occurs between age thirty and fifty and is like the wrinkling of our skin and graying of our hair.

It is the case that in this process of degeneration, some discs will herniate and some others will become painful *without* herniating.

In answer to your question, though, having been told that you have two or three degenerating discs is no reason to be alarmed that your whole spine is going to become diseased, painful, inadequate, and in need of a great deal of treatment.

Chapter XI

The Future of Back Care

Some Predictions, Speculations, and Hopes

IF YOU'RE battling chronic backache, you probably wonder how the future will deal with man's most important non-life-threatening ailment. Will backache one day be wiped out like smallpox or bubonic plague? Or will we merely get more adept at diagnosing and treating it? Will our diagnostic tests and surgical procedures become less painful or risky? Will epidemiologists be able to predict—with the statistical accuracy of, say, cereal manufacturers pinpointing their markets—exactly who's at risk, and why? Will spine consultants tell us precisely how to revamp our life-styles to spare out backs?

The predictions you'll read here are conservative, and may seem less than earthshaking to the uninitiated. On the other hand, anyone intimate with the puzzles of idiopathic back pain (and if you've read this whole book, you're included) may find the projections overly optimistic, even fantastic. Yet I believe most of the following forecasts will come true in your lifetime.

Epidemiology

Epidemiology is the study of the incidence of a disease in a particular population, with reference to recognizing the cause of the disease. The population is usually characterized according to age, sex, occupation, race, religion, geography, and socioeconomic standing.

- There will be more studies of the role of vibrations as a cause of disc herniation. We will learn more about why certain cars may be causing disc problems.
- One thing we've neglected up to now are studies to determine what sort of person is *unlikely* to develop serious back problems, and I think before long we'll have his/her demographic portrait. When we do, the rest of us may learn to imitate these backache-free types by simulating the way they live and work.
- Being in shape may prove to be one of the factors that characterize those who are unlikely to develop serious back pain.

Emotions/Psychology/Socioeconomics

You've learned that your state of mind is intricately intertwined with the state of your back.

- We can look forward to more accurate psychological tests to gauge which people could benefit most from counseling or psychotherapy, and which would be better off with another form of treatment, such as medication or exercise. We'll learn even more accurately to identify patients who are likely to be helped by surgery.
- Stress, depression, and other mental states affect your body's physiology and biochemistry. As we refine our understanding of exactly how your altered biochemistry changes your spine's mechanical behavior so as to cause pain, we'll learn to protect against or even undo the damage.
- Your brain and central nervous system can produce and respond to chemicals that modify your perception of pain. Specifically, we now know our bodies produce internal opiates, called endorphins, that block pain. They aren't the only naturally produced pain-modifying "drugs" in our bodies. As we explore the biochemistry of pain, we'll be able to unlock the body's pain mechanisms. With the current knowledge explosion in the field of endorphins and related substances, we'll almost certainly develop new methods of stimulating their secretion.

- We know that psychological factors in the workplace may affect the prevalence of low back pain problems. Future studies will identify these factors more clearly. We will discover methods and techniques for improving the psychological environment of the workplace.
- Physicians and therapists will have more psychologically based skills and methods designed to motivate, engender cooperation from, and therefore provide better results for our patients. Behavioral psychologists will help to provide the new knowledge for these skills.
- This issue may be too complex to handle succinctly here, but here is a try, as I believe that it will be useful to present it: There is considerable evidence that compensation laws—among other things, of course—play a significant role in the clinical problem of low back pain. I *am not* addressing the topic of malingering. True malingering in my opinion is very rare. However, there is evidence that some compensation laws and some policies and practices tend to perpetuate pain and pain behavior. These laws and practices will be revisited first in Sweden, with the goal of improving them so that they are fair to the back-pain sufferer as well as just and appropriate for the overall society. At present there is a great deal of human suffering and disability, as well as health care and administrative costs, all of which could be significantly reduced if the laws and practices could be justly improved. We may witness some serious attempts at this in the not-so-distant future.

Medication

- I predict we'll see safer and more effective drugs to combat stress and improve our moods. These futuristic drugs may enable us to nip many a backache in the bud.
- New drugs will fight inflammation—or the tissues' response to it—better than current anti-inflammatory drugs.

Muscles/Fascia/Discs

- Future studies and refinements of MRI techniques will help us to recognize when back pain is due to muscle and/or fascia injury or disease. The clinical science of various muscle fascia and tendon conditions that may cause pain will be discovered and described. The elusive and protean problem of "muscle spasm" will be analyzed.

The clinical science of muscle development, strengthening, and conditioning, and the quantitative monitoring of muscle function will be greatly advanced. The therapeutic benefit of muscle rehabilitation for low back pain will be more clearly delineated.

I also look forward to being able to distinguish scientifically and clinically between actively painful discs and those that are simply wearing out.

- Not all herniated discs are painful. We will learn why some are and some aren't. We will better delineate how, when, where, and why some cause inflammation and/or pain and others do not.

Biomechanics

Biomechanics are crucial to your back. No matter what your back disease, properly controlled biomechanics can minimize pain and improper biomechanics can aggravate it. Much future progress lies in the study of the "B and the B of the I.V.D."—that is, the Biochemistry and the Biomechanics of the Intervertebral Disc.

- New information will permit us to improve the mechanics of work and play so as to cut down on spine stresses and prevent injury. Back-pain schools will become more numerous and effective, back-care information more accurate and better disseminated.
- Disease-prevention courses will enter our school systems; students will learn the rudiments of back protection. Medical students will be taught more about back pain and encouraged to do spine research.
- In industry, tests of body strength and body mechanics will match workers with appropriate jobs and protect them from spine-endangering tasks. These and other screening tests will be used to instruct employees in back-saving precautions. Employers will design workplaces to minimize back stress and injury. For example, the design and selection of seats will be based on back protection first, and only secondly on aesthetics. (The two are *not* mutually exclusive.) It has been shown that appropriate design in the workplace can prevent one-third of compensable low back injuries. Equipment in the working

and/or lifting areas will be constructed to the proper height to limit bending. In my opinion, no new work environment should be built without informed and thorough consideration of the biomechanics involved in protecting the back. On-the-job information and exercise programs will emphasize general conditioning and back care.

- And what about conditions on the home front? The future will transform design there, as well. We'll institute painless vacuuming methods and special exercise and back-care programs for home workers. Cleaning and upkeep of floors, furniture, beds, and clothes will be revamped to minimize back strain.
- New designs in automobile seats and suspension will attenuate the bump-bump-bump punishment to your back. The future consumer will choose a new car as much on the basis of "vibes-per-mile" as on miles-per-gallon. New seat designs will also enhance public-transportation vehicles and airplanes.
- Improvements in athletic equipment, coaching, training techniques, and, yes, maybe even rule changes—with tradition deferring to human health—will benefit athletes' backs.
- The problem of spinal instability as we have traditionally looked at it will change radically during the next decade. One or more mechanical derangements of the spine, which can be recognized and reasonably correlated with back pain, will be discovered. Percutaneous transpedicular immobilization of the spine as a means of identifying spinal instability will be further developed and will help in the understanding of this clinical problem.

Biochemistry

The analysis of the spine's structure ultimately leads us all the way down to the chemical molecules that make up our anatomy. The intervertebral disc and cartilage, for example, are composed mainly of water, collagen, and proteoglycans. Bone is made up of collagen and calcified hydroxy appetite crystals. The physiology and nutrition of the disc, and its water content, probably have a lot to do with backache.

- We'll learn about the normal or abnormal chemical makeup of the disc and facet joints. Circulatory, nutritional, and hormonal changes can affect the disc's biochemistry, causing pain. We know, for example, that pregnancy and menstruation often aggravate backache, probably via biochemical changes.

- Clearly, stress can provoke or worsen back pain. The following excerpt from a letter from a back patient who is also an orthopaedic surgeon illustrates the delicate interplay between psychological trauma and disc disease:

> I had two episodes of moderately severe low back pain . . . and muscle spasm with no sciatica, each of which lasted about four or five days. The episodes were severe enough to make me miss work and required me to be recumbent. . . . The first episode occurred about the time I was to take my Orthopaedic Boards in September of 1978. The second episode, which was practically identical to the first, occurred just over a year later at a time of major personal stress within my family. . . . In the summer of 1980, I separated from the Air Force . . . and returned to my hometown of Little Rock, Arkansas, where I went into the private practice of orthopaedics. The week before I started in my new position [I developed a fresh case of severe backache].

The future will most likely *prove* that stress, such as this young doctor suffered, does indeed cause back pain. New medication to prevent or reverse the stress process will come to our aid.

- Smoking and prolonged riding or driving in cars, trucks, or buses, epidemiologists say, can spell backache. In the next few years we'll learn whether nicotine or road vibrations change the spine's circulation and blood supply, hampering disc nutrition.
- Several important breakthroughs in disc biochemistry may revolutionize our understanding of disc disease. Biochemical tests may reveal a hereditary abnormality in the disc. Or we may turn up abnormal biochemical irritants in the disc that cause nerve irritation and pain. This leads us directly into the neurology of low back pain.

Nerves and Pain

The extremely complex and sophisticated science of neurophysiology has not yet told us much about backache.

- Future research is likely to identify just which nerves are transmitting pain in the back, and why. What is it that starts the chain of events that stimulates a nerve ending, and goes to the spinal cord, and the brain, to culminate in the brain's reasoning cortex saying to itself, "My back hurts"? Is it a push, a pull, a squeeze, a shear force, a chemical, an electrical charge, too little oxygen, too much acid—or what? We'll find out whether it takes place in the disc, muscle, facet joint, bone, cartilage, or at several sites.
- We'll also learn how to better manipulate the pain-control mechanisms of the brain and spinal cord, perhaps by regulating natural painkillers like endorphins. The upshot is that you may be trained in techniques to control your own pain without drugs.

Diagnostic Tests

- The imaging capabilities and techniques based on MRI will improve, and biochemical labeling is likely to help in clinical evaluations.
- I also envision using more dynamic imaging tests—that is, tests that image the spine in different positions with different stresses.
- Improvements in electrical diagnostic techniques will permit them to be used more effectively.
- The idea of a "trial" of fixation of two or more vertebrae in the low back to determine whether or not pain is eliminated may prove to be a useful procedure. If so, don't be put off by the fact that there will temporarily be metal inside the vertebral bone that extends out through the skin to the outside. Sounds dramatic, and it is, but it's also quite reasonable, provided studies show it to be useful. The idea is that this technique can thoroughly fix the vertebrae, and if this reliability eliminates the pain, then a spinal fusion may benefit the patient.

Treatment

- Advances in the selection, precision, and efficacy of many surgical treatments will help back sufferers. New percutaneous discectomy techniques and instrumentation techniques will be developed and utilized. We'll have new and different surgical methods for pain arising from the facet joints. Severe arthritis will be relieved with an internally implantable spine prosthesis.

- Better painkillers and anti-inflammatory drugs will join our arsenal.
- Exercise and ergonomic programs will improve and we will learn precisely which exercises are best. The equipment will be developed to guide and nurture these therapeutically appropriate exercises.
- Spinal manipulation won't stay in a "Who knows?" limbo. Scientific analysis will tell us unequivocally whether it works or not.

Of course, no progress will occur through natural evolution alone. All these advances depend on extensive research in several medical and scientific fields.

What can you do about it? You can, of course, contribute to a university, medical school, hospital, or researcher of your choice. Or you can use your influence in a corporation, insurance company, foundation, or labor union. *Advocate preventive programs in your sphere of influence.*

It's estimated that two billion people will have backache this year and that two million doctors will treat them, but that only about twenty people on earth will be carefully researching back disease. We have a long way to go.

So ends the proselytizing part of this book. I hope you won't think a couple of brief paragraphs, *to support your local back-pain researcher,* too much of an imposition.

The Compensation Issue

There is a very serious, expensive, and complex game that's played in our society. The players are the patient (worker or professional), lawyer, doctor, employer, union, insurance company, and our society. In any given game there may be any combination of winners and losers. Unfortunately, the patient and/or our society is often the loser. Our compensation laws, labor practices, employee policies, insurance and legal systems all somehow work in such a way as to potentiate, foster, and perpetuate pain behavior and disability. In the future our society will improve this current counterproductive situation in the following manner: A multidisciplinary panel of experts—economists, lawyers, clinicians, psychologists, psychiatrists, ethicists, labor leaders, insurance and corporate leaders—will convene. The purpose will be to study the problem with the goal of rewriting the compensation laws so that justice is assured to the individual back-pain sufferer and to our society. It is possible to devise fair, humanitarian laws and practices that *do not* perpetuate illness and engender a great deal of nonproductive expenditure of time and money on the part of doctors, lawyers, judges, therapists, insurance personnel, employers, etc. This we can look forward to in the future.

CONCLUSION

If you have journeyed through this book from start to finish, thanks for staying with me. I sincerely hope that the information here has diminished your pain, frustration, and confusion and enhanced your strength, optimism, determination, and ability to beat the backache and get on with your life!

Glossary*

AIDS: Acquired immunodeficiency syndrome. A fatal viral infection in which the body's ability to combat infection and cancer is reduced to the point that the patient succumbs to one or both.

AEROBIC EXERCISE: Any of a variety of sustained exercises, such as jogging or rowing, that stimulate and strengthen the heart and lungs thereby improving the body's utilization of oxygen.

ANALGESIC: Pain-controlling medication such as Tylenol, aspirin, Darvon, Darvocet, Demerol, codeine.

ANKYLOSING SPONDYLITIS: An inflammatory disease of the spine that causes pain and leads to bony ankylosis of the vertebral articulations.

ANNULUS: The tough outer fibrous portion of the intervertebral disc (see Figures 2–3 and 2–6B).

ANTI-INFLAMMATORY: Drugs such as Feldene (piroxicam), Motrin (ibuprofen), Naprosyn (naproxen), Voltaren (diclofenac sodium), etc., that tend to reduce swelling, inflammation, and pain.

ARACHNOIDITIS: Inflammatory disease leading to fibrosis that binds the roots of the cauda equina.

ARTHRITIS: Inflammation and irritation of the joints. It is associated with swelling, secretion of fluid, and usually pain.

ARTHRODESIS: A synonym for fusion (see Fusion).

AXIAL ROTATION: Twisting of the spine about the long axis of the body. Figure 2–8D.

BENDING MOMENT: When a load is applied to a long structure that is not directly supported at the point of application of the load, the structure deforms, and this deformation is called bending. The bending moment is a product of the force applied times the distance between the point of application and the point of attachment of the long structure.

BEHAVIOR MODIFICATION: The utilization of one or more of a number of techniques based on learning theory and the principles of learning

* This glossary was prepared with the help of *Dorland's Medical Dictionary* and the *American Academy of Orthopaedic Surgeons' Glossary of Spinal Terminology.*

to effect specific changes in behavior. In this context we want the patient's pain behavior (hurting and suffering) to change.

BIOFEEDBACK: A process whereby one or more physiological systems is monitored, usually electronically, and the information is fed back to the individual in a usable form so that he/she can learn to exercise voluntary control over the physiological system. The aim is to reduce or remove unpleasant experiences associated with bodily functions.

BONE SCAN: A scan in which an image of the bone is produced after the patient is given a radioactive material. The material then collects in the bone, with an increased concentration in areas where there is an increased blood supply to the bone. This is done by moving a detector with a sweeping beam across the area of interest. An image of the bone in any area of concentrated activity can be developed and interpreted.

CAT SCAN: A computerized tomogram (an X-ray image) that can be reconstituted by a computer to depict bone and soft tissues in several planes. It provides visual slices of the material from several perspectives. One important point for readers here is that it allows one a view of the spinal canal and evidence of soft-tissue encroachment, such as a herniated disc, into it.

CENTER OF GRAVITY: The point in a body where the body mass is centered.

CHEMONUCLEOLYSIS: A process through which biological or biochemical substances are placed in the intervertebral disc in order to break down the chemical substances within the disc. Enzymes are placed within the disc in order to achieve this effect. Chymopapain and collagenase are commonly used enzymes for this purpose.

CLIMAX: A synonym for orgasm.

CLINICAL STABILITY: The ability of the spine under physiological loads to limit patterns of displacement so as not to damage or irritate the spinal cord or nerve root and, in addition, to prevent incapacitating deformity or pain due to structural changes. This is commonly measured as excessive motion on X rays with the patient in full flexion and full extension.

COCCYX: The structure at the very tip of the spine—tailbone. This structure is connected to the bottom of the sacrum.

COMPENSATIONITIS: Medical jargon for pain behavior that may be subconsciously influenced by issues of compensation and/or litigation.

COMPRESSION: The normal force that tends to push together material fibers. The unit of measure is newtons (poundforce).

CONSCIOUS: That part of a person's psychological functioning of which he/she is generally aware.

DAMPING: A material property that constitutes resistance to speed.

DEGENERATION: A change of tissue from one form and function to another. Commonly used to describe changes in the intervertebral disc. The disc is transformed over many years from an elastic, resilient, strong structure with a jellylike center and firm periphery to a dried-out structure with a relatively inelastic, fragmented periphery. Usually in this process the disc loses some of its height (see Figure 3–1).

DEGENERATIVE DISC DISEASE: A situation in which disc degeneration produces clinical symptoms and signs.

DEGENERATIVE JOINT DISEASE OF THE ZYGAPOPHYSEAL JOINT: Degenerative changes in the facet joints characterized by cartilage thinning and osteophyte formation (see Figure 3–5).

DENIAL: A defense mechanism whereby the individual rejects certain aspects or interpretations of external reality. They may be replaced by unrealistic or wish-fulfilling ideation.

DEPRESSIVE NEUROSIS: An excessive reaction of depression due to an internal conflict or to an identifiable event, such as the loss of a loved object or cherished possession.

DISC DEGENERATION: The loss of the structural and functional integrity of the disc. This may or may not be a cause of pain (see Figure 3–1).

DISC NARROWING: A situation in which a disc is degenerating. It loses its height and the two vertebral bodies come closer together as a result of the narrowing of the disc (see Figure 3–1).

DISC SCARRING: Medical jargon for soft tissue that is sometimes seen on an X ray to surround a nerve root in the region or at the level of a previously operated-on herniated disc.

DISCECTOMY: The removal of all or part of the intervertebral disc.

DISCOGRAPHY: The introduction of radio-opaque fluid into the nucleus pulposus for purposes of identifying disc configuration. This may include evaluation of the amount of fluid injected or the resistance to fluid injected. Some clinicians also assess the pain response to injection of radio-opaque media and/or other substances designed to either stimulate or relieve pain.

DISPLACED DISC: A situation in which fragments of disc are moved away from each other (see Figure 2–6B).

DRUG DEPENDENCE. This category is for patients who are addicted or dependent on drugs other than alcohol, tobacco, and ordinary caffeine-containing beverages. Dependence on medically prescribed drugs is also excluded, so long as the drug is medically indicated and the intake is proportionate to the medical need. This diagnosis requires evidence of habitual use or a clear sense of need for the drug.

DURA: The strongest and outermost of three membranes that protect the spinal cord and nerves of the cauda equina (see Figure 2–6B).

ELASTICITY: The ability of a material or a structure to return to its original form following the removal of the deforming load.

ENERGY-ABSORPTION CAPACITY: The mechanical energy absorbed by a structure when loaded (pressed, bent, or twisted) to failure. The unit of measure is newton meters (foot poundforce).

EPIDEMIOLOGY: The science that concerns itself with the study of factors that influence the frequency and distribution of various human diseases within a defined community.

EQUILIBRIUM: The body is said to be in a state of equilibrium if it is at rest or in uniform motion under a given set of forces and moments.

ERGONOMICS: The scientific and clinical study of the most healthy use of the body in a work, sports, or recreational setting.

EXERCISE, AEROBIC: See Aerobic Exercise.

EXERCISE, LOW-IMPACT AEROBIC: Aerobic exercise in which at least one foot must be kept on the floor at all times.

EXTENSION: Backward bending of the spine (see Figure 2–8B).

FACET JOINTS: Located behind the vertebral body, these paired joints connect the posterior elements of the vertebra. They have a slick surface and a lubricating substance, and are covered by a capsule of sinewy tissue (see Figure 2–2).

FACET RHIZOTOMY: Denervation of a zygapophyseal joint by destruction of capsular and pericapsular tissue.

FACETECTOMY: Excision of the articular process that contains the facets of a zygapophyseal joint.

FASCIA: A sheet or band of fibrous tissue that separates various muscles and organs within the body. Analagous to files in a file cabinet, where our body is the file cabinet, the various organs and muscle groups are the individual files, and the fascia are the manila folders, separating each of these files.

FATIGUE (MECHANICAL): A process of birth and growth of cracks in structures subjected to repetitive load cycles. The load is generally below the failure load of the structure.

FLEXION: Forward bending of the spine (see Figure 2–8A).

FORCE: Any action that tends to change the state of rest or motion of a body to which it is applied. The unit of measure for the magnitude of force is newtons (poundforce).

FRACTURE: A break in the continuity of bone; a failure of the bone. There are two types of fracture. A regular fracture occurs with one particular episode of force, loading, or energy input. A fatigue fracture occurs as a result of repeated loading at a level that does not cause fracture in a single episode, but rather after repeated episodes finally cause the bone to fail.

FRIGIDITY: A term applied to a female who is unable to become sexually aroused or experience an orgasm.

FUNCTIONAL SPINAL UNIT: Also referred to as the motion segment. This biomechanical term is defined as two adjacent vertebrae and their intervening soft tissue.

FUSION: A process in which a bone graft either from the patient or from another human being, or from an animal, is selected and processed and preserved, and then placed in and about the bone of a patient in such a manner as to achieve a solid union between the bone graft and the bone to which it is attached; through that coupling the two bones are united ("welded together"—like grafting a limb onto a tree). As a consequence the region is considerably immobilized. A spinal fusion is the process by which two or more vertebrae are connected with a bone graft to reduce motion and eliminate pain (see Figure 7–11).

HEMILAMINECTOMY: Removal of a vertebral laminae on one side only (see Figure 7–2).

HEPATITIS: An infection and inflammation of the liver that prevents the organ from performing many of its important functions.

HERNIATED DISC: Displacement of nuclear material and other disc components beyond the normal confines of the annulus (see page 304). Four degrees of displacement are recognized:

1. Intraspongy nuclear herniation.
2. Protrusion: The displaced material causes a discrete bulge in the annulus, but no material escapes through the annular fibers.
3. Extrusion: The displaced material is present in the spinal canal through disrupted fibers of the annulus, but remains connected to material persisting within the disc.
4. Sequestration: Nuclear material escapes into the spinal canal as free fragments that may migrate to other locations.

HYPOCHONDRIACAL NEUROSIS: A condition dominated by preoccupation with the body and with fear of presumed diseases of various organs. Those fears are not of delusional quality as in psychotic depressions; they persist despite reassurance. The condition differs from hysterical neurosis in that with hypochondria there are no actual losses or distortions of function.

HYSTERIA: An abnormal psychological condition in which symptoms observed in the patient are due more to the dynamics of the emotions than to identifiable changes in organs or tissues.

HYSTERICAL NEUROSIS: A neurosis characterized by an involuntary psychogenic loss or disorder of function. Symptoms characteristically begin and end suddenly in emotionally charged situations and are symbolic of the underlying conflict. Often they can be modified by suggestion alone. The disorder is limited to the voluntary musculature or the organs of special sense.

TYPES OF INTERVERTEBRAL DISC DISPLACEMENTS

Terms	*Definition*	*Example*
Bulging annulus fibrosis Intra spongy nuclear herniation Bulging disc	General extension of disc beyond boundary of adjacent vertebral body end plates.	Figure 7–5
Protrusion Prolapsed disc	*Distinct* bulge in annulus, created by displaced material beyond the margin of the vertebral end plate. Nuclear material may or may not have extended through the annulus. But, though herniated, it remains in continuity with the more central nuclear material.	Figure 7–5
Extrusion Extruded disc	*Large* displacement of the portion of the disc material into the spinal canal with persistent connection of extruded material with the more central nucleus with the disc.	Figure 2–6A and B 3–3 7–2
Sequestration Free Fragment	*Complete* displacement of nuclear material into the spinal canal with no connection to remaining disc. This sequestrated fragment may migrate to locations away from the level of the disc.	7–3 (but with fragment completely separated)

Comments: Clearly this is a spectrum of severity as one moves from the top to the bottom of this chart; there is some clinical relevance to this grouping of degrees of disc herniation. This is more cogent now that MRI technology makes it possible to identify the various types of disc displacements. Generally, the more severe the type of herniation bulge, protrusion, extrusion to sequestration, the more severe the symptoms. All should be initially treated conservatively. Chemonucleolysis and percutaneous nucleotomy are feasible only in those types in which the herniation is in continuity with the central nucleus (bulge, protrusion, extrusion). Surgery will work for any of the four, but should not be done for a mere bulging disc. The selection of treatment is not based just on the imaging studies of the type of disc displacement but on the entire clinical picture of the patient.

HYSTERICAL NEUROSIS, CONVERSION TYPE: In the conversion type the special senses or voluntary nervous system are affected, causing such symptoms as blindness, deafness, anosmia, anesthesias, paresthesias, paralysis, ataxias, akinesias, and dyskinesias. Often the patient shows an inappropriate lack of concern or indifference about these symptoms that may actually provide secondary gains by winning him sympathy or relieving him of unpleasant responsibilities. This type of hysterical neurosis must be distinguished from psychophysiologic disorders, which are mediated by the autonomic nervous system; from malingering, which is done consciously; and from neurological lesions, which cause anatomically circumscribed symptoms.

IMPOTENCE: Loss of the ability of the male to attain and maintain an erection up until the point of ejaculation.

INFERIOR ARTICULAR PROCESS: Part of the back of the vertebra, this is a projection which articulates with a similar structure on the vertebra below. This structure also forms part of the bony spinal canal. The bony projection is partially covered with cartilage that forms part of the small paired facet joints in the back of the spine. (Figure 2–2.)

INTERNAL FIXATION: The binding together of two or more vertebrae with implants of metal and other material.

INTERVERTEBRAL DISC: An energy-absorbent structure that lies between the cylinderlike vertebral bodies in the spine. It is made up of a jellylike center and a sinewy arrangement of crossing tissues (see Figure 2–3).

JOINT REACTION FORCE: If a joint in the body is subjected to external forces in the form of external loads and/or muscle forces, the internal reaction forces acting at the contact surfaces are called the joint reaction forces. The unit of measure is newtons (poundforce).

KINEMATICS: That division of mechanics (dynamics) that deals with the geometry of the motion of bodies—displacement, velocity, and acceleration—without taking into account the forces that produce the motion.

LAMINECTOMY: A surgical procedure in which a portion of the lamina (the platelike configuration of bone that lies posterior to the vertebral canal) is removed (see Figure 7–2).

LAMINOTOMY: Creating an opening in one or more lamina (see Figure 7–2).

LATERAL BENDING: Bending of the spine to either side (see Figure 2–8C).

LEVEL: This is often seen as "spinal level," and for the purposes of this book it would be "lumbar spinal level." It relates to the number of the vertebra to which one is referring. There are five lumbar vertebra; the fifth sits on top of the sacral vertebra that is the next level down, the fourth sits on top of the fifth, and the third on the fourth, etc., up to the first. When people describe a herniated disc that is between the L4 and L5 level, they say it is located at the L4–5 level (see Figure 3–4). Similarily, a herniated disc between L5 and S1 is said to be located at the L5–S1 level (see Figure 8–1).

LOAD: A general term describing the application of a force and/or moment (torque) to a structure. The units of measure are newtons (poundforce) for the force and newton meters (foot poundforce) for the moment.

LUMBAR LORDOSIS: The position of the vertebra of the lumbar spine in which the convexity of the curve as we look from the side is anterior (see Figure 8–1).

LUMBOSACRAL SPRAIN: A ligamentous injury of the lumbosacral region. This term is imprecise but frequently used when localized pain follows a specific moderately traumatic injury.

LUMBOSACRAL STRAIN: A musculature injury about the lumbosacral region. Like the preceding term this is imprecise and used in a similar fashion.

MALINGERING: Consciously feigning illness or pain.

MASOCHISM: A state in which pleasure is derived from suffering physiological or psychological pain. The reason is usually unconscious and usually has some sexual basis, either apparent or concealed.

MASS: The quantitative measure of inertia for linear motion. The unit of measure is kilograms (pounds).

MOTION: The relative displacement with time of a body in space, with respect to other bodies or some reference system.

MOTION SEGMENT: A unit of the spine representing inherent biomechanical characteristics of the ligamentous spine. Two vertebrae, the intervertebral disc, and all the connecting ligaments are included in the motion segment. (See also Functional Spinal Unit.)

MUSCLE SPASMS: Involuntarily contracted, intensely painful muscles.

MYELOGRAM: A radiologic test in which X rays are taken after a radio-opaque medium has been placed into the dural sheath with the cauda equina. This allows visualization of the spinal cord, cauda equina, and nerve roots. A water-soluble myelogram is done with a contrast medium that is absorbed by the body. A fat-soluble myelogram involves a contrast medium that is not absorbed by the body and must be removed.

NARCOTIC: A drug that tends to put one in a state of narcosis—that is, a stupor or sense of insensibility. Narcotics tend to combat pain more by causing the patient to become indifferent to it than by actually reducing the sensation of pain. Unfortunately, these drugs are clinically addictive.

NEUROLOGIC DEFICIT: Loss of a reflex, such as a knee-jerk reflex (the patella tendon in front of the knee is hit with a hammer and the patient involuntarily kicks the leg). Loss of normal motor strength, or loss of ability to feel light touch or pain, would also be a neurological deficit.

NEUROLOGIC PROBLEM: A situation in which the patient and/or physician is aware of an abnormality due to some malfunction of the nerves. Obvious examples would be weakness, numbness, and loss of reflexes.

NERVE ROOT: The portion of the nerve as it leaves the dural sheath, goes through the foramen, and out just beyond the vertebra. (Figure 2–6B.) It combines with other nerve roots to form a larger nerve such as the sciatic nerve.

NUCLEUS PULPOSUS: The central gelatinlike component of the intervertebral disc (see Figure 3–4).

OCCULT DISC: A small, sometimes overlooked, discrete disc herniation that may be difficult to diagnose and may require several different imaging studies to characterize it.

ORGANIC: Used in medical jargon to describe disease or pain that can be recognized to be related to some physical abnormality in the body. This is in contradistinction to *function;* a term which is used to describe disease or pain in which there is unlikely to be any physical explanation and the implication is that the disease or pain could have a psychological or emotional component. Such disease or pain is no less "worthy" and no less "real," however.

ORGASM: A peak of sexual excitement, and/or culmination of an episode of sexual excitement.

OSTEOMALACIA: Reduction in the physical strength of bone due to its decreased mineralization.

OSTEOPENIA: Any state in which bone mass is reduced below normal.

OSTEOPOROSIS: Diminution in both the mineral and matrix components of bone. A condition in which the bone loses its strength and the various materials of which it is composed.

PARS INTERARTICULARIS: The part of the neural arch between the superior and inferior articular processes (see Figure 3–4).

PEDICLE: A tubular bony structure that connects the vertebral body to the posterior elements (see Figure 2–2).

PLACEBO: A substance or procedure that is given as treatment but that has no known or recognizable therapeutic effect. This is sometimes used to satisfy a patient's psychological need for medicine or treatment. More often it is used in controlled experimental studies as a standard of comparison to measure the efficacy of some drug or treatment modality that is thought to be specifically useful in combating a disease or condition.

PREMATURE EJACULATION: Ejaculation that occurs prior to the time that the sexual partner has achieved satisfaction.

PSEUDARTHROSIS: A situation in which there has been an attempt to create an arthrodesis of the spine, and this has healed in such a way that there is not complete bony continuity across the region in which the bone graft was applied in order to achieve the fusion. A defect in bone secondary to failure of union in either a bone or bone graft.

PSYCHOLOGICAL TESTING: The employment of various standardized techniques in which an individual responds either verbally or behaviorally to various commands. The manner in which he/she responds tends to reveal significant information about him/her that is not obtained through physical examination or interview.

PSYCHOTHERAPY: The use of learning, conditioning methods, and emotional reactions in a professional relationship to assist persons to modify feelings, attitudes, and behaviors that are intellectually, socially, or emotionally maladjustive or ineffectual.

RADICULITIS: Inflammation of a spinal nerve in the spinal or neural canal.

RANGE OF MOTION: Quantities that indicate two points at the extremes of the physiological range of translation and rotation of a joint for each of its six degrees of freedom. The units of measure are meters (feet) and degrees, respectively.

RETROLISTHESIS: Posterior displacement of a vertebra in relation to the one below.

RUPTURED DISC: See Herniated Disc.

SACROILIAC JOINT: The connection of the sacrum to the pelvis on each side (see Figure 3–7).

SCIATICA: The name given to a situation in which a patient complains of pain in the region of the body that is supplied by the sciatic nerve. This pain is usually in the buttock, posterior thigh, and lateral aspect of the leg and/or the foot. The most likely cause of sciatica, although certainly not the only cause, is a herniated disc (see Figure 2–6A and B).

SCOLIOSIS: An abnormal curvature of the spine (see Figures 3–4 and 5).

SECONDARY GAIN: An external, situational gain derived from any illness.

SPINAL NERVE ROOT: Those neural structures (motor nerve and sensory root) that combine to form a single entity that begins at the emergence from the dura and extends to the level of the sensory ganglion, and are invested by an extension of the common dural sac (see Figure 2–6B).

SPINAL STENOSIS: Reduction in the size of the spinal canal or regions thereof to a pathological degree (see Figure 3–3). The classifications:

A. Congenital stenosis: Malformation present at birth.
B. Developmental stenosis: Malformation of genetic origin.
C. Acquired stenosis: Malformation developed after birth; a lateral stenosis of the nerve canal (lateral recess entrapment).

SPINE: The midline and posteriormost portion of the vertebra, the tips of which can be felt as the line of bones just beneath the skin going down the middle of your back. Also the entire group of articulated bones which connect to the skull and end with the coccyx (see Figure 2–1).

SPONDYLOSIS: Degenerative disease of both the disc and the facet joints.

SPONDYLOLYSIS: A defect in the pars interarticularis (see Figure 3–4).

SPONDYLOLISTHESIS: Anterior displacement of a vertebra on the adjacent vertebra below, which occurs in one of several ways (see Figure 3–4). The ones that are most important for us, are described here:
A. Isthmic: Fibrous defects are present in the pars interarticularis, permitting forward displacement of the upper vertebra and separation of the anterior aspects of that vertebra from its neural arch. This is the one we think occurs as a birth defect.
B. Degenerative: Anterior displacement of a vertebra arising from erosive degenerative changes in the facet joints. These occur in the elderly and may be associated with spinal stenosis.
C. Traumatic: Anterior displacement of a vertebra due to traumatic injury to its restraining structures. This is what we see in the gymnast, weight lifter, or sumo wrestler.

STRESS: The force per unit area of a structure and a measurement of the intensity of the force.

SUBLUXATIONS AND DISLOCATIONS: A subluxation may be defined as a partial dislocation. It is any pathological situation in which there is not a normal physiological juxtaposition of the articular surfaces of a joint. Such situations should be reliably demonstrable radiographically.

SUPERIOR ARTICULAR PROCESS OR SUPERIOR ARTICULAR FACET: This forms part of the facet joint, which connects it to the posterior parts of the vertebra above (see also Figure 2–2; see also Inferior Articular Process).

SYMPTOM: A complaint from a patient regarding something that is wrong as perceived by the patient. This could be pain, as it commonly is, or some other bodily function that the patient perceives as abnormal, such as weakness, burning, or numbness.

TENDON: A fibrous cord that attaches a muscle to a particular bony structure or joint.

TENSION: A normal force that tends to elongate the fiber of a material. The unit of measure is newtons (poundforce).

TORQUE: When we twist something with a force, we apply a torque. We apply a torque when we use our steering wheel to turn a corner. When we wring out our T-shirt (after our vigorous trunk-strengthening exercises), we apply a torque.

TORSION: Same as a torque. A type of load that is applied by a couple of forces (parallel and directed opposite to each other) about the long axis of a structure.

TRANSVERSE PROCESS: Winglike projection at the side of the vertebra. (Figure 2–6B.)

TRIGGER POINT: A localized area of pain or tenderness that reproduces pain symptoms on application of mechanical pressure, and that results from referred pain.

TRUNK MUSCLES: The abdominal and back muscles, including the iliopsoas (see Figure 2–4).

UNCONSCIOUS: That part of an individual's psychological functioning of which he/she is not aware.

VERTEBRAL BODY: A large cylindrical portion of vertebra attached to the disc above and below (see Figure 2–1C).

VERTEBRAL CANAL: Sometimes called spinal canal. The tunnel that runs down the spine just behind the vertebral bodies and just in front of the vertebral arch (base of spinous process and lamina). Above the lumbar spine (low back), the spinal cord lies in this tunnel and ends at the level of the first lumbar vertebra (L1). Below that zone in the low back, the spinal nerves run in that tunnel and we call them the cauda equina (see Figure 2–6A and B).

VERTEBRAL OSTEOMYELITIS: Infection in the bony structures of the spine.

X RAY: Electromagnetic radiation that has a wavelength capable of penetrating, among other things, the human body, and providing a differential simulation of a photographic plate, giving a picture of bone and other structures within the body.

Bibliography

Chapter I

General Epidemiology

Cervical Dorsal and Lumbar Spine Syndromes. L. Hult: *Acta Orthop. Scand.* 17. (Suppl.) 1954. (This publication provides reliable information about the natural course of the disease.)

The Clinical Biomechanics of Spine Pain. Chapter 6, *Clinical Biomechanics of the Spine.* A. A. White, and M. M. Panjabi: J. B. Lippincott, 1990, second edition. (This chapter provides an illustrated overview of the epidemiology and treatment of spine pain.)

Demographic Characteristics of Persons with Acute Herniated Lumbar Intervertebral Disc. J. L. Kelsey and A. M. Ostfeld: *J. Chronic Disease.* 28:37, 1975. (A high-quality epidemiological study done in Connecticut.)

Epidemiology and Impact of Low Back Pain. J. L. Kelsey and A. A. White: *Spine* 5(2):133–42, 1980. (This publication summarizes the effects of back pain on society through a review of most of the cogent epidemiological studies.)

Symposium on Idiopathic Low Back Pain. A. A. White and S. L. Gordon, eds.: C. V. Mosby, 1982. (This book includes several publications by world authorities on the epidemiology of back pain.)

Occupational Factors

Investigation of the Relationship between Low Back Pain and Occupation. Four physical requirements: Bending, rotation, reaching, and sudden maximal effort. A. Magora: *Scand. J. Rehabil. Med.* 5:186, 1973. (This important study showed that, among other things, back pain may be caused by a sudden unexpected exertion while carrying a heavy object.)

Low Back Pain in Industry. A position paper. M. L. Rowe: *J. Occup. Med.* 11:161–69, 1969. (One of the first industrial epidemiological surveys of back problems. This was a long-range study of Kodak employees in Rochester, New York, with back disability.)

Low Back Pain in Industry. Updated position. M. L. Rowe: *J. Occup. Med.* 12:476–78, 1971.

Low Back Pain Sick Listing. A nosological and medical insurance investigation. C. G. Westrin: *Scand. J. Soc. Med. Suppl.* 7:1, 1973. (An enlightening and important study. For the laborer, the supervisor, and the high-level executive.)

Driving and Back Pain

Driving of Motor Vehicles as a Risk Factor for Acute Herniated Lumbar Disc. J. L. Kelsey and R. J. Hardy: *Am. J. Epidemiology.* 102:63, 1975. (This was probably the first study to show the relationship between driving and back problems.)

Epidemiological Studies of Low Back Pain. J. W. Frymoyer, M. H. Pope, M. C. Costanza, M. C. Rosen, J. E. Goggin, and D. G. Wilder: *Spine.* 5:419–23, 1980. (This study shows the association of back pain with driving and also with smoking.)

Vibration as an Etiologic Factor in Low Back Pain. M. H. Pope, D. G. Wilder, J. W. Frymoyer: *Engineering Aspects of the Spine.* Proceedings of conference. Joint meeting of the British Orthopaedic Association and the Institute of Medical Engineering, Westminster, May 7–9, 1980.

Pregnancy

Pregnancy and the Syndrome of Herniated Lumbar Intervertebral Disc. J. L. Kelsey, R. A. Greenberg, R. J. Hardy, and M. F. Johnson: *Yale Journal of Biol. Med.* 48:361, 1975. (This is a report on part of a very large yet well-conceived epidemiological study done in Connecticut.)

CHAPTER II

Low Back Pain. *CIBA Clinical Symposia.* 32(6): 1980. H. A. Keim and W. H. Kirkaldy-Willis: Summit, New Jersey, 1980. (Beautifully illustrated and well-labeled color drawing by the great medical illustrator Dr. Frank Netter.)

Measurements of Loads on the Lumbar Spine. G. B. J. Anderson: *Symposium on Idiopathic Low Back Pain.* A. A. White and S. M. Gordon, eds.: C. V. Mosby, 1982. (A thorough review of the forces exerted on the spine with various activities.)

Physical Properties and Functional Biomechanics of the Spine. Chapter 1, *Clinical Biomechanics of the Spine.* A. A. White, and M. M. Panjabi: J. B. Lippincott, 1990, second edition. (This is advanced reading for those seeking detailed data and theory, as well as in-depth knowledge of the biomechanics of the spine as it relates to back pain.)

CHAPTER III

Acute Low Back Syndrome—A study from general practice. J. B. Dillane, J. Fry, G. Kalton: *Br. Med. J.* 2:82–84, 1966. (This study showed that a large majority of patients presented with backache could not be diagnosed.)

The Aging Athlete. D. Menard, W. D. Stanish: *Am. Jour. Sports Med.* 17:187–196, 1989.

Back Pain and Sciatica. J. W. Frymoyer: *N. Engl. J. Med.* 318 + 5:291–300, 1989.

Camptocormia. C. A. Rockwood and R. E. Eilert: *J. Bone and Joint Surg.* 51A:553, 1969. (A good synopsis and a clear description of a very interesting hysterical-disease process.)

The Etiology of Spondylolisthesis. L. L. Wiltse: *J. Bone and Joint Surg.* 57A:17, 1975. (A thorough review of most aspects of this disease.)

Lumbar Spinal Stenosis and Nerve Root Entrapment Syndromes: Definition and Classification. *Clin. Orthop. Related Res.* 115:4, 1976. (A clear description of the disease and all the situations that can cause it.)

New Perspectives on Low Back Pain. J. W. Frymoyer and S. L. Gordon: American Academy of Orthopaedic Surgeons, 1989. (The latest "state of the art" scientific document on low back pain. A must for the reader who wants experimentally documented facts and references.)

Pain In the Back and the Neck. J. J. Mankin and R. D. Adams. Chapter 7, pp. 38–48, *Principles of Internal Medicine.* K. J. Isselbacher, R. D. Adams, E. Braunwald, R. G. Petersdorf, J. D. Wilson, eds.: McGraw-Hill Book Co., 1980. (*The* textbook of medicine.)

Prevention of Involuntary Bone Loss by Exercise. J. F. Aloia, S. H. Cohn, J. A. Ostuni, R. Cane, K. Ellis: *Ann. Intern. Med.* 89:356–358, 1978.

The Relation of Facet Orientation to Intervertebral Disc Failure. H. F. Farfan, J. D. Sullivan: *Can. J. Surg.* 10:179, 1967. (A good discussion of the associations of facet joint position and disc herniation.)

Ruptures of the Intervertebral Disc with Involvement of the Spinal Canal. W. J. Mixter and J. S. Barr: *N. Engl. J. Med.* 211:210, 1934. (This is the article that put the focus of the medical world and its surgeons on the disc as a cause of back pain.)

The Vertebral Columns of Monkeys, Apes, and Men. B. L. O'Connor: *Symposium on Low Back Pain.* A. A. White and S. M. Gordon, eds.: C. V. Mosby, 1982. (An expert on comparative anatomy reviews the problem and lays to rest the hypothesis that our backs hurt because we don't walk on all fours.)

Chapter IV

Acute Back Pain in Industry: A controlled prospective study with special reference to therapy and confounding factors. M. Bergquist-Ullman and U. Larsson: *Acta Orthop. Scand.* 170 (Suppl), 1977. (This study demonstrates the effectiveness of the low back school.)

Cultural Components on Responses to Pain. M. Zborowski: *Journal of Social Issues.* 8(4):16–30, 1952. (This interesting work studies pain responses among patients of Jewish, Italian, and "Old American" [Anglo-Saxon] cultural origins.)

Exercise for Backache. A double blind controlled trial. P. H. Kendall and J. M. Jenkins: *Physiotherapy.* 54:154, 1968. (This study shows the value of isometric abdominal exercises.)

Industrial Injuries of the Back and the Extremities. R. K. Beals and N. W. Hickman: *J. Bone and Joint Surgery.* 51A:1593–1611, 1972. (This gives some concrete information showing the effect of compensation factors on the problem of back pain.)

Introduction to Ergonomics. W. T. Singleton: World Health Organization, 1972. (A good synopsis and thorough explanation of ergonomics.)

Human Strength Capacity and Low Back Pain. D. B. Chaffin: *J. Occup. Med.* 16:248, 1974. (This shows the possible benefits of strength testing for selection for certain jobs.)

Life Change and Illness Susceptibility: Separation and Depression. S. H. Holmes and M. Masuda: *AAAS Publication No. 14,* p. 161, 1973. (A fascinating and thoroughly documented demonstration of the relationship between the onset of life crises and disease.)

An Occupational Biomechanics of Low Back Injury. D. B. Chaffin: *Symposium on Idiopathic Low Back Pain.* A. A. White and S. M. Gordon, eds.: C. V. Mosby, 1982. (An excellent summary of all the practical considerations of back mechanics as it relates to the worker.)

Pain Mechanisms: A New Theory. R. Melzack and P. D. Wall: *Science.* 150:971, 1965. (This, dear readers, is the classic exposition on the important gate-control theory of pain. Highly recommended for those who wish to study it in detail. Moreover, this article contains an excellent review of the literature on the pathophysiological aspects of pain.)

People in Pain. M. Zborowski: Jossey-Bass Inc., Publishers, San Francisco, 1969. (Several intergroup statistical comparisons among individuals from Jewish, Italian, Anglo-Saxon, and Irish cultures in their response to pain.)

Psychiatric Considerations in Pain. D. Blummer: Chapter 18, *The Spine,* Vol. 2. R. H. Rothmann and F. A. Simeone, eds.: W. B. Saunders, Philadelphia, 1975. (One of the most comprehensive works on the psychopathophysiological aspects of spine pain.)

Psychological/Psychiatric Factors in the Low Back Patient. A. F. Poussaint: *Symposium on Idiopathic Low Back Pain.* A. A. White and S. M. Gordon, eds.: C. V. Mosby, 1982. (This publication gives a thorough review of the important emotional aspects of low back pain.)

A Quantitative Study of Back Loads in Lifting. B. J. G. Anderson: *Spine.* 1:178–185, 1976. (This shows in the real world the importance of lifting objects close to the body.)

Relation of Lumbar Spine Disorders to Heavy Manual Work and Lifting. J. D. G. Troup: *Lancet.* 1:857, 1965. (A good synopsis and excellent review of the biomechanics of lifting.)

The Relaxation Response. H. Benson with M. Klipper: Avon Books, 1975. (A neatly and interestingly written exposition of a skill that may help not only your backache, but other aspects of your life as well.)

The Role of Abdominal Pressure in Relieving the Pressure on the Lumbar Intervertebral Disc. D. L. Bartelink: *J. Bone and Joint Surg.* 37B:718, 1957. (Discussion of the mechanism of the protection of the spine by the abdominal muscles.)

SAS In-the-Chair Exercise Book. F. Mossfledt and M. S. Miller: Bantam Books, Inc., 1979. (Recommended for the frequent sitter or traveler.)

Secondary Gain as a Factor in Results of Treatment. C. H. Epps. Chapter 8, *Complications in Orthopaedic Surgery,* Vol. 1. C. H. Epps, ed.: J. B. Lippincott, 1978. (Here we have a frank discussion of how patients, therapists, doctors, and lawyers can consciously conspire for profit from someone's back.)

Strength and Fitness and Subsequent Back Injuries in Firefighters. L. D. Caddy et al: *J. Occup. Med.* 21(4):269–272, 1979. (This is a well-done study showing that physical fitness helped prevent back injuries in these workers.)

Chapter V

Bed Design and Its Effect on Chronic Low Back Pain. S. R. Garfin and S. A. Pye: *Pain.* 10:87, 1981. (A neat, very-much-needed study on an immensely important topic. Probably the first and only research on an environment in which we spend approximately one-third of our time.)

How Many Days of Bed Rest for Acute Low Back Pain? A randomized clinical trial. R. A. Deyo, A. K. Diehl, and M. Rosenthal: *N. Engl. J. Med.* 315:1064, 1986.

Chapter VI

Acute Back Pain in Industry: A controlled prospective study with special reference to therapy and confounding factors. M. Bergquist-Ullman and U. Larsson: *Acta Ortho. Scand.* 170 (Suppl), 1977. (This justifies the back school.)

Auto-traction for Treatment of Lumbago-Sciatica: A multicentre controlled investigation. U. Larrson, U. Choler, A. Lidstrom, G. Lind, A. Nachemson, B. Nilsson, and J. Roslund: *Acta Orthop. Scand.* 51:791–798, 1980. (This study shows the value of auto-traction treatment over that of a corset and bed rest alone.)

Back Pain: A randomized clinical trial of rotational manipulation of the trunk. J. R. Glover, J. G. Morris, and T. Khosla: *Br. J. Industr. Med.* 31:59, 1974. (An important, informative, well-designed, and well-executed study.)

Chemonucleolysis: Experience with 2000 cases. *Clin. Orthop. Related Res.* 146:128–135, 1980. (A comprehensive report of one surgeon's experience. This explains indications for and complications of the procedure.)

Chymopapain: A case study in federal drug regulations. P. Sampson: *JAMA.* 240:195–219, 1978. (A superb review of the question, with good illustrations.)

The Clinical Biomechanics of Spine Pain. Chapter 6, *Clinical Biomechanics of the Spine.* A. A. White, and M. M. Panjabi: J. B. Lippincott, 1990, second edition. (This contains a detailed review of the various studies of spinal-manipulative therapy.)

A comparative analysis of lumbar disc disease treated by laminectomy or chemonucleolysis. E. J. Nordby and G. L. Lucas: *Clin. Orthop. Related Res.* 90:119, 1973.

Comparison of Internal Mammary Artery Ligation and Sham Operation for Angina Pectoris. E. G. Dimond, C. F. Kittle, and J. E. Crockett: *Amer. J. Cardiol.* 5(4):483–486, 1960. (A fascinating and classical ethical study demonstrating some powerful placebo effects from surgery.)

Conservative Therapy for Low Back Pain: Distinguishing useful from useless therapy. R. Deyo: *JAMA.* 250:1057, 1983. (A milestone publication.)

The Herniated Intervertebral Disc: An analysis of 400 verified cases. J. L. Poppen: *N. Engl. J. Med.* 232:211. 1945. (This shows the serious complications of spinal manipulation in the patient with a herniated disc.)

The Immobilizing Efficiency of Back Braces. P. L. Norton and T. Brown: *J. Bone and Joint Surg.* 39A:111, 1957. (A good study of the assets and limitations of braces.)

Lesions of the Lumbrosacral Spine. Part two. Chronic traumatic (postural) destruction of the lumbrosacral intervertebral disc. P. C. Williams: *J. Bone and Joint Surg.* 19:690, 1937.

Lumbar Traction Theory. Elimination of physical factors that prevent lumbar stretch. B. D. Judovich: *JAMA.* 159:549, 1955.

Manipulating the Patient: A comparison of the effectiveness of physician and chiropractor care. R. L. Kane et al.: *Lancet.* 1:1333, 1974. (This is the study demonstrating that patients responded favorably to certain personality characteristics in their therapists.)

Manipulation in Treatment of Low Back Pain: A multicenter study. D. M. L. Doran and D. J. Newell. *Br. Med. J.* 2:161, 1975. (This is one of the studies that shows quick but rapidly fading pain relief with manipulation.)

The McKenzie program: Exercise effective against low back pain. A. Dimaggio and V. Mooney: *The Journal of Musculoskeletal Medicine.* December 1987. (A preliminary study.)

The Natural Course of Low Back Pain. A. Nachemson: *Symposium on Idiopathic Low Back Pain.* A. A. White and S. M. Gordon, eds.: C. V. Mosby, 1982. (This gives a detailed statistical account of what you can expect to happen to your back pain in a variety of different circumstances.)

Objective Assessment of Spine Functioning Following Industrial Injury: A prospective study with comparison group and a one-year follow-up. T. G. Mayer, R. J. Gatchel, N. Kishino: *Spine.* 10:48–58, 1985. (A milestone study in the clinical science of low back pain rehabilitation.)

Physical Therapy for Lumbar Disc Disease. C. P. Jackson: *Seminars in Spine Surgery.* Vol. 1. No. 1:28–34, 1989. (A cogent, concise, well-referenced, useful review.)

Position Paper on Chiropractic. The National Council Against Health Fraud, Inc.: Box 1276, Loma Linda, CA 92354, 1985.

Report of a Case of Ruptured Intervertebral Disc Following Chiropractic Manipulation. E. D. Fisher: *Kentucky Med. J.* 41:14, 1943. (This is why we discourage manipulations when you haven't had an adequate medical diagnostic evaluation.)

The Research Status of Spinal Manipulative Therapy. M. Goldstine, ed.: HEW Publication No. 76, p. 998. Bethesda, 1975. (This publication does an excellent job of presenting a large amount of information on this topic, including several points of view. The document does not answer the question of effectiveness of spinal-manipulative therapy, nor does it resolve controversy.)

A Scientific Test of Chiropractic Theory. E. S. Crelin: *Am. Sci.* 61:574, 1973. (Professor Crelin of Yale Medical School has been an outspoken opponent of chiropractic theory for many years. Some of his views are expressed in this publication.)

Spinal Braces: Functional Analysis and Clinical Application. Chapter 7, *Clinical Biomechanics of the Spine.* A. A. White, and M. M. Panjabi: J. B. Lippincott, 1990, second edition. (There's probably as much here as any of you would like to know about bracing.)

A Study of the Results Following Rotatory Manipulation in the Lumbar Vertebral Disc Syndrome. O. D. Chrisman, A. Mittnacht, and G. A. Snook:

J. Bone and Joint Surg. 46A:517, 1964. (An informative clinical study of spinal-manipulative therapy.)

Symposium: Percutaneous Nucleotomy. M. B. Stern, ed: *Clin. Orthop.* pages 1–106, 1989. (This is the best synopsis of our current knowledge of this important new development.)

Transient Hypercorticism after Epidural Steroid Injection: A Case Report. J. L. Stambough, R. E. Booth, and R. H. Rothman. *J. Bone and Joint Surg.* 66–A: 1115, 1952. (This case is accompanied by a superb review and summary of the complications associated with the use of epidural steroids.)

Vascular Accidents to the Brain Stem Associated with Neck Manipulation. D. Green and R. J. Joynt: *JAMA.* 170:522, 1959. (This time the complication was death when an undiagnosed disease was manipulated.)

Vertebral Manipulation. Third edition. G. D. Maitland: London, Butterworth, 1973. (Spinal manipulation is viewed differently in various countries. This is the way the English see it.)

CHAPTER VII

Biomechanical Considerations in the Surgical Management of the Spine. Chapter 8, *Clinical Biomechanics of the Spine.* A. A. White, and M. M. Panjabi: J. B. Lippincott, 1990, second edition. (This chapter includes a brief description and illustrations of virtually all the operations done on the lumbar spine.)

Duration of Disability Following Lumbar Disc Surgery. V. V. Surin.: *Acta Orthop. Scand.* 48: 466–471, 1977. (Some good data to help in the decision "to operate or not to operate, and when.")

The Effects of Delayed Disc Surgery on Muscular Paresis. H. Weber. *Acta Orthop. Scand.* 46:631, 1975. (This study tells what happens to moderate leg weakness without surgery—answer: You can get over it even without surgery.)

End-Result Study of the Treatment of Herniated Nucleus Pulposus by Excision with Fusion and without Fusion. Res. Com. Amer. Orthop. Surg., I. W. Nichlas, chairman: *J. Bone and Joint Surg.* 34A:981, 1952. (Some evidence to suggest that routine fusion is not necessary with a routine disc operation.)

Low Back Pain: A joint neurosurgical and orthopaedic project. B. R. Selecki: *Med. J. Aust.* 2:889, 1973. (A detailed study comparing the results and frequency of surgery done by a group of orthopaedic surgeons and neurosurgeons in Australia.)

The Lumbar Disc Herniation: A computer-aided analysis of 2,507 operations. E. V. Spangfort: *Acta Orthop. Scand.* 142 (Suppl), 1972. (This shows how the results of disc surgery are very much related to the findings of abnormality at the time of surgery.)

The Lumbar Spine, an Orthopaedic Challenge. A. L. Nachemson: *Spine.* 1:59, 1976. (Some good guidelines for expected results of disc surgery with various preoperative findings.)

Percutaneous Radiofrequency Lumbar Rhizolysis (Rhizotomy). J. A. McCullough: Int. Symp. Radiofrequency Lesion-Making Procedures, Chicago, Ill., 1976: *Appl. Neurophysiol.* 39:87–96, 1976–77. (A very good explanation of the procedure and its rationale. The procedure, however, has not yet distinguished itself.)

A Program for the Evaluation and Management of the High-Performance Athlete with Acute Low Back Pain: A. A. White, R. Voy, E. Ryan, R. Beeten. *Athletic Training. In press,* 1990.

A Program for the Evaluation and Management of the High-Performance Athlete with Acute Low Back Pain: A. A. White, R. Voy, E. Ryan, R. Beeten. *Clin. Sports Med. In press,* 1990.

A Prognosis in Sciatica: A clinical follow-up of surgical and nonsurgical treatment. A. Hakelius: *Acta Orthop. Scand.* 129 (Suppl), 1970. (This gives some idea of outcomes in disc disease patients with and without surgery. The study is difficult to interpret, especially when one tries to apply it to an individual patient. Discuss it with your surgeon.)

Results of Surgical Intervention in the Symptomatic Multiply Operated Back Patient: Analysis of sixty-seven cases followed for three to seven years. W. J. Finnegan, J. M. Fenlin, J. P. Marvel, R. J. Nardini, and R. H. Rothman: *J. Bone and Joint Surg.* 61A:1077–1082, 1979. (This article demonstrates the complexity of evaluating a patient with back pain after several operations have been done.)

Sexual Complications of Anterior Fusion of the Lumbar Spine. J. C. Flynn and C. T. Price: *Proceedings, 49th Annual Meeting of the American Academy of Orthopaedic Surgeons.* New Orleans, 1982. (This study suggests that the complications of fusions from the front for low back pain, though quite rare, can be serious for the male.)

CHAPTER VIII

The Cradle of Erotica. A. Edwards and R. E. L. Masters: The Julian Press, Inc., New York, 1963. (A marvelous study of Afro-Asian sexual expression—certain to stimulate your imagination and feed your ingenuity.)

Frequency of Sexual Dysfunction in "Normal" Couples. E. Frank, C. Anderson, D. Rubinstein: *N. Engl. J. Med.* 299:111–115, 1978. (This study showed that roughly fifty percent of men and women had some problem.)

The Joy of Sex: A Gourmet Guide to Love Making. A. B. Comfort, ed.: Crown Publishers, Inc., New York, 1972. (This book should help you to establish communication with your lover about lovemaking. There are enough options on the menu to suit the taste of just about all you good readers.)

Sexual Adjustment and Chronic Back Pain. D. Osborne and T. Maruta. *Medical Aspects of Human Sexuality.* 14: 104–113, 1980. (A good discussion of some of the problems that may relate to medications you may be taking and long-standing disability.)

Sexual Consequences of Disability. A. B. Comfort, ed.: G. F. Stickley Co., 1978. (This is a description of severe sexual disabilities. Several chapters are potentially relevant, however.)

Sexual Problems Among Family Medicine Patients. J. T. Moore and Y. Goldstein: *Journal of Family Practice.* 10:243–247, 1980. (This piece shows that even without backache, sexual problems are present in over fifty percent of couples.)

Chapter IX

Backache in Oarsmen. M. C. Stallard: *British J. Sports Med.* 14:105–108, 1980. (An excellent exposition on this subject.)

A Chronicle of Injuries of an American Intercollegiate Football Team. S. T. Canale, E. D. Cantler, T. D. Sisk, B. L. Freeman: *The Jefferson Orthopaedic Journal.* 9:34–42, 1980. (This publication and its references give a good idea of the various injuries sustained by players on a college football team.)

The Effects of Torsion on the Lumbar Intervertebral Joint: The role of torsion in the production of disc degeneration. H. Farfan et al: *J. Bone and Joint Surg.* 52A:468, 1970. (This explains in biomechanical terms why there's so much talk here about twisting.)

Injury Rates Vary with Coaching: Football injury survey. C. S. Blyth and F. O. Mueller. *Physician and Sports Medicine.* Vol. 2:45–50, 1974. (This shows that coaching *can* make a difference.)

Measurement of the Intra-Abdominal Pressure in Relation to Weight Bearing of the Lumbar Spine. N. Eie and P. Wehn: *J. Oslo City Hosp.* 12:205, 1962. (This is an interesting, informative study that would be particularly useful for the weight lifter.)

A New Consideration in Athletic Injuries: The classical ballet dancer. E. H. Miller et al.: *Clin. Orthop. Related Res.* 111:181–191, 1975. (This shows the importance to the dancer as well as the athlete of special attention in matters of backache and other clinical problems.)

Physical Properties and Functional Biomechanics of the Spine. Chapter 1, *Clinical Biomechanics of the Spine.* A. A. White, and M. M. Panjabi: J. B. Lippincott, 1990, second edition. (This contains some detailed analyses of the mechanics that go into causing damage to the spine.)

Spinal Cord Injury Resulting from Sport Diving. R. J. DiLibero and A. Pilimanis: *Proceedings, 49th Annual Meeting of the American Academy of Orthopaedic Surgeons.* New Orleans, 1982. (This describes an unusual yet serious mechanism of back pain from scuba diving.)

Spondylolysis in the Female Gymnast. D. W. Jackson, L. L. Wiltse and R. J. Cirincione: *Clin. Orthop. Related Res.* 117: 68–73, 1976. (An excellent review of the cause and treatment of this problem.)

A Study of Changes in the Spine in Weight Lifters and Other Athletes. M. D. Aggragal et al.: *British J. Sports Med.* 13: 58–61, 1979. (Shows frequency of backache and describes some of the associated X-ray irregularities in the spine.)

Use Your head in Tennis. Revised edition. Bob Harman and Keith Monroe: Thomas Y. Crowell Company, 1974. (This book will help you to enjoy your tennis so much more that you will forget about your backache.)

Chapter X

Acupuncture Treatment of Chronic Back Pain: A double blind placebo controlled trial. G. Mendelson, T. Selwood, H. Kranz, et al.: *Am J. Med.* 74: 49–55, 1983.

The Effects of Mammary Hypertrophy [large breasts] on the Skeletal System. G. Letterman and M. Schurter: *Annals of Plastic Surgery.* 5,6:425–431, 1980.

Scientific Approach to the Assessment and Management of Activity-Related Spinal Disorders. W. O. Spitzer: *Spine.* 12 (Suppl 1), 1987. (A milestone publication on the clinical care of spine problems. Cuts through all the B.S. [Bold Speculation].)

Chapter XI

New Perspectives on Low Back Pain. J. W. Frymoyer and S. L. Gordon, eds.: American Academy of Orthopaedic Surgeons, 1989. (A superb scientific "state-of-the-art" reference with extensive bibliography.)

Symposium on Idiopathic Low Back Pain. A. A. White and S. M. Gordon, eds.: C. V. Mosby, 1982.

Miscellaneous

Radiological Perspectives on Idiopathic Low Back Pain. D. Kido. 1982.

Occupational

Low Back Pain in Industry. S. Snook. 1982.

On Occupational Biomechanics of Low Back Pain. D. B. Chaffin. 1982.

Pain Mechanics

Endogenous Mechanisms of Pain Modulation. H. Fields. 1982.

Pain Pathways and Mechanisms in the Central Nervous System with Special Reference to Low Back Pain. K. L. Casey. 1982.

Glossary

Dorland's Illustrated Medical Dictionary. Twenty-fifth edition. W. B. Saunders, Philadelphia, 1974.

Glossary of Spinal Terminology. American Academy of Orthopaedic Surgeons, Park Ridge, Ill., 1985.

High-Resolution MR Imaging of Sequestrated Lumbar Intervertebral Discs. T. J. Masaryk, J. S. Ross, M. T. Modic, H. Bohlman, G. Wilber: *AJNR* 9:351, 1988.

Index

ABOUT THE AUTHOR

Dr. Augustus A. White III is a scientist who has distinguished himself on many fronts, most notably orthopaedics. He is Orthopaedic Surgeon-in-Chief at Boston's Beth Israel Hospital and Professor of Orthopaedic Surgery at Harvard Medical School and the Harvard-MIT Division of Health Sciences and Technology. Dr. White's career goals shifted from psychiatry to orthopaedics as a result of his experiences on the football team while an undergraduate at Brown University. A star athlete as well as a scholar, he became fascinated by orthopaedic treatment of sports injuries, and went on to specialize in orthopaedic surgery. While he was a medical student at Stanford University School of Medicine he became interested in the complex problem of back pain. After graduation, his skills were further honed at Yale Medical Center, where he had his orthopaedic residency, and subsequently at Karolinska Institute in Sweden, where he received his doctorate in medical science for his research on the biomechanics of the spine. He returned to Yale Medical School, where he subsequently became a Professor of Orthopaedic Surgery. He continued to concentrate much of his teaching, research, and patient care on problems of the spine. While his professional life has drawn him to classroom, laboratory, and lecture hall, he is most committed to direct patient care.

Dr. White is an avid researcher whose major efforts are directed at study of the spine and fracture healing. He has written and collaborated on more than one hundred and thirty scientific publications, including the highly regarded definitive work, *The Clinical Biomechanics of the Spine.* This book, now in the second edition, was the first of its kind, designed to present scientific material about spine mechanics in a way that can be directly applied to the comprehensive care of patients with spine problems. He has edited a book for scientists and physicians entitled *Symposium on Idiopathic Low Back Pain.* This work emanated from a meeting chaired by Dr. White. It was the first multidisciplinary broad-based international meeting organized for the purpose of reviewing current knowledge and suggesting future research on the scientific aspects of the cause of back pain.

Dr. White is a recipient of the United States Jaycees' "Ten Outstanding Young Men" Award and the Martin Luther King, Jr., Medical Achievement Award, and in 1982 was named an

Exceptional Black by the CIBA-GEIGY Corporation. Among his credits are the Kappa Delta Award, a national honor awarded for outstanding orthopaedic research, and the Eastern Orthopaedic Association's Award for Spine Research. Dr. White is a member of Brown University's Board of Fellows and a past trustee of Northfield–Mount Hermon School. He is a recipient of the Bronze Star, earned while stationed as a Captain in the U.S. Army Medical Corps in Vietnam, where he also did extensive volunteer work in a leper colony.

Dr. White lectures often in this country and abroad, and his work is frequently reported in the national lay press and on television.

Dr. White is listed in *Who's Who in America, Who's Who Among Black Americans, American Men and Women in Science,* and the *Town and Country* magazine list of Outstanding Medical Specialists in the U.S. He is a member of the American Academy of Orthopaedic Surgeons, the American Orthopaedic Association, the Orthopaedic Research Society, the Scoliosis Research Society, the International Society for the Study of the Lumbar Spine, the American Orthopaedic Society for Sports Medicine, and the Cervical Spine Research Society of which he has been a past President. He has served the National Institutes of Health as a member of the Advisory Council of the National Institute on Arthritis, Diabetes, and Digestive and Kidney Diseases.